Rx for Health Care Reform

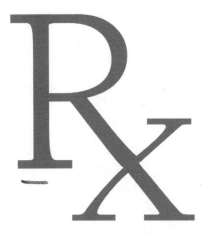

for Health Care Reform

Ken Terry

Foreword by Paul B. Ginsburg

Vanderbilt University Press • Nashville

First Edition 2007
11 10 09 08 07   1 2 3 4 5

This book is printed on acid-free paper
made from 50% post-consumer recycled paper
Manufactured in the United States of America

Library of Congress Cataloging-in-Publication Data
Terry, Ken, 1948-
Rx for health care reform / Ken Terry.—1st ed.
p. ; cm.
Includes bibliographical references and index.
ISBN 978-0-8265-1570-4 (cloth : alk. paper)
ISBN 978-0-8265-1571-1 (pbk. : alk. paper)
1. Health care reform—United States.
2. Medical policy—United States.
3. Medical care—United States. I. Title.
[DNLM: 1. Health Care Reform—United States.
2. Health Care Sector—United States.
WA 540 AA1 T329r 2007]
RA395.A3T455 2007
362.1'04250973—dc22
2007007055

To Lisa,
whose love sustains me every day

Contents

Part IV
Rx for Health Care Reform

Acknowledgments

It is impossible to acknowledge the contributions of everyone who made this book possible. But I would like to thank Marianne Mattera, the former editor *of Medical Economics Magazine*, for giving me the time and space to pursue my dream. Also, Leslie Kane, our current editor and former articles editor, supported my project from the beginning. So did Joseph Scherger, MD, a professor of family medicine at the University of California, San Diego, who devoted many hours to reading and critiquing my book in its formative stages. I also received valuable feedback from Paul B. Ginsburg, president of the Center for Studying Health System Change; Jacque Sokolov, MD, a health care consultant and former member of the Clinton health care task force; and Robert Berenson, MD, a fellow at the Urban Institute whose sharp criticisms of the prevailing paradigm undergirded my own. These experts, and many others, gave me faith that I was going in the right direction.

Many friends and colleagues also supported my work. Among them are Jeff Burger, Wayne Guglielmo, Robert Lowes, Charles Paikert, and Ken Schlager.

Finally, I'd like to thank my family—and particularly my children, Selene, Alycia, Justin, and Adam—for their love and support. Without them, and without the love of Lisa Lucas, I would never have had the courage to complete this book.

Foreword

The shortcomings of U.S health care—high costs, uneven quality, and inadequate access for many Americans—are well known to health-policy experts and researchers. The reasons for these shortcomings are also well known. Our health system is fragmented, making coordination of increasingly complex care extremely difficult. Most insured consumers are sheltered from high health care costs to a large extent and consequently there is no groundswell of support for efforts to make the system more efficient and economical. Providers are paid for services on a piecework basis, creating incentives for them to generate patient demand for services and not to invest in developing the systems to treat patients efficiently. Providers advertise the latest medical technologies directly to consumers, who in turn demand more services paid for by a third party. Neither consumers nor regulators have adequate tools to measure the quality of care, so providers are under little pressure to improve. The combination of advances in technology and lack of efficiency gains in service provision has caused health care spending to rise more rapidly than either workers' earnings or government tax revenues, making health insurance unaffordable to an increasing proportion of employers and employees, crowding out other government services, and ultimately leading to higher tax rates.

Periodically, initiatives surface to reform health care. Many focus on how government can take steps to increase the proportion of the population covered by health insurance. Today, the politically feasible course to achieve near-universal coverage is a combination of expanding means-tested public insurance programs, providing employer subsidies to cover lower-income workers, creating exchanges where small employers and individuals can buy insurance more efficiently and benefit from risk pooling, and mandating individuals to obtain coverage. Massachusetts enacted such a program in April 2006 with support from both political parties and major stakeholders—and this initiative has inspired policymakers elsewhere.

These efforts to reform health care, however, often seem to be mere patches and do not include powerful steps to address the systemic problems summarized above. Our leaders would like us to believe that steps such as expansion of information technology, quality reporting, and pay for performance will solve our problems, but to me it confirms a long-standing impression that they would rather not deal with the real problems. This is why when Ken Terry began sending me early chapters of *Rx for Health Care Reform*, I was struck not only by his understanding of the underlying problems of the health care system but also by his intriguing ideas about how to change the system. I agreed to read his drafts and give him constructive feedback.

The book begins with an analysis of what is leading to failure in our health care system. When Terry measures current "solutions," such as consumer-directed health care, pay for performance, and health information technology, against what is causing failure in our system, he understandably concludes that they are not up to the job; good ideas, perhaps, but they do not attack the real problems. Terry's own plan has two unique elements: First, he would induce primary-care physicians to form groups and assume risk for the costs of all professional services. Second, he would reduce insurers' roles to that of public utilities—one per region with regulated profits. In this role, insurers would not negotiate provider payment rates or manage care. They would only collect premiums, pay claims, and measure physician-group quality of care. Consumers would choose among groups on the basis of quality of care and cost.

Terry brings something unique to this analysis—his years of experience as a reporter and editor for *Medical Economics Magazine*. Terry knows physician practices to a degree that few other health care analysts do. I know this from my experience being interviewed by him on market and policy developments affecting physicians. His questions are always among the most insightful.

—Paul B. Ginsburg
President of the Center for Studying Health System Change

Introduction

What would happen if we all had to buy our own health insurance? My friend Bill found out when he was laid off from his editorial job at a national magazine. The federal COBRA law required his former employer to maintain his group coverage for eighteen months after termination, but Bill had to pay 100 percent of the premium. That came to about $12,000 a year for himself and his family. If he hadn't found a job before his COBRA coverage ran out, a nongroup insurance policy would have cost him $20,000.

George and Rita, a suburban couple in their fifties, have to buy insurance on their own because George, a lawyer, is self-employed. Rita is fairly healthy, but her husband has a heart condition. So they pay $12,000 a year for a plan with a $3,000 deductible. Rita has gone back to work as a substitute teacher to pay their medical and insurance bills.

At least Bill, George, and Rita have health coverage, which means they have better access to care than the uninsured do.[1] But other middle-class people who believe that they'll always have solid health insurance may be in for a shock. For one thing, the number of uninsured is expected to rise from 46.6 million today[2] to 56.0 million by 2013[3]—a warning sign for anybody who might get laid off in these days of job insecurity. And, as health costs soar, employers are pushing more of those costs onto their employees. So, gradually, the plight of the uninsured will start to become the nightmare of the insured.

Rising deductibles, coinsurance, and copayments have already resulted in higher out-of-pocket costs for many insured people. One study found that 16 million adults were underinsured in 2003[4]—and that doesn't include Medicaid recipients, who have very limited access to care.

The result, in human terms, is deeply troubling. When the uninsured and underinsured get sick, they tend to go without needed care, avoiding

doctor visits and not adhering to their medications.[5] One in seven families and nearly 40 percent of adults have difficulty paying their medical
bills, and medical costs are responsible for about 30 percent of personal
bankruptcies.[6] Notably, many of those who go bankrupt because of illness or injury have insurance. A *New York Times* article tells the heart-
breaking story of a young, middle-income couple, Sharon and Arnold
Dorsett, who were unable to pay the medical bills for treating their son
Zachery's immune system disorder. Although the Dorsetts were insured,
the noncovered portion of their medical expenses was so high that they
had to declare bankruptcy to avoid losing their home.[7]

Meanwhile, fewer people can afford coverage, because the cost of
health insurance has continued climbing at or near double-digit rates.
In 2006, the average price of family coverage was $11,480, more than
the annual earnings for a minimum-wage worker. While employers still
paid about the same percentage of the premium that they had in previous years, the average worker contribution to family coverage jumped
83 percent from $1,620 a year in 2000 to $2,973 in 2006—far faster than
the rate of inflation or the increase in workers' pay.[8]

Are Employers Going to Bail Out?   By 2015, it's forecast,
U.S. spending on health care will total $4 trillion, or $12,320 per person,
and health care will devour 20 percent of our GDP.[9] Between now and
then, forecasts Uwe Reinhardt, a health economist at Princeton University, a third of U.S. wage earners will probably lose their health insurance.[10] Donald Crane, president and CEO of the California Association
of Physician Groups, believes that if costs keep rising, most employers
will drop insurance. If that happens, he predicts, we're going to get a
government-run health care system by default.

While things aren't that bad yet, there are signs that employer-
provided insurance is unraveling: From 2000 to 2005, the percentage
of employers offering health benefits dropped from 69 percent to 60
percent.[11] Most of those dropping coverage were smaller employers,
but big corporations are also taking a harder line. For example, in 2005
General Motors extracted concessions from the United Auto Workers
Union that were expected to knock $1 billion off its annual health care
bill of nearly $6 billion.[12] Retirees and active workers now have to pay
more for coverage, and current employees are forgoing raises to pay for
the retirees' care.[13] The ailing car company has also trimmed medical
benefits for its nonunion retirees.

The autoworkers still have relatively generous insurance compared with that offered by many employers. For example, the percentage of small companies requiring a deductible of $1,000 or more jumped to 34 percent in 2004 from 31 percent the previous year.[14] Some big employers with low-wage workers either don't offer insurance or restrict it to only some employees. Fewer than half of Wal-Mart's 1.2 million employees, for example, are eligible for health coverage, and many of those can't afford their part of the premium. Consequently, many Wal-Mart workers are on Medicaid.[15]

A growing number of companies are offering workers inexpensive "mini-medical" policies that cover drugs and doctor visits, but little hospitalization.[16] However, a coalition of big employers that tried this approach found that few uninsured workers bought this limited coverage. The others either couldn't afford it or didn't think it was worthwhile.[17]

Some companies are even looking outside our borders for solutions. In southern California, employers are sending their workers down to Mexico for annual checkups, medications, and even surgeries. Health care costs south of the border are 40 to 50 percent lower than they are in California, and U.S. and Mexican HMOs cover "Baja care" for as little as $100 per employee per month.[18]

An Unsustainable Trend   Some health economists assert that the United States can afford to keep spending more and more of its national wealth on health care.[19] They say that we can cut expenditures on other goods and services, that medical advances extend life and improve worker productivity, and that it doesn't matter how much is spent on health care as long as the poor get their fair share. But many other experts, employers, and health care providers don't believe we can simply raise health care's portion of the GDP from the current 16 percent to 20 or 30 percent.

In July 2004, the National Coalition on Health Care (NCHC), representing a hundred big corporations, unions, health care providers, insurers, and consumer groups, called for price controls on health care. In its little-noticed report, the NCHC said, "The escalation of health care costs is not only a health care issue; it is also a major national economic problem." Not only does it reduce investment in new industrial capacity and reduce the global competitiveness of American businesses but it also holds down wage increases and makes it harder for employers to create new jobs.[20]

Meanwhile, the public has had about enough. According to a 2006 Commonwealth Fund survey, three-quarters of American adults said the U.S. health care system "needs either fundamental change or complete rebuilding." About half of the respondents said they worried about the affordability of care if they or their families needed it.[21]

As I explain in Chapter 1, there have been repeated warnings of health care calamity since 1970. But the difference this time is that medical costs as a percentage of GDP are more than twice what they were thirty-five years ago; if that percentage doubles again by 2040, we'll be spending a third of our income on health care. Medicare is projected to go broke by 2020; to make it actuarially sound in the long run, we'd have to double Medicare taxes or halve benefits immediately.[22] And Medicaid is in such bad shape that two-thirds of the states tax providers to help fund it.[23]

Despite the enormous challenges faced by government programs, health care leaders across the country no longer believe that free-enterprise reforms can solve the problems of the health care system without more government intervention.[24] Alain Enthoven, a Stanford University economist, has even forecast that "Medicare for all"—a government-run health care system—might be in the platform of the winning candidate for President in 2008.[25]

Free Enterprise Uber Alles   While that's unlikely, the suggestion shows that health care reform efforts in this country are still stuck in the same rut. For the past century, there has been a tug of war between those who favor a government-controlled or highly regulated system that provides universal health care, like those of Western Europe, and supporters of a free-enterprise approach that rations care by income. Time and again, the free-enterprise advocates have won, and they remain firmly in control.

The American way of life is solidly rooted in private enterprise; and, although the government pays about half of our national health care bill through Medicare, Medicaid, and other programs, the political process usually favors entrepreneurs and profit-making activities. Thus, it came as no surprise that when Congress finally passed a Medicare drug bill in 2003, it forbade the Centers for Medicare and Medicaid Services (CMS) from negotiating prices with the drug companies.[26]

Pharmaceutical firms are, of course, not the only ones that want to maximize their profits. So do device manufacturers, health plans, hospitals, physicians, and other health care providers. "The American health system is often described as a nonsystem," Uwe Reinhardt says. "But it's actually one of the most finely honed systems in the world. It's like a Mercedes-Benz. Its purpose is to maximize the amount of money that can be sucked out of the rest of society. And it does that with uncanny efficiency."[27]

So, on one hand, there is a growing recognition that the rise in health care costs is unsustainable; on the other hand, we have a society utterly dedicated to free enterprise, innovation, and personal choice. It is clear that unless we put a brake on the rapid escalation in new technology and health care profits, the train is going to run off the tracks. And it's equally clear that our current system of financing and delivering health care must be radically restructured to prevent that train wreck. Yet politicians and special interests still resist any suggestion of a greater role for government.

A New Deal for Health Care   While Americans rejected the Clinton health care reform plan a decade ago, they might be more amenable today to a Rooseveltian New Deal for the health care that they see slipping away from them. Like the 1930s social reforms, the solutions proposed in this book are radical and far-reaching. But they could provide universal coverage and reduce health costs by 30 percent or more if we can just make a few adjustments in our thinking about health care.

To start, we need to drop our resistance to government intervention. Although local control of most elements of health care is preferable to central direction, only the federal government, working with the states, has the power and the authority to implement the changes that need to be made. Moreover, as I point out in the final chapter, restraining future cost growth will require a national organization to assess the value of new technologies.

Some observers will attack this approach as a form of socialism that places intolerable constraints on health care entrepreneurs. But this route to universal, comprehensive, affordable coverage would preserve much of the free-enterprise system. It would add just enough government intervention to make the system work properly. And while it would produce wrenching changes in the short run, it would put us on the path toward better health care at a price we can afford.

We also have to stop thinking in terms of choosing among insurance companies when we buy coverage. Since most plans include the majority of local health care providers, the competition should be among provider groups instead. That, of course, would require more physicians to join groups, and it would relegate insurance carriers to a secondary role. Many insurance jobs would be lost, and doctors would have to take financial responsibility for their own services. But these reforms would restore control over health care to doctors and patients, where it belongs, and it would give every patient a free choice of physicians.

For this solution to succeed, we would have to stop believing that more care is always better or that every insured person is entitled to everything that health care providers can possibly deliver. This goal would be the trickiest to achieve, given the entitlement mentality of the public and the ceaseless drumbeat of publicity about the latest medical advances.

Here, physicians would have to lead the way. They would have to learn how to manage care and how to explain to patients why they cannot have everything they want. No doubt, many people will object; but since we don't have unlimited resources, there must be a budget, whatever kind of health care system we have.

"Our system is going to continue in a death spiral until we come to the grips with the fact that we can only afford so much," says Jonathan Weiner, a professor of health policy at the Johns Hopkins Bloomberg School of Public Health. "We need a fixed budget like every other system in the world. And then we need to figure out how to meet our needs within that budget, or collectively we have to add to the budget. Morally, we're on very shaky ground until everybody gets at least basic health care. Giving some people wasteful health care and others, none, is completely untenable. If we gave everyone decent health care, and others wanted to pay more to get more, that would be fine."

The Floor Plan   This book is divided into four parts. In Part I, I explain how we got into this mess, starting with a history of health care reform and finishing with a roundup of current reform proposals. Part II provides a detailed critique of government and private initiatives to change the system. In Part III, I show how the "medical-industrial complex"—the interlocking colossus of health care providers and drug and device manufacturers—is driving up health costs. In the final part, I present a set of proposals for restructuring health care financing and delivery and for restraining the medical-industrial complex.

However daunting the problems of health care seem to be, Americans have shown an unparalleled resilience and an ability to overcome even the thorniest challenges. I am sure that we can find a way to ensure good health care for all, if that is what we want to do. Our most difficult challenge is to recognize that we're all in this together. Unless we give our weakest and most vulnerable citizens access to decent health care, one day we could all find ourselves out in the cold.

Part I
Whither Health Care Reform?

1 How We Got into This Mess

Since the nineteenth century, Americans have been divided between those who believe that the purpose of government is to protect individual liberties and those who believe that government should also serve the interests of society at large.[1] This not a simple conflict between advocates of free enterprise and advocates of regulation, or between capitalists and socialists. It reflects the dualism in the very ideals of liberal democracy: The egalitarianism that produced a meritocracy opposed to the old European concept of inherited class also led to the progressivism of the early twentieth century and the social welfare reforms of the 1930s.

In the health care reform debate that has persisted for more than a century, the key difference between these two strains of egalitarianism can be summarized as follows: The conservatives hold that there must be winners and losers in society, and that it's up to the winners to decide how much health care the losers should get. The liberals maintain that everyone is entitled to at least basic health care.

The majority of Americans support the idea of health care as a right.[2] But, as the history of the Clinton health care reform plan shows, the middle class is not willing to spend very much to expand access to health care. The Clinton plan collapsed mainly because middle-class people believed that, if it were adopted, their own coverage would suffer or they'd have to pay more for insurance. So America was and continues to be torn between self-interest and the ideal of universal coverage.

Our current health care crisis is closely intertwined with the peculiar public-private structure of the U.S. health care system, which allows millions of people to be uninsured and permits providers to shift costs between the government and private payers. Other advanced countries don't have these problems, because they have universal coverage. Moreover, their government-run systems provide care that, in many ways, is as good as ours at a fraction of the cost.

Why haven't we adopted national health insurance? The answer is complex, but I believe that three factors are chiefly responsible: entrepreneurial ambition, physician resistance to outside interference, and escalating consumer demand for services. The last factor wasn't important until after 1950, when private insurance became widespread. But the other two factors had a unique and remarkable effect on the early development of the U.S. health care system.

During the first U.S. attempt to enact compulsory health insurance during World War I, for example, unions, employers, and physicians all fought it for various reasons. So did insurance companies, even though they didn't sell medical coverage. Why were they against it? Because the proponents of national health insurance had foolishly included funeral benefits in their package. Since the insurers made a lot of money from funeral benefits, they helped kill the bill.[3]

Doctors and Health Insurance   In the early twentieth century, physicians and the American Medical Association (AMA) opposed not only national health insurance—which they said would lead to "socialized medicine"—but also voluntary, private health insurance.[4] They did so mainly because they viewed prepaid care and organized financing systems as intrusions on their right to determine their own fees and practice medicine as they saw fit. So, in the 1920s and 1930s, the AMA fought "contract practices" that competed for a share of workman's comp business and warned doctors not to join the prepaid groups then springing up in the West.[5]

When the Depression arrived, the incomes of both physicians and hospitals fell sharply. Some hospitals responded by forming nonprofit "service-benefit" plans that later became Blue Cross. For a modest monthly fee, employees of local companies could obtain insurance for most hospital services; no matter what these cost, the members would not be liable for any additional charges. Moreover, the early Blue Cross plans charged all of the employee groups the same "community rate"; the healthy subsidized the sick, and workers in small businesses were not disadvantaged compared with those in large firms. Together, these "socialistic" innovations constituted a mighty leap forward for the insured, and millions of people joined these plans.[6]

The AMA took a dim view of the prepaid Blue Cross plans. But consumers were demanding insurance for physician services as well, and some state and county medical societies organized service-benefit plans that would later be called Blue Shield. The AMA cautiously endorsed these efforts, but with a few qualifications: First, it argued that the physician plans should be separate from the hospital plans and under the control of medical societies. Second, the AMA wanted the health plans to reimburse patients, who would still pay cash to the doctors under what is known as an "indemnity" policy. And third, the medical society remained unalterably opposed to compulsory health insurance, which it termed "bureaucratic, inefficient and potentially harmful to the quality of American health care."[7]

The AMA's opposition to national health insurance was the main reason President Franklin Roosevelt did not include it in his package of New Deal social reforms.[8] And the AMA's preference for indemnity insurance helped steer Blue Shield plans toward that type of coverage, which kept the doctors independent of the financing organization.[9] By the 1950s, under pressure from rising costs and competition from commercial insurers, most Blue Cross plans also abandoned their service-benefit orientation and started paying limited cash benefits. And, since the majority of Americans were insured by then, the argument for national health insurance was much weaker than it had been a decade earlier. So the physicians had helped block national health insurance by accepting private insurance, and their endorsement of indemnity policies had staved off the threat of third-party control.

At the same time, the big commercial insurance companies were becoming prominent in health care. While they had initially avoided health insurance because it seemed too risky, the success of the Blues forced them to join the fray. They challenged the nonprofit plans by offering cheaper indemnity insurance and also by segmenting the market into different risk groups. In place of community rating, they used "experience rating" to charge employee groups different premiums, depending on how much health care they used. This meant lower rates for healthier groups; and as the better risks were pulled out of Blue Cross and Blue Shield plans, they had to abandon community rating in order to compete.[10] Once again, entrepreneurial ingenuity won out over social solidarity.

Health Care Becomes Big Business   Several factors contributed to the rapid growth of the health care industry in this period.

First, during World War II, many employers had begun to offer health insurance to their workers. They did so because of the labor shortage and government controls that prevented them from attracting workers with higher wages. The government accelerated this trend by making employee benefits tax-deductible to the employers. After the war, labor unions began to bargain with companies for health benefits, and some cosponsored plans with employers.[11]

The expansion of insurance was accompanied by rising health costs. Between 1935 and 1946, for example, hospital admissions more than doubled, from 2.2 million to 4.7 million.[12] But insurance was not the only driver of spending growth. New technologies added considerable expense, especially in hospitals. So did federal government programs aimed at spurring medical innovation and the availability of health care to the population.

The discovery of penicillin and other "wonder" drugs in the 1930s inspired a great upwelling of public support for medical research. In 1948, Congress created the National Institutes of Health (NIH), starting with the Heart Institute and soon adding five other research centers. Large sums of money followed, and after the successful trials of the Salk vaccine, which eradicated polio, the NIH was assured of continued political support.[13]

In 1946, Congress also passed the Hill-Burton Act, which authorized federal aid to the states for hospital construction. The goal was not only to build more hospitals but to generate jobs and business. Between 1947 and 1971, the government disbursed $3.7 billion in Hill-Burton funds, generating another $9.1 billion in matching state and local funds.[14]

Together, the medical research and hospital funding laws helped turn health care into a big business. Government-funded basic research provided essential support for the budding pharmaceutical and medical device industries, and the spread of community hospitals greatly increased the number of beds that physicians could fill with patients who might benefit from the new technologies.[15] So, while insurance created demand and a way to pay for new services, the availability of those services gave providers a reason to use them.

Medicare Proves a Bonanza   Reformers had been unable to pass national health insurance in the late 1940s, even with the support of President Harry Truman, and their efforts had stalled in the 1950s. But as the 1960s began, a new emphasis on providing insurance to the elderly and the poor started picking up political support. As usual, the AMA opposed this reform and tried to co-opt it with a plan for privately sponsored coverage. But supporters made Medicare politically attractive by turning hospital insurance into an extension of Social Security while patterning medical coverage for the elderly after private policies. At the same time, Congress expanded existing welfare aid to the states into the Medicaid program.[16]

The Blues plans, which already covered millions of seniors, stood to lose from the enactment of Medicare. But they adapted by winning a key role as Medicare intermediaries, processing claims, paying providers, and helping the government do utilization review.[17]

Physicians soon discovered that Medicare was a bonanza, because it guaranteed government payments of the "usual and customary" fees prevailing in their areas. These averages were determined by the Blue Cross and Blue Shield carriers, which were still close to the health care providers that had created them. Hospitals also benefited greatly from Medicare, partly because they'd persuaded Congress to have Medicare pay them on the basis of their costs, rather than negotiated rates.[18]

Nixon Co-Opts the Reformers   With the introduction of the government health programs, it might have seemed that the health care reform impulse would subside. But in the early 1970s, the country came closer to adopting national health insurance than it ever had—or would again. Moreover, this movement occurred under a Republican President, Richard Nixon, and his successor, Gerald Ford, also a Republican.

Rapidly rising costs were the catalyst for action. From 1960 to 1970, per-capita health expenditures had more than doubled, and Medicare and Medicaid had greatly accelerated that growth. Nixon predicted that the system would break down unless action was taken, and the majority of people believed that health care was in a state of crisis. In 1970, Senator Edward Kennedy (D-MA) issued his first call for "Medicare for all." Labor unions and some corporate leaders supported the idea of national health insurance.[19]

But in the end, Nixon proposed a free-enterprise plan to subsidize and promote HMOs, which he viewed as a way to contain costs without having the government take over health care. Nixon also countered the Democrats' campaign for a government-run "single-payer" system with a plan that would have required all employers to cover their workers through private insurers.[20] Representing a decisive break from previous proposals for national health insurance, this approach would set the direction for several subsequent efforts to achieve universal coverage.[21]

Kennedy and Representative Wilbur Mills (D-AR), the broker of Medicare, embraced Nixon's plan with some modifications, but Mills was unable to work out a congressional compromise this time around. Not only was the plan too big for the public to digest but many Democrats also continued to favor the single-payer alternative. In the wake of Watergate, they decided to wait for a more commanding majority after congressional elections. So in 1974, the reform effort died.[22]

It is tempting to speculate about what might have been if Nixon had led the reform effort more strongly or if the final bill hadn't been introduced in the shadow of the Watergate scandal. But all that happened was more spending. In 1974, after Nixon's wage and price controls ended, health care costs shot up 12 percent, three points more than general inflation. And by 1980, health care accounted for nearly 9 percent of GDP, compared with 7.3 percent in 1970.[23]

Watershed in Reform   As Paul Starr points out in his classic book *The Social Transformation of American Medicine*, the early 1970s marked a watershed in health care reform.[24] From World War II until then, the government had focused on building the health care infrastructure and encouraging the provision of more care. But starting with Nixon's HMO crusade, the government took measures to control the rate of spending growth. Public alarm over high costs was partly responsible; but so too was the government's newly vested interest in holding down Medicare and Medicaid spending.

This fiscal restraint did not mean that the government cut off support for health care growth. It continued to support the NIH and increased aid to medical schools, which helped raise the number of doctors by 40 percent from 1970 to 1980.[25] But the early 1970s also saw the passage of laws that encouraged the growth of HMOs, established peer-review organizations to evaluate the medical necessity of physician services, and required states to adopt "certificate of need" laws to check the explosion of new health care facilities.[26] All of this legislation had one purpose: cost containment.

In the long run, none of it really worked. One example, which I return to later, is the 1974 health-planning statute that mandated certificate of need (CON) regulations. The consensus of experts is that CON laws have done little to limit industry growth because they are too easy to get around. But in some states, they have prevented overbuilding of certain kinds of facilities, and health planning has recently been revived in Rochester, New York (see Chapter 21).

What's indisputable is that the deregulatory tide that started in the 1980s has swept away most health planning agencies and prompted many states to repeal their CON laws. Over the years, business interests and conservative politicians have managed to block nearly all government efforts to plan the growth of health care so that the supply of resources matches the need for them.

Hospitals Do an End Run   Hospitals have also been fairly adept at getting around government regulations. A classic example was their response to Medicare's prospective payment system (PPS). Introduced in 1984 when soaring hospital costs threatened to bankrupt Medicare, prospective payment replaced reimbursement for individual services with prepayment for "diagnosis-related groups" of services.[27]

This change in reimbursement methods was initially effective. The growth in Medicare expenditures, which had averaged 16 percent a year from 1970 to 1984, dropped to half of that rate from 1985 to 1989.[28] But the hospitals still managed to maintain their profit margins by charging other payers more, according to the health economist Stuart Altman of Brandeis University. "Hospitals," he wrote in 1994, "have also sought to recoup lost revenues by providing services that pay higher Medicare rates, such as open-heart surgery, and by providing services not controlled by PPS payments, such as expanded outpatient services."[29]

In 1989, Medicare imposed a physician fee schedule based on a complex "relative-value" system.[30] Later, when doctors responded by ratcheting up the volume of services, Medicare began to calibrate annual payment increases to the growth in volume and other factors. But this approach proved to be very crude and contentious, and Congress has had to revisit the issue of physician reimbursement repeatedly.[31]

Employer Self-Funding: A One-Time Fix   Back in the 1980s, meanwhile, employers were also trying to mitigate the pain of skyrocketing health costs, which were consuming up to half of their profits.[32] One strategy was to self-insure. Under the federal Employee Retirement Income Security Act, that approach exempted companies from state benefit requirements. Self-funding also gave firms more control over their cash flow and lowered their expenses if they had a healthy workforce.[33]

But as costs continued to rise, more and more employers turned to the new managed-care organizations to administer their health benefits.[34] These entities included not only HMOs but also PPOs, which offered networks of doctors and hospitals that had agreed to accept discounts in return for patient volume.

Neither Medicare prospective payment nor eighties-style managed care had a long-term impact on cost growth. While increases in the national health tab briefly dipped into single digits in mid-decade, by the early nineties, health costs were rising at 12 percent a year and devouring 14 percent of GDP—twice the amount that they had consumed in 1970—and the number of uninsured people was rapidly rising.[35] In other words, the ingredients for a new stab at health care reform were all present. And soon a new President named Bill Clinton would try to turn them into a recipe for success.

The Clinton Plan: More Government

Although Clinton was elected in 1992 with only 43 percent of the vote, he and his advisers felt they had a mandate to turn the dissatisfaction of the public with out-of-control health costs into a sweeping transformation of the system that would, at long last, provide universal coverage. What they came up with was a combination of market-based "managed competition" and "backup" price controls that would have capped the annual growth in insurance premiums. As in the Nixon plan, employers would have been required to cover their workers, and the government would have subsidized coverage of the poor and of companies with low-wage workers.[36]

Under Clinton's brand of managed competition, HMOs, PPOs, and fee-for-service plans would have competed for the business of employees and self-employed individuals through regional health insurance purchasing alliances.[37] All plans would have had to offer standard, community-rated benefit packages. Only large companies were allowed to self-insure; smaller firms would have had to use the alliances to buy insurance.[38] Some observers immediately pointed out that, since employer contributions in the alliances were capped at 7.9 percent of payroll, even the large companies would have been forced to join them sooner or later.[39] Moreover, experts noted that the payroll limit would mean that government subsidies would be substantial to start and would certainly rise, since health costs were increasing faster than wages.[40]

Because taxes had already been raised to reduce the federal deficit,

Clinton did not suggest increasing them further. Cutting Medicare and Medicaid "waste" was part of the financing formula, and so was the employer mandate.[41] If the government had to limit premiums to contain costs, a national health board was to set a national budget and allocate spending among the regional alliances, which would have negotiated premiums with the health plans.[42]

The lead architect of managed competition, Alain Enthoven of Stanford University, complained that the Clinton administration had transformed his model into a single-payer system. While Enthoven favored two key features of the Clinton plan—universal health insurance and an employer mandate—he criticized the reform proposal for relying on price controls, rather than market forces, to contain costs. And he noted that the regional purchasing alliances would have so much power that they'd be likely to turn into regulatory agencies, rather than the neutral market makers he'd proposed.[43]

There was another key difference between the Clinton approach and that of Enthoven, Paul Ellwood, and other managed-competition theorists who were collectively known as the Jackson Hole Group. Whereas the Clinton plan, at its core, relied on increasing competition among health plans, the Jackson Hole Group wanted to change how health care was delivered as well. They wanted insurers and providers to be combined in competing "integrated delivery networks" that were patterned after Kaiser Permanente and other "group-model" HMOs. This process of integration did occur to a limited extent, first in anticipation of the Clinton plan's passage and later, as a result of market forces. But it fell apart as HMOs declined and insurers were forced to broaden their networks to include more physicians and hospitals.

Why the Plan Collapsed   The public had only a limited grasp of these issues. In fact, in August 1994, nearly a year after the Clinton plan was unveiled, fewer than 20 percent of respondents in a national survey said they understood it. The Clinton plan lost support, the pollster Daniel Yankelovich reported, "because its opponents found it easy to raise the public's fears about reforms people did not understand."[44]

In October 1993, right after Clinton introduced his program, 60 percent of the public endorsed it. But by the following April, according to polls conducted by Robert Blendon of Harvard and his colleagues, "most Americans did not see themselves as better off if the plan became law." Loss of support for the proposal was especially acute among Democrats and the elderly. The majority believed it would hurt quality and raise the cost of care to them.[45]

It would have also meant higher overhead for small companies that weren't currently covering their employees. So, despite the initial support for the plan from big business and even the U.S. Chamber of Commerce, the small business lobby fiercely attacked the proposal.[46] In this effort, they received support from both Republicans in Congress and the Health Insurance Association of America, which produced the memorable "Harry and Louise" television ads that questioned whether there wasn't "a better way."

One of Clinton's top health care advisers, Walter Zelman, believes that the administration's approach to an employer mandate was widely misinterpreted. Its subsidies to small businesses would have made insurance affordable for those who did not already offer it and would have cut costs for those who did, he says. "What we were saying to many small, low-wage businesses was, 'We're going to give your employees health insurance, and you have to pay only 20 percent for it.' At the low end of the scale, for 20 percent of the premium cost, they could offer their employees health insurance. It was an enormous boon for them."

But the Princeton economist Uwe Reinhardt believes that the employer mandate was the nail in the coffin of the Clinton plan. While there's nothing wrong with using private companies to pool insurance risk, he notes, "the minute you mandate coverage, you effectively have imposed a huge payroll tax, which is very regressive. That's why I came out against the Clinton plan. The First Lady actually asked me, 'Why are you against it?' And I told her, 'I think this employer mandate is going to be the killer of your plan,' and it was.' "

Managed Care Triumphs   After the collapse of Clinton's legislation, health care reform didn't go away; it was simply privatized. With government no longer taking the lead, employers increasingly looked to managed-care plans to ease their financial pain, and doctors and hospitals started consolidating to increase their leverage with insurers. Within a few years, the transition from traditional indemnity plans to HMOs, PPOs, and their variants was nearly complete.

Meanwhile, the insurance companies showed how adept they are at gaming the system. In the early 1990s, some states and business coalitions had formed small-business insurance purchasing groups. Homegrown versions of the Clintonites' more elaborate regional alliances, these were insurance "markets" that allowed qualified plans to offer one or more standard benefit packages to employees of member companies. While some alliances, such as California's, used their size to bargain with carriers on rates, others, such as Florida's, relied exclusively on price competition among the plans. For a time, insurance rates in these alliances were as much as 25 percent lower than those outside for comparable plans—and workers had a choice.[47]

But it didn't take the insurers long to figure out how to undercut the alliances. Some refused to participate in them or offered insurance agents lower commissions on alliance business. Other carriers simply used low rates to lure healthy firms away from buying groups or offered multiple-choice plans of their own. A 2002 study by Milliman USA, an actuarial firm, said most of these small-business alliances failed because their premiums were substantially higher than those of policies that small firms could obtain outside.[48]

The managed-care companies showed similar savvy as they pursued larger clients. After getting companies to switch from an indemnity plan to an HMO or a PPO for a substantial one-time saving, they often priced their premiums just below those of the traditional plans. But as competition among managed-care plans heated up, and they fought fiercely for market share, rates did drop for a time. In 1994, employers' cost of providing health benefits actually dipped below that of the previous year.[49]

Backlash Destroys Market Discipline   Since the managed-care plans had very low co-payments back then, they relied mainly on discounting and provider management to keep costs down. Their bag of tricks is well-known: selective contracting, utilization review, pre-authorization, and the use of primary-care physicians as "gatekeepers" to restrict specialty referrals and hospital admissions. In many parts of the country, they used capitation—a form of prepaid care—to give doctors an incentive to hold down utilization. This tactic was most effective in California, where capitated physician groups significantly cut hospital admissions and lengths of stay.[50]

While some of these groups did well under capitation, doctors as a whole rebelled against the health plans' reimbursement cuts and the intrusion of corporate interests into their practices.[51] They communicated their unhappiness to their patients, who were also displeased with managed care. One reason: many employers offered only one plan, and if it was an HMO, some workers felt they were being cheated.[52] Consumers also resented denials of payment for care that they or their doctors felt was necessary, and they feared what might happen if they got really sick. The media fed this disquiet with a steady stream of HMO "horror" stories.

Because HMOs tended to be the most restrictive plans, this managed-care backlash prompted many employers to offer and many employees to sign up with PPOs, which now dominate the market.[53] Companies also demanded that health plans or administrators of self-funded plans provide them with a broad range of doctors and hospitals, because that's what their employees wanted.[54] Meanwhile, in response to the market and to state "patient rights" laws, HMOs began dropping utilization review and referral restrictions and covering more services.[55] As a result, managed care soon lost its ability to save money, except by paying providers less. And, while plans have continued cutting payments to physicians in some areas, hospital consolidation has made it difficult or impossible for insurers to hold the line on inpatient costs.[56]

On to "Consumer-Driven" Care   Although some experts believe that the retreat of managed care helped bring back high rates of spending growth,[57] nobody is talking about returning to the much-vilified HMO approach of the mid-1990s. Rather than relying on providers to keep health care affordable, we're now moving toward a "consumer-driven care" model that will allegedly motivate consumers to reduce spending. But as Paul Ginsburg, president of the Center for Studying Health System Change, observes in a 2005 essay, we're still stuck in a no-man's-land between the demise of managed care and the advent of the new order.[58] Meanwhile, the health care bill keeps rising, and employers keep shifting more of the cost to consumers—a trend that's likely to accelerate with the growth of consumer-driven care.

In 2002, Lewis Sandy, MD, then executive vice president of the Robert Wood Johnson Foundation, wrote that our predicament was exactly the same as it had been in 1990, before the Clinton reform plan and the rise of HMOs. Despite incremental reforms that had given workers the right to keep insurance when they changed jobs and had provided federal aid to cover poor children, health care, he pointed out, was still in crisis.[59]

The central problem, according to Sandy, is that "our collective demand for health services is greater than our collective willingness to pay for them, both from public and private sources." Thus, in the future, he expected most people to have only limited access to care. "With health care costs increasingly being passed on to workers and with income inequality increasing, the costs of broad health care coverage will increasingly be unaffordable for all but the wealthiest."

The Public Clinic Will Serve You   More recently, the health-policy expert Donald Moran predicted that "employer-based insurance . . . will continue to thin out and could amount to a 'catastrophic only' insured benefit before we are too far into the next decade." As more and more people lose insurance or can buy only limited coverage, the government might open public clinics staffed by employed physicians. Rather than just taking care of low-income patients, as federally funded community health centers do today, he says, these clinics would also serve the middle class.[60]

Taking a more optimistic view is Thomas Bodenheimer, MD, of the University of California, San Francisco. A self-described liberal, Bodenheimer hopes that the current policies promoting high-deductible plans will be short-lived and that the government will eventually meet what he sees as its obligation to ensure that everyone has access to decent health care. He points to a few areas of agreement across the political spectrum, including bipartisan support for quality improvement and the expanded use of health information technology.[61]

Quality improvement is like motherhood: Who could be against it? But other health care reform options are far more contentious, because they reflect the basic philosophical split between the rugged individualists and the social reformers. Thus, as the next chapter explains, the differences between the political parties over health care greatly outweigh their agreements. So, while several states are trying to enact or implement meaningful reforms, Congress remains gridlocked. Meanwhile, the possibility of comprehensive care for all Americans is quietly slipping away.

2   'Round and 'Round on the Reform Carousel

Karen, a pleasant, middle-aged woman, cleans houses for a living. She's in good health, but her husband, Jack, recently died of bladder cancer. Jack, a Vietnam War veteran, drove trucks until he was laid off. For eighteen months, he was able to extend his former employer's group coverage through COBRA insurance that cost about $800 a month. That paid for most of his expensive chemo and radiation treatments. Then COBRA ran out, and he couldn't afford to buy individual insurance. Shortly before he died, he went to a Veterans Administration hospital for free care. His widow remains uninsured.

Karen is part of the swelling tide of the uninsured, which increased by 6 million people between 2000 and 2004.[1] The ease with which she and her husband slipped into a precarious financial situation explains why so many other people are afraid of losing their own health coverage. In 2005, 41 percent of nonelderly Americans with incomes between $20,000 and $40,000 were uninsured for at least part of the year—up from 28 percent in 2001.[2]

Unfortunately, as Donald Moran points out, all of the current economic forces are moving in the opposite direction from universal coverage;[3] and, as time goes by without action, comprehensive insurance is also becoming endangered.

What are Congress and the administration doing about this? Much less than you'd expect, considering the importance of this issue to the public. In President George W. Bush's first term, he proposed only minor changes—relatively small tax credits, association plans, and tax deductions for certain individually purchased policies—that would do little to reduce the number of uninsured.[4] Early in 2007, Bush announced a much broader plan that would give all individuals tax breaks for buying insurance and make all employer-paid health insurance taxable. But this risky leap into the unknown would extend coverage to only 3 million to 5 million people.[5] The administration also supports the expansion of "health savings accounts," which are tax-favored vehicles that must be combined with high-deductible insurance policies. But as I show in a later discussion, these are more likely to benefit the affluent than to cover the uninsured.

Since the Democratic sweep in the 2006 midterm elections, the climate for real health care reform has markedly improved. But the ideas being advanced nationally are still irreconcilable, and neither party is expected to make much progress before the next Presidential election.[6] Here's a quick rundown of the current proposals, plus some that have been hanging fire for the past few years.

The Democratic Agenda

As always, Democrats want to expand government programs, while Republicans want to cut or privatize those programs, limit insurance, and shift costs from employers to consumers. Both sides want to tinker with quality improvement and health information technology without understanding much about either. Some reformers want to change how the system is financed, but nobody wants to tackle major restructuring of health care delivery. That's partly because of the fate of the Clinton plan, which relied heavily on HMOs, and the subsequent public backlash to managed care. But, as we see later, there's really no way to save the system without overhauling it completely.

The most radical proposal from the left—that the United States switch to a single-payer system—deals exclusively with financing. This version of national health insurance would preserve private ownership of health care facilities and physician practices. As in the Canadian system, the government would pay most doctors on a fee-for-service basis. All patients would have a free choice of health care providers and would be covered for all "medically necessary" services. Proponents claim that this approach would guarantee universal coverage for much less than we pay today, mainly through savings in administrative costs.[7] And, while employers as well as individuals would have to pay taxes for national health insurance, companies would no longer have to cope with escalating premiums.[8]

This is not the place to analyze the plusses and minuses of a single-payer system. But in brief, some experts question whether the claimed administrative savings would be as significant as single-payer advocates claim.[9] They also cite the problems that many people encounter in gaining access to health care services in government-run systems. And they point out that a single-payer approach would ration care in ways that Americans would find difficult to accept.[10]

For a number of reasons, including a nationwide distrust of government and devotion to free enterprise, health policy experts think it's unlikely that the United States will adopt a single-payer system in the foreseeable future. According to Paul Ginsburg, "Virtually all health policy people in Washington feel that it's infeasible politically."

Congressional Health Plan   Other liberal proposals would build on the current system. Karen Davis and Cathy Schoen, president and vice president, respectively, of the Commonwealth Fund, have devised a plan to achieve near-universal coverage, partly by increasing eligibility for Medicare, Medicaid, and the State Children's Health Insurance Program.[11] Like Senator John Kerry during his 2004 presidential campaign, Davis and Schoen would also offer the uninsured access to the same health plans that federal workers have. This Congressional Health Plan, as they call it, would include all of the insurance plans now participating in the Federal Employees Health Benefit Program, although it would be separate from the federal employees program. Besides the uninsured who lack access to group coverage, self-employed people and small businesses with fewer than fifty employees could buy insurance from these plans at lower rates than they could get on their own.

The main problem with the Congressional Health Plan—which echoes many earlier Democratic proposals—is that nobody would be required to join it. This is the same defect, Ginsburg points out, that was the Achilles' heel of Kerry's proposal: If small employers and individuals could get coverage wherever they liked, the plans participating in the national insurance pool would likely attract a disproportionate number of sick people, while other insurers would cherry pick the healthiest firms and individuals. If that happened, premiums would rise faster in the congressional plans than in the market as a whole.

Moving Toward Individual Insurance   To finance their plan, Davis and Schoen would rely on tax credits and an employer mandate to cover their workers. In contrast, Jeanne Lambrew and Teresa Shaw of the Center for American Progress, and John Podesta, who was White House chief of staff under President Jimmy Carter, favor an individual mandate—that is, everyone not covered by Medicaid or their employer would either have to buy insurance or pay an "income-related assessment." To ensure that nobody paid more than a certain percentage of their income for insurance, they'd offer refundable tax credits indexed to earnings. And, since the deficit-plagued federal government isn't about to subsidize insurance out of its general funds, they'd impose a value-added tax (VAT)—a tax on goods and services at each stage of production—to cover the cost of their plan.[12]

Victor Fuchs, a Stanford University health economist, and Ezekiel Emanuel of the National Institutes of Health also advocate a VAT, which they'd use to raise money for "universal health care vouchers." With these vouchers, people could buy "basic" insurance on a guaranteed basis, regardless of health status. While the federal government would have a much larger role in running the system than it does now, consumers would choose among private health plans and would be able to buy coverage for additional services beyond the standard benefit package. A VAT would inevitably be passed on to consumers in the form of higher prices; and, like any consumption tax, it would take a higher portion of income from the poor than from the middle and upper classes. But Fuchs and Emanuel say that a VAT doesn't have to be regressive if it excludes goods like food and utilities.[13]

In the real world, Massachusetts enacted legislation that required all state residents to purchase health insurance by July 1, 2007. While the goal is near-universal coverage, this program does little to prevent employers from dropping insurance and, in fact, might encourage more of them to do so (see Chapter 18). Nevertheless, the Massachusetts approach has had a major impact on state and national policymakers.

An individual mandate to buy insurance forms the core of two recent national reform proposals. Representative Ron Wyden (D-OR) has proposed a universal coverage plan that would combine an individual insurance mandate with a requirement for employers to increase wages by an amount equivalent to what they now pay for insurance. Companies that don't offer coverage would pay into a premium reduction fund. Wyden's program would incorporate the Congressional Health Plan approach, allowing individuals to choose among standardized plans and deduct insurance premiums from their taxes. He'd provide government subsidies to people making up to 400 percent of the federal poverty level and would limit tax deductions for the affluent.[14]

Former North Carolina Senator John Edwards, who's seeking the 2008 Democratic presidential nomination, also favors an individual mandate combined with a "pay or play" system that requires employers to cover their workers or pay into an insurance fund.[15] Edwards would also provide new tax credits and expand Medicaid and the State Children's Health Insurance Program. The subsidies required to reach universal coverage by this route would cost up to $120 billion a year.[16] Edwards proposes to finance his plan by raising taxes on the wealthy, among other methods.

Edwards also wants to create regional "health markets" for individuals who don't get insurance at work, as well as businesses that choose to participate. Under this proposal, the federal government would help states and groups of states form purchasing pools that would offer a choice of plans, including a public plan patterned after Medicare. These health markets, Edwards asserts, would drive down rates by negotiating with insurers and by reducing the high administrative costs of individual and small-group coverage.[17]

While this approach resembles the Congressional Health Plan in some respects, the idea of having the government itself sell insurance to individuals and companies would be a step toward a single payer system. It would be a giant step if public plans undercut private ones on price, encouraging employers to buy insurance through the government.[18] "Over time, the system may evolve toward a single-payer approach if individuals and businesses prefer the public plan," states Edwards' campaign.[19]

The Republican Agenda

In general, Republicans don't favor government mandates on businesses, and they abhor the idea of a single-payer system. Although some of them support the individual mandate, most Republicans are less interested in universal coverage than in cutting costs and reducing the burden on employers. To achieve those goals, they want to reduce coverage for everyone and get more people to buy their own insurance. But Republicans don't want to do this in such a way that it would destroy job-based insurance, because that would pave the way for a government takeover of health care.

A few years ago, the AMA suggested a way to decouple insurance from the workplace without abandoning the employer-based system. Under the AMA plan to attain universal coverage, the employer-paid portion of insurance premiums would become taxable to employees, and everyone would receive tax credits, inversely proportional to income, for buying required health coverage on their own. Private insurance markets or state-run insurance pools would be established to help individuals purchase coverage at affordable rates.[20]

Since higher-paid people would see their taxes go up more than they'd receive back in tax credits, this would mean a major transfer of income from the affluent to the less affluent—not a politically popular idea.[21] Nevertheless, the idea of ending the tax exclusion of employer-provided insurance has a lot of support on the right. For example, when Bill Frist was Senate Majority Leader, he said that the tax exclusion insulates people from the true cost of health care and thus drives up costs.[22] Other conservatives maintain that it's unfair for individuals who buy their own insurance not to be able to deduct the cost from their taxes if those with work-related coverage can.[23] But until recently, nobody dared to tamper with a tax preference that has been in place for 60 years and benefits the majority of Americans.

That all changed with President Bush's 2007 State of the Union address. In his speech, Bush proposed that everyone pay taxes on the cost of health insurance after a $7,500 standard deduction for single people and a $15,000 deduction for families.[24] This means that those with employer-provided insurance worth more than the deduction would have to pay taxes on some of their insurance benefits. While Bush describes such policies as "gold-plated," critics point out that many people of modest means, including teachers, nurses, and factory workers, would face a tax increase unless they chose leaner health plans.[25] Bush's program would mean a tax decrease for people with policies worth less than the deductible; but for 30 million others, it would result in a tax hike.[26]

The proposal *would* lower the cost of buying coverage for the uninsured. But some experts note that the poor and the near-poor, who make up the bulk of the uninsured, would still be unable to afford coverage.[27] Middle-class people would also find it hard to find affordable, comprehensive policies in the individual market, where insurance costs much more than group coverage and people in poor health are often shut out.

Some critics maintain that the President's plan would accelerate the decline of employer coverage. For example, Sara Rosenbaum, chair of the health policy department at George Washington University in Washington, DC, argues that the ability of individuals to take a tax deduction for buying insurance on their own would give some employers an excuse to terminate coverage.[28] Other observers predict that the tax deduction for insurance would encourage younger, healthier employees to buy individual coverage, driving up premiums for a company's other workers.[29] But the White House denies that it's trying to move people away from job-based insurance.[30]

'Moral Hazard' and Consumer-Driven Care   The other goal of Bush's plan, some observers say, is to reduce the amount of health insurance that people have.[31] This is a very credible argument, both because people would have to pay taxes on the value of expensive insurance policies and because many Republicans believe that comprehensive coverage drives health costs up.[32] If they had their druthers, we'd all be in catastrophic, high-deductible plans.

Conservatives oppose coverage for ordinary medical bills because they view it as a source of "moral hazard"—meaning that people are motivated to overuse health care when they are insured. The 2004 *Economic Report of the President* states, "Over-reliance on health insurance as a payment mechanism leads to an inefficient use of resources in providing and utilizing health care."[33] Of course, uninsured and underinsured people who use fewer services also tend to be in poorer health[34]—but that isn't a concern of those who worry about moral hazard.

The main Republican gambit for cost containment, health savings accounts (HSAs), reflects this bias. Created by the 2003 Medicare Modernization Act but available only to those who aren't enrolled in Medicare, HSAs are similar to flexible spending accounts, except that they can be rolled over from year to year and can be funded by employers as well as employees. The pretax money in an HSA can accumulate and be invested tax free, and it remains tax free if it's withdrawn to pay medical expenses.[35]

HSAs must be coupled with insurance plans that have a deductible of at least $1,000 for a single person and $2,000 for a family. Members of these plans are at financial risk for the difference between the amount employers place in their HSAs and the deductible, which is usually much higher. Proponents of HSAs say they will hold down health costs by encouraging people to avoid unnecessary care. Detractors argue that HSAs benefit mainly the healthy and the wealthy.[36] If you're sick, they note, you'll quickly use up the funds in your health spending account and have to pay out of pocket until you meet the deductible.[37] Critics also point out that only a small percentage of enrollees in these "consumer-directed health plans" (CDHPs) were previously uninsured.[38] So it doesn't look like these plans will do much to expand coverage.

Employers are showing some interest in CDHPs, whether the high-deductible plans are coupled with HSAs or health reimbursement arrangements (HRAs). (The latter is a variation on the theme that allows companies to hold onto health funds when employers leave or are laid off.) A 2005 Deloitte and Touche survey of large, self-insured corporations found that 22 percent had a CDHP in place, and 21 percent intended to offer one in the following year.[39] However, only 7 percent of all employers that provided health benefits in 2006 included a consumer-directed plan, and only 4 percent of workers were enrolled in one.[40] While 3.2 million people were in high-deductible plans that were eligible for HSAs or HRAs,[41] just 1.3 million people had health savings accounts.[42]

CDHP Targets Minority of Costs   If CDHPs were widespread, would they restrain growth in health care costs? Insurers and conservative pundits say yes. Some companies that sell CDHPs say they've seen physician office visits and drug costs drop substantially when patients feel their own money is at stake.

But John Erb, a benefit consultant with Deloitte & Touche, notes that the majority of health care expenses are not discretionary and are determined by physicians. Partly for that reason, Marilyn Moon, a health-policy expert at the American Institutes for Research, doubts that consumer-directed plans will save much money. "The first $500 or $1,000 of expenditures is a drop in the bucket compared to total health spending," she says. "Ten percent of the population accounts for 70 percent of the cost. And those people aren't in a position to be changing how they use health care, except now and then to be using less, which I'm not sure we want them to. So there's not very much to be gained."

Avoiding Necessary Care   A 2005 survey found that 35 percent of people in CDHPs delayed or avoided necessary health care, compared with 17 percent of those in comprehensive health plans.[43] Other evidence also suggests that CDHPs motivate consumers to skip care. For example, patients in one CDHP visited their doctors 20 percent less often than they did before.[44] What portion of those missed visits should have been made?

A report from the Commonwealth Fund concludes that CDHPs discourage patients from seeking needed preventive care and treatment for chronic conditions.[45] Other CDHP opponents note that, even with the new Web-based tools that insurers are making available, most consumers don't know enough about medicine or the health care system to make good decisions about what care they need and from whom they should seek it (see Chapter 6).

Donald Berwick, MD, president of the Institute for Healthcare Improvement and a leader of the health care quality movement, lambastes consumer-directed plans on moral grounds. "I do not believe that making the individual American patient more 'cost-sensitive' has any rationale in science, ethics or evidence," he says in a published interview. "It will fail, and it will fail miserably. It will result in a shifting of care away from the people who need it the most."[46]

Paying Again for Quality   Observers all along the political spectrum agree that higher-quality care would cost less. That's partly because there is so much waste in the system, and partly because of all the unexplained variations in care that result in unnecessary spending (see Chapter 8). If doctors delivered only appropriate, scientifically justified care, and available resources were used more wisely, patients would benefit and costs might drop by 30 to 40 percent, Berwick and other experts estimate.

That's the rationale for the growing "pay-for-performance" (P4P) trend, which has been embraced by employers, health plans, and the government. The advocates of P4P believe that if you pay doctors extra to do particular things, such as making sure that patients with diabetes get hemoglobin A1c tests, they'll be more likely to do them. That seems obvious, and there's some evidence that P4P can change physician behavior.[47] But P4P also has some unintended consequences, which are explained in Chapter 4. Moreover, it mainly tackles the underuse of services, so it will probably cost more money, not less, in the short run.

P4P does little about the misuse and overuse of services, which not only endanger patients but also drive up costs.[48]

Information Technology   Another key plank in the Republican health care platform is the use of health information technology to improve care and reduce medical errors. President Bush's campaign to computerize health records began with his 2004 State of the Union address. Information technology experts applauded his initiative but scratched their heads when he allocated only $100 million to the effort in fiscal 2005.[49] In April 2004, Bush announced the health care equivalent of landing a man on the moon (or Mars): He proposed that most Americans should have access to electronic health records within ten years. He also named a national health information technology coordinator, David Brailer, MD, to lead this Herculean effort.[50] Later, the Republican-dominated Congress trimmed the $50 million allocated for Brailer's office from the budget.[51] Although the Department of Health and Human Services found money to keep it going, Congress also cut Bush's modest request for health information technology funds in fiscal 2006, and Congress failed to pass bipartisan bills to promote EHR adoption.[52]

President Bush, former Senator Frist, Health and Human Services Secretary Mike Leavitt, and former House Speaker Newt Gingrich have hailed health information technology as if it were a magic elixir. There's no doubt that electronic health records would improve quality, and it has been estimated that full clinical data automation could save more than $80 billion a year by increasing efficiency and safety.[53] But there's tremendous resistance among physicians and hospitals to making the investment in information technology, which would financially benefit government and private payers much more than providers. Only about 15 percent of doctors had electronic health records (EHRs) in 2005, and fewer than 10 percent of hospitals had computerized order entry systems.[54] If current trends continue, one study predicts, it will be twenty years before EHRs are widespread.[55]

Public Reporting   In the administration's game plan, the acceleration of EHR adoption is closely linked with public reporting of data on physician and hospital performance. These "report cards" are supposed to help members of consumer-directed plans select health care providers.

To make this vision come true, President Bush in August 2006 signed an executive order that requires all federal agencies involved in health care—including Medicare, the Departments of Defense and Veterans Affairs, and the Office of Personnel Management—to start offering provider quality and cost information to people enrolled in their health care programs and, if the agency wishes, to the public. Private insurers will have to report this data to the Federal Employee Health Benefits Program and to the Center for Medicare and Medicaid Services (CMS), if they operate Medicare HMOs.[56]

Most of the quality data is not yet available, and the cost data will merely show what the plans pay each doctor, hospital, and other provider for particular services. Since Medicare sets its own prices, and most physicians have little leeway to bargain with private insurers,[57] these cost comparisons won't really help insured people or Medicare patients choose a doctor. But in this administration, facts seem to be less important than ideology.

The Real Challenges

Michael Fleming, MD, former president of the American Academy of Family Physicians, likes to tell medical students about a thirty-three-year-old man he encountered a few years ago. One night, the patient woke up feeling chest pain. "He was taken to the emergency room, where he had every test known to man done," Fleming says. "He had a CT scan of his chest; everything was negative, except on the periphery of the CT scan they saw a calcified nodule in his neck. They did a CT scan of his neck to make sure. He went to an ENT surgeon who opened his neck, and it turned out to be a calcified carotid bulb, which you can't live without, so the surgeon left it alone. Then the man went to a cardiologist, who did a treadmill stress test. That was equivocally positive, so he had a heart cath, which was cold normal. So now this man has a hole in his groin, a scar on his neck, two CT scans, and he still has chest pain.

"So he came to my office, and I said, 'What do you do?' We have an Air Force base in town, and he's a civilian employee of that Air Force base, and he works on jet engines. And he raised his arm up and said, 'Oh, that's it.' And it turns out that his power scaffolding had broken, and they'd gotten him a new one, and it didn't go as high as the old scaffolding. I reached across and squeezed a muscle—his anterior axillary fold—and he said, 'That's where it hurts.'

"He had a ton of medical bills, plus he put himself at risk for two procedures, because no one asked him how it hurt, and no one examined him. The reason is that no one gets paid for examining and asking questions, but you get paid for CT scans and surgery.

"My office visit that day cost $60, and his bills added up to $128,000. That tells me that there's a lot of money in the system that we're wasting. We could be providing good quality care and we're not doing it."

Too Many Specialists   Fleming's tale contains several lessons about what's wrong with the system. First, in both hospitals and outpatient settings, people are consulting or being referred to specialists much more often than they were a decade ago, when managed-care plans restricted access to these consultants. Many people believe that specialists are better diagnosticians than primary-care physicians, but it ain't necessarily so. And every trip a patient makes to a specialist is likely to lead to a cascade of tests and procedures.

Second, the cognitive work that primary-care physicians do is undervalued by comparison with the high-tech tests and procedures that specialists do.[58] For example, in 2006 Medicare paid primary-care physicians $50 for a medium-level office visit by an established patient. In contrast, CMS paid cardiologists $383 for a catheterization on the left side of the heart, and that doesn't include the additional amount cardiologists could net if they owned their own cardiac cath lab.[59] Not surprisingly, specialists earn much more than primary-care physicians, and fewer young doctors are going into primary care as a result.

Many specialists have joined large single-specialty groups. This move gives them more clout in negotiating with health plans and enables them to buy expensive diagnostic equipment and set up imaging centers, cardiac catheterization labs, and other income-generating facilities.[60] Some groups have even invested in specialty hospitals, many of which perform only lucrative cardiology or orthopedic procedures. These institutions drain off the best-paying business from general hospitals that still have to maintain emergency rooms and care for the uninsured.[61]

Too Much Money to Be Made   Not that most hospitals are ailing. In fact, they're now in the midst of what's probably their biggest building boom since the government phased out its Hill-Burton subsidies in the 1970s.[62] Also, in 2004, hospitals enjoyed their largest profit margin ever,[63] and it rose even further the next year.[64] One reason is that in many markets, the consolidation of facilities into multihospital systems has given them an edge in negotiating fees with insurers.[65] The average net income of multihospital organizations jumped 44 percent in 2005.[66]

Also riding on the health care gravy train are pharmaceutical companies, which harvest immense profits from the system. The big drug companies argue that they have to charge Americans high prices to finance research on new life-saving drugs. But in fact, they spend twice as much on marketing and administration as on research, and most of their products are "me-too" variants on rival companies' medications. The drug industry now rakes in well over $200 billion a year in U.S. sales, more than three times as much as in 1980.[67] And despite some recent setbacks, pharmaceuticals remains one of the most profitable businesses in the nation.

The insurance industry, too, is riding high. Profits for the nation's HMOs jumped 10.7 percent in 2004;[68] UnitedHealth Group, one of the largest insurance companies, had net profit growth of 28 percent in 2005.[69] Now the insurers are seizing the twin opportunities of government-subsidized Medicare drug plans and the management of financial assets for people in consumer-directed health plans.[70] Meanwhile, insurance premiums continue to soar, and more than a million people lose their insurance every year.

Perverse Incentives   One thing that liberals and conservatives agree on is that the U.S. health care system provides little incentive for physicians and other health care providers to improve quality. In fact, when doctors and hospitals try to do the right thing, they're often punished financially. One stunning example occurred in New York. According to the *New York Times*, four of the city's hospitals set up diabetes centers to teach patients how to manage the disease and check their blood-sugar levels. After seven years, three of the four centers had been shut down because they'd lost money. While there is no money in preventive care, the article notes, it's very profitable to treat complications of diabetes, such as kidney failure and loss of circulation in extremities, which leads to amputation.[71]

Despite the perverse incentives in the system, reformers like Donald Berwick have persevered in pushing the quality agenda. Berwick and his Institute for Healthcare Improvement (IHI) recently announced that three thousand hospitals across the country had saved an estimated 122,000 lives by making certain process changes advocated by IHI. Among the hospitals' goals are to ensure that antibiotics are administered before surgery to prevent infections. Another goal, designed to prevent adverse drug events, is to guarantee that someone find out what medications a patient is on when he or she is transferred from one care setting to another.[72]

Donald Fisher, president of the American Medical Group Association, praises Berwick's initiative. But he points out that unless the financial incentives change, it will have little impact on the system as a whole. "Every time a hospital avoids that adverse event, that's a loss of revenue for that institution," he says. "And if you're a small community hospital, how long can you reduce your revenue stream by $5 million every year? It's terrific that you're saving lives and money, but the fact is that these folks have fixed costs."

Fragmented Delivery System   Another reason health care is dysfunctional is that it's highly fragmented. The majority of physicians work in small practices that have no business relationship with one another. Patients see a primary-care physician and are referred to a specialist, handed off to another consultant, admitted to a hospital, discharged to a nursing home or rehab facility, and then sent back to the hospital. Along the way, they may have tests at different labs and may pick up prescriptions at multiple pharmacies. And every time they move from one care setting to another, information about their previous care is lost.

Wouldn't the administration's campaign to expand the use of health information technology help overcome this problem? Undoubtedly. But as mentioned earlier, the prevalence of small practices and the lack of financial incentives militate against the rapid spread of EHRs. Moreover, even if every doctor and hospital in the country were computerized, fragmentation and the scarcity of organized care systems would still impede communication among providers. Finally, primary-care physicians are not paid to coordinate care, although they're the only ones who could do so.

Rapidly Advancing Technology No matter how we reform health care financing and delivery, the explosion in medical knowledge will confound our efforts to contain costs. William Schwartz, MD, in his book *Life without Disease: The Pursuit of Medical Utopia*, points out, "In 1950 costs of health were relatively low, because, for a large percentage of patients, doctors couldn't really do very much."[73] Now they can do a whole lot more, and the health care portion of GDP has shot up from 4.4 percent in 1950 to 16 percent today. Organ transplants, kidney dialysis, cardiac surgery, neonatal intensive care units, biologic drugs, new imaging techniques, and other medical advances have saved and improved countless lives. But as George Halvorson and George Isham note in their book *Epidemic of Care*, "Miracles cost money."[74]

This is not a reason for despair, however. When we recognize that not everyone can have everything, learn how to distinguish what's truly beneficial, and devise a socially responsible way to distribute the fruits of technology, we should be able to sustain comprehensive, affordable health care. But we can't build such a system until we replace our mindless devotion to ever-bigger profits with a dedication to universal coverage as a social good.

Avoiding the Politically Unpalatable The two sides in the health care debate agree that current spending growth is unsustainable. But they cannot agree on how to reduce the waste in the system. While conservatives recognize that the current incentives are wrong, they believe they can change provider behavior with pay for performance. At the same time, they say that reducing insurance coverage will induce consumers to spend less. But neither of these initiatives will get spending under control, because they don't address the structural problems listed above. They won't stop physicians from providing inappropriate care; they won't overcome the basic incentives of fee-for-service to do more, rather than provide better quality; they won't improve care coordination; they won't take the profit out of "me-too" drugs and MRI machines; and they won't limit the amount of money that insurance companies can drain from the system.

Liberals are just as myopic about the need for structural changes. Those who support a single-payer system would have us believe that a top-down government solution can control costs without restricting the freedom of providers or patients. They talk about doctors being paid more for doing more in the same breath that they speak about imposing global budgets.[75] Those who believe we can achieve universal coverage by simply expanding government programs and subsidizing the cost of insurance aren't proposing changes in health care delivery, either. Yet unless we alter how care is delivered, it won't matter how we finance it. We'll still go broke.

All parties would also prefer to ignore the fact that, with technology inexorably advancing, no solution can succeed without some kind of rationing. The real question is how we want to ration care. Do we want to follow the Republican prescription, which is to preserve comprehensive services for the affluent, while skimping on care for everyone else? Or do we want to provide comprehensive care for everyone, as the Democrats' proposals aim to do? And if we choose the latter course, how much would we be willing to pay in health insurance premiums and taxes? Are we willing to limit certain kinds of very expensive care of marginal value? If so, who will be able to obtain those services?

These are some of the questions that are addressed later in the book. But first, let's take a closer look at what's wrong with the current paradigm of health care reform, starting with disease management, which is the forerunner and substratum of pay for performance.

Part II
The Emperor's New Clothes

3   The Two Faces
of Disease Management

Chronic diseases account for about three-quarters of all health care spending. Nearly half of the U.S. population has at least one chronic disease, and half of those have more than one.[1] The number is growing as boomers age and as more and more people—including children—begin to suffer from obesity.[2] Not only do chronic diseases generate the majority of doctor visits and drug prescriptions, but the treatment of these illnesses is driving up hospital costs. In 2004, the hospitalization of people with coronary artery disease, congestive heart failure, chronic obstructive pulmonary disease, mental health disorders, diabetes, hypertension, and asthma cost $94.3 billion. Among Medicare patients alone, inpatient treatment for those seven diseases cost $58.8 billion.[3]

Many of these hospitalizations could have been avoided if patients had received better care. According to a landmark RAND Corp. study published in 2003, adult patients in this country get only about half of the preventive, chronic, and acute care recommended by best-practice guidelines.[4]

What that figure means is that every day people are dying who might have been saved. For example, only 65 percent of people with hypertension in the study received all of the recommended care. Down the line, uncontrolled hypertension can lead to heart attacks and strokes. "Poor blood pressure control contributes to more than 68,000 preventable deaths annually," the researchers note.

The RAND study also found that only 24 percent of diabetic patients had received three or more glycosylated hemoglobin tests in a two-year period. More reliable than the self-testing methods that diabetics use, these HbA1c tests, as they're known, are the best way to measure blood-sugar levels. When people aren't tested, their diabetes can get out of control. Long-term consequences may include amputations, blindness, kidney failure, and death.

If patients receive appropriate care at an early stage in the course of a chronic disease, its progression can be slowed and its adverse effects minimized. But physicians don't always provide the right care, and patients don't always seek it or comply with doctors' orders. So they get worse. That's why a technique called disease management was invented in the mid-1990s.[5]

Originally devised by pharmaceutical companies,[6] disease management has evolved into a variety of methods for controlling the progress and minimizing the impact of chronic ailments. Employers and health plans have embraced disease management, and Medicare is trying it out in demonstration projects. Many state Medicaid programs are also using disease management. Together, public and private payers spent $1.12 billion on disease-management programs in 2005, up from $900 million in 2004.[7]

Continuous Quality Improvement   Disease management started out with a grand vision. The idea was to apply the industrial principle of continuous quality improvement to the whole spectrum of care for a particular condition, including inpatient and outpatient care and ancillary services. By persuading physicians to follow practice guidelines, measuring the results, and feeding those results back to the doctors, health plans and medical groups hoped to reduce variations in care and produce better outcomes. Proponents also maintained that optimum use of drug therapies would reduce emergency room visits and hospitalization, thus cutting overall costs.[8]

It was a great concept, but it quickly ran into major obstacles. First, except in some large medical groups that were integrated with hospitals, there was not enough structure in local medical communities to monitor patients across the continuum of care settings. Also, information systems were rudimentary, even in the most advanced groups, and so it was hard to keep track of what was being done for each patient. And, as this chapter shows, the evidence that disease management saves more than it costs is still fairly shaky.

Some Early Breakthroughs   Nevertheless, some groups and HMOs did achieve significant results in their pioneering work in disease management. The Harvard Community Health Plan (now Harvard Pilgrim), for example, made strides in pediatric asthma care. A diabetes care coordination program at Group Health Cooperative showed how patient education and disease registries (data on patients with a particular disease) could improve diabetes care.[9] And the Lovelace Clinic in Albuquerque, New Mexico, reported a 34 percent reduction in hospital admissions of children with asthma. Improvements in prenatal care and an enhanced focus on complicated patients helped reduce the rate of premature births, saving $440,000 in neonatal intensive care costs in the first year. Among the other conditions addressed by the three-hundred-doctor group were attention deficit hyperactivity disorder, allergic rhinitis, breast cancer, cardiac revascularization, congestive heart failure, depression, diabetes, hyperlipidemia (high cholesterol), hypertension, low back pain, pneumonia, and stroke.[10]

The success of Lovelace's disease-management program can be attributed to the involvement of clinicians in all phases of its design and execution. First, multidisciplinary teams of specialists, primary-care physicians, nurse case managers, and pharmacists worked together to design clinical guidelines. Second, these guidelines were boiled down to simple checklists that doctors could refer to in the exam room. Third, physician champions went from one Lovelace office to another, preaching the value of the guidelines. And fourth, doctors received data showing how their own work diverged from best practices, as defined by the group. The other key ingredient was financial support from a pharmaceutical company that underwrote the program's costs.

Meanwhile, Group Health Cooperative, a group-model HMO in Seattle, was creating what later became known as the "chronic-care model." Conceived by a team under the leadership of Edward Wagner, MD, who heads a research institute that's part of Group Health Cooperative, the chronic-care model calls for mobilizing community resources to meet patient needs; reorganizing the delivery system to create quality incentives and to promote communication among primary-care physicians, specialists, and other clinicians; teaching patients how to manage their own care; providing individual case management for complex patients; ensuring regular follow-ups by the care team; promoting adherence to evidence-based guidelines; and integrating disease registries and other decision support tools into practice with the help of information technology.[11]

Devolution of Disease Management   While big groups like Lovelace and Group Health Cooperative pressed forward with their versions of disease management, health plans and independent practice associations also began to apply approaches loosely called "disease management" to small practices. Some of the more sophisticated independent practice associations (IPAs), such as Brown and Toland and Hill Physicians in northern California, created fairly advanced programs similar to those of the large group practices. But what most HMOs did was quite different.

Instead of engaging physicians in their disease-management programs, the insurers farmed the programs out to firms that specialized in helping the sickest patients with particular conditions.[12] While there have been some advances in the field since then, the basic formula is still the same: The disease-management vendors employ nurse case managers who call and pay home visits to patients and keep track of their health status, sometimes with the aid of remote monitoring devices. They involve physicians only if a patient is having an acute episode or needs to have his or her medication adjusted.

Big Turnover Is Key Factor   How did disease management depart so far from its original focus? First, it's important to understand that the main goal of health plans in this endeavor is to save money. Second, because their membership has an average turnover of around 20 percent a year, long-term savings are as likely to benefit their competitors as themselves. So most plans address only conditions that are widespread and expensive and in which interventions can yield substantial short-term savings. The most popular candidates are asthma, diabetes and high-risk pregnancy.[13]

To avoid losing money on disease management, HMOs have also concentrated on patients with severe disease, typically comprising about 3 percent of their members.[14] Because these are the patients who are most likely to visit the ER or be admitted to the hospital, keeping their conditions under control can produce a quick return on investment. For example, if a patient with congestive heart failure alerts a care manager immediately that his weight has risen by a few pounds, a costly hospitalization can sometimes be averted.[15]

Meanwhile, attempts by health plans to get doctors to follow guidelines have been mostly ineffective. The most important reasons are that most physicians distrust the HMOs, feel that guidelines impinge on their clinical autonomy, and cannot deal with multiple guidelines for the same condition from different plans.[16]

No Financial Incentive   Another major barrier to involving physicians in disease management is that they have no financial incentive to do so. "Sure, doctors should coordinate care better, take calls from the durable equipment company, make sure the oxygen gets delivered, but nobody does any of that because they don't get paid to do it," says David Nash, MD, a disease-management expert and chairman of the health policy department at Jefferson Medical College in Philadelphia.

"The disease-management industry consists of about one hundred companies, including maybe ten worth knowing about," he continues. "These ten deliver coordinated chronic care. What's doctors' role? Basically, to stay out of the way. This is too important to be left to primary-care physicians. They're too busy; they don't have any incentive to do any of this; they're not paid to do it; and the reality is they're not good at it, anyway."

Julie Sanderson Austin, vice president of quality management and research for the American Medical Group Association, agrees that most physicians have no financial reason to do disease management. "If they're paid fee-for-service, it's hard to make the argument that they should be at risk for the outcomes of their patients. The incentives are all wrong for them. They get paid less for quality care than for care that causes problems. The more patient visits and the more procedures they do, the more they get paid."

Lack of Organization   Large prepaid groups can do disease management properly and also have an incentive to coordinate care because they're financially accountable, Nash notes. But he doubts that doctors in small practices could do the same job, even if they were economically motivated to take on the task.

He cites his own faculty practice, which, with twenty internists, is far bigger than most primary-care practices. The group lacks an electronic medical record, and its nurses don't have time to call sick patients at home regularly. "We refer everybody with severe disease to specialists, and we have no idea what happens until they come back to us," he says. "It's not coordinated in any way.

"Compare my practice to that of a typical internist at Kaiser Permanente. Kaiser has its own hospitals, pharmacies, and practice guidelines, its own electronic medical record, and a Web portal to e-mail with patients. We don't do any of that. So it's apples and oranges in terms of where we are. Or maybe it's current and future practices."

Hospital Incentives Vary   Hospital executives may have a hard time seeing how disease management will help them, since hospitals lose money when fewer people are admitted. But they also lose money on Medicare patients with chronic conditions, because Medicare pays flat rates for episodes of acute care. So some hospitals have started programs for asthma and other chronic diseases. Sutter Healthcare, a large integrated delivery system in northern California, takes full-risk capitation from HMOs, giving it another incentive to do disease management. Its programs for heart failure, diabetes, and asthma have paid off. ER visits for enrollees in these programs are about half of what they are for the general patient base, and Sutter saves an average of $600 a month for each patient enrolled in these programs.[17]

The Department of Veterans Affairs (VA) health care system has also been running disease-management programs for several years. In its diabetes program, it has steadily increased the percentage of patients who have received recommended screening tests and have reached the goals for controlling their disease. As a result, it has far surpassed the national average on those measures and has reduced the rate of diabetes-related amputations by half.[18] By integrating care coordination services with daily in-home monitoring and clinical information tools, the VA has also decreased hospital admissions by 60 percent among patients in its disease-management programs.[19]

Looking Below the Surface   Why can't Medicare or commercial health plans do the same thing? To begin with, the VA hospitals and clinics form the largest integrated delivery system in America. Like Kaiser, the VA has its own pharmacies, labs, and guidelines—and, unlike HMOs that contract with independent physicians, it can tell its employed doctors to use those guidelines. It has a large workforce of nurses who can be deployed to educate chronic-disease patients. And the VA has a systemwide electronic health record that enables physicians to coordinate care, track patients' progress, and measure their own performance much better than they could on paper.

The American College of Physicians, in a 2004 public policy paper, says it prefers the chronic-care model used by the VA and Kaiser to conventional disease management, partly because it enhances the role of physicians: "The chronic-care model is much more encompassing, and includes direct patient care and self-care support, as well as care oversight for one or more chronic conditions plus all existing co-morbid conditions."[20]

Only very large physician groups, however, have the resources and the infrastructure to attempt such an ambitious project. Most small practices don't even have the capability to build an electronic registry of their chronic-disease patients, which is a cornerstone of the chronic-care model.[21]

Newer Approaches   Conventional disease management has a lot of shortcomings. It's fine to help the sickest patients, but other patients who have mild or moderate forms of a disease might someday get sicker, and they're not receiving any special help to prevent that. Also, elderly people frequently have multiple conditions, such as cardiac disease, arthritis, and osteoporosis, and patients with a chronic disease often have more than one ailment. A patient with diabetes, for example, is likely to have hypertension and is at high risk for developing heart disease. Yet most disease-management programs still focus on particular conditions, rather than the whole person. So the patient may be dealing with multiple care managers who work for different programs or even different disease-management companies.

In an effort to improve the care of the sickest and costliest patients, some health plans and employers have recently shifted their emphasis from traditional disease management to "predictive modeling"—computerized forecasting of who will get sick—and high-risk case management. "By identifying high-risk patients prospectively, plans and employers hope to lower future health costs by avoiding delays in needed care, improving care coordination, eliminating redundant care, and encouraging self-management of health conditions," researchers from the Center for Studying Health System Change note.[22]

The coordination of care for patients with multiple chronic-care conditions is a top priority for the managed-care industry.[23] While 10 percent of the population accounts for 70 percent of health spending, the sickest 1 percent accounts for a staggering 27 percent.[24]

Cost Savings Are Uncertain   Some health plans have reported dramatic savings from disease management. CIGNA, for example, saw a 26 percent decrease in hospital admissions of patients enrolled in American Healthway's disease-management program for diabetes. Overall, the plan estimated, it saved nearly 15 percent on treating these patients.[25] Aetna reported a 3:1 rate of return on disease management for very sick patients, such as those with congestive heart failure. A Cornell University study also showed savings from programs for congestive heart failure, but mixed results on asthma and diabetes.[26]

A 2004 report by the Congressional Budget Office raised doubts about whether disease management as a whole saves more than it costs. Based on its examination of studies of programs for congestive heart failure, coronary artery disease and diabetes, as well as other literature reviews, the government agency stated, "To date there is insufficient evidence to conclude that disease management programs can generally reduce the overall cost of health care services."[27]

Similarly, a survey of disease-management programs in twelve markets across the country concluded that "evidence of their clinical and cost effectiveness remains limited." The researchers found that the experience of health plans was "too preliminary to assess how well they work." Even plans that found the programs improved care for some conditions had difficulty showing a return on investment.[28]

A large, randomized controlled trial in Texas found that a conventional disease-management program using nurse case managers did not reduce the costs of treating heart failure patients. They had just as many office visits, ER visits, and hospitalizations as those in the control group. This finding is surprising because a number of previous studies had indicated that disease management could decrease hospitalizations of these very expensive patients. But as the study's authors point out, the earlier studies (including a few randomized trials) were much smaller and briefer; they also used patient cohorts that were less representative of the general population.[29]

Addressing Underuse Costs Money   Even large, sophisticated organizations that have advanced disease-management programs may not save money on them. For example, Bruce Fireman and his colleagues in Kaiser Permanente's northern California HMO examined the results of four programs—for coronary artery disease, congestive heart failure, diabetes, and asthma—from 1996 to 2002.[30] Kaiser's state-of-the-art approach included clinical guidelines, patient self-management education, disease registries, proactive outreach to patients, coordination of hospital and community services, reminders to doctors, multidisciplinary care teams, and performance feedback to providers.

By 2002, 20 percent of Kaiser's patients with coronary artery disease, 24 percent of those with congestive heart failure, 23 percent of those with diabetes, and 14 percent of those with asthma had participated in these programs. Physicians provided more of the recommended care to these patients than they'd received before. Partly as a result, median LDL cholesterol levels dropped significantly among the patients with heart disease and diabetes, and more patients got their blood pressure under control.

Net costs for patients with these conditions, however, rose between 19 and 27 percent during the study period, after adjusting for general inflation. An analysis of the data showed that, contrary to expectations, Kaiser's disease-management programs had failed to reduce hospital utilization. "Diabetes and asthma patients had fewer hospitalizations in 2002 than in 1996, even as hospital days stayed about the same," the study notes. "Heart failure and CAD patients had more hospital days in 2002 than in 1996."

Based on their research, the study's authors said they doubted reports of big cost savings in disease-management programs. "When DM [disease-management] programs remedy under-use of effective treatments, DM cannot be cost-saving unless the recommended treatments are," they wrote. "Most of the treatments recommended for the targeted conditions are cost-effective but not cost-saving. They increase the length and quality of life at a cost that is reasonable—a good value compared with other services—but higher than the savings that accrue when exacerbations and complications are prevented."

Better Care for the Same Money   Joel Hyatt, MD, an assistant medical director in Kaiser Permanente's southern California unit, believes the Fireman study demonstrates that comprehensive disease management saves as much as it costs and delivers better value than conventional care. After adjusting for the general growth in chronic-disease spending, he says, "We've not seen absolute cost savings, but we haven't seen cost increases. The return has been managing more patients and getting better results for no increase in cost."

Kaiser's disease-management figures do not appear to include its massive investment in information technology. But it would be impossible to achieve what Kaiser has without the giant HMO's level of clinical data automation. While independent disease-management firms are also highly computerized, they lack Kaiser's access to detailed clinical data. In the fragmented delivery systems that dominate most of the country, it's unclear how these companies have achieved their claimed savings. "We should all be skeptical about the outlandish return on investment these companies are claiming," Hyatt says.

Al Lewis, president of the Disease Management Purchasing Consortium, a consulting firm based in Wellesley, Massachusetts, agrees that some vendors and benefit consultants overestimate savings. But Lewis, who advises insurers and employers, rejects the reports and studies that question the economic value of disease management. Noting that corporate investment in disease management tripled from 2001 to 2005, he says, "You can't argue with the marketplace." In other words, the fact that more plans and employers are spending more on this approach means that it must work.

So how much does it save? According to Lewis, the return on investment for conventional, telephone nurse–based disease management falls between 1.5:1 and 2:1. He adds that he's referring to the more intensive variant that targets not only high-risk patients but also their multiple diseases.

Why Disease Management Falls Short of Potential   Studies provide some evidence that the chronic-care model—because it involves physicians in multidisciplinary teams—is more likely to cut costs than disease-management programs that rely mainly on the telephone support of nurse case managers.[31] But, in the short term, neither approach will make a dent in the growth of health spending. Even if one accepts Lewis's estimate that disease management can save twice what it costs, that means that in 2005, it saved only about $1 billion—less than 1 percent of the growth in health spending from the previous year.[32]

The long-term effects might be much greater, at least for diseases like diabetes and hypertension; but the employers and plans that are currently pouring large sums into disease management can't wait that long. They need results now.[33] The question is how long they'll continue to support disease management without a significant reduction in health costs.

There is no question that disease management is helping to improve care for many people today.[34] But as studies show, the conventional approach addresses only high-risk patients who are expected to run up a big health tab. And the chronic-care model, while more comprehensive, cannot succeed in the settings where most physicians practice. So the two faces of disease management remain averted from the majority of patients who need its help.

Meanwhile, most physicians aren't directly involved in either type of disease management—a significant reason it falls short of its potential. "The optimal form of disease management for both high- and low-risk patients," says Lawrence Casalino, MD, a health-policy expert at the University of Chicago, "would have the doctors deeply involved with it in their offices, and that isn't usually the case today."

Instead, patients are stuck in a system that doesn't reward doctors for taking good care of them, and physicians are stuck doing piecework at an ever-increasing rate to keep their incomes up. What's the solution? Why, pay for performance, of course. But, as the next chapter shows, pay for performance is more of a band-aid than a solution.

4　Paying for Performance

The past few years have seen a vast upwelling of support for pay-for-performance (P4P) programs that reward physicians and hospitals for meeting specific goals in the domains of quality, efficiency, and information technology.

By November 2005, health plans, employers, and other organizations were sponsoring more than a hundred P4P programs, up 25 percent from the previous year.[1] The majority of the nation's fifty-one Blue Cross and Blue Shield plans have launched P4P initiatives.[2] More than half of commercial HMOs had some kind of P4P program in 2005,[3] and a *Medical Economics* survey of office-based physicians revealed that about a quarter of respondents contracted with at least one health plan that offered pay-for-performance incentives.[4]

Meanwhile, the Centers for Medicare and Medicaid Services (CMS) plans to implement P4P on a broad scale. It has launched a pilot program for large physician groups,[5] has announced a three-year pilot involving small practices,[6] and has nearly completed a large-scale demonstration project for hospitals.[7] If Congress gives CMS the go-ahead to adopt P4P, private-sector efforts will undoubtedly accelerate.[8]

"Report cards" on doctors and hospitals are also becoming widespread (see Chapter 6), and many of these are associated with P4P programs. A 2005 survey of sponsoring organizations found that about 30 percent were publishing data on health care providers (mostly hospitals and large physician groups), and that 43 percent of respondents planned to implement scorecards within a year or two.[9]

Pay-for-performance programs proceed from the assumption that paying physicians more for doing well on a small number of measures will improve overall care and lead to lower costs. "We're going to be paying for better care, not just for more procedures and visits," said then CMS administrator Mark McClellan, MD, at a 2005 press conference announcing the large-group P4P project. "There are chances to save money here."

The Bush administration is not alone in its optimism about P4P. "Most agree that the existing financial incentives in health care need to be realigned," Karen Davis, president of the Commonwealth Fund, said in commenting on early results of several P4P programs funded by the Robert Wood Johnson Foundation. "These projects add to the mounting evidence that rewarding good performance can encourage doctors to provide appropriate care to patients to help them live longer and healthier lives."[10]

Some evidence indicates that P4P can improve quality, but it's still sketchy. Even if P4P does result in better care, there won't be much short-term cost savings, says Robert Berenson, MD, a health-policy expert at the Urban Institute and a former senior manager at CMS. "There's no evidence that disease management saves money," he notes. "Disease management is using a third-party vendor to try to work with patients, whereas P4P is an approach to improve the performance of the physicians providing the care. But I think the same sort of logic is there. For example, P4P might improve the quality of care for diabetes, which is increasing in prevalence, and the cost associated with diabetes is well known. But most of the savings happen down the road, many years later."

Alice Gosfield, a leading health care attorney and former chair of the National Committee on Quality Assurance, explains the problem another way: Current P4P programs, she points out, are oriented mainly to correcting underuse of services. "That means, by definition, that they're paying for something that hasn't been going on. If Elizabeth McGlynn and her colleagues at RAND are right, and Americans are getting only 55 percent of the care they should get, we have a 45 percent under-use problem, which means that health care is going to cost more."

Many P4P programs also try to address overuse and misuse of services by including extra payments for generic drug prescribing and more efficient use of resources—a standard approach of HMOs that has never gone away. But, like the quality incentives, these efficiency rewards are unlikely to change the basic physician motivation to earn more by doing more.

"Pay for performance provides marginal incentives that would likely be ignored if they go counter to the underlying incentives in the system," Berenson says. "In a fee-for-service system, which has basic incentives to drive volume up, it's hard to imagine that pay-for-performance is going to be successful at holding down costs."

Physician Resistance Spreading   Despite the grand plans of public and private payers, a December 2005 paper published by the Center for Studying Health System Change found that "most P4P initiatives are still on the drawing board." Of the twelve communities that the center surveyed, the researchers discovered, only two—Orange County, California, and Boston—had significant P4P programs. "In the other 10 communities, where almost no physicians have received quality-related payments to date, physician attitudes about P4P ranged from skeptical to hostile."[11] Among the reasons for their skepticism, the researchers found, is a widespread belief that health plans will use pay for performance to redistribute money from some doctors to others.

Some health plans are playing this "zero-sum" game by withholding money from all physicians' reimbursement and paying bonuses to top performers out of that "withhold" pool.[12] The Medicare Payment Advisory Commission recommended a similar approach to Congress,[13] as did the prestigious Institute of Medicine,[14] and some P4P bills have reflected that recommendation.[15] Moreover, the CMS hospital demonstration project will penalize the lowest-scoring facilities in the pilot's third year.[16]

Medical associations strongly oppose this punitive approach. "The reason some hospitals and practices don't perform well is that they lack the resources to improve," says William Jessee, MD, president and CEO of the Medical Group Management Association. "So if you transfer resources from poorer performers to better performers, you end up exacerbating the problem rather than solving it."[17]

The American College of Physicians, representing internists, argues in a 2005 press release that Medicare should share cost savings from reduced hospitalizations and emergency room (ER) visits with physicians.[18] If that were done, Robert B. Doherty, one of the group's senior vice presidents, points out, the P4P program could be budget-neutral while raising overall physician payments.[19] But current Medicare policy prohibits the commingling of hospital and physician funds.

The American Medical Association (AMA), like the American College of Physicians, would like to see physicians participate in any P4P savings. But its paramount goal is to change Medicare's formula for reimbursing physicians. In 2005, this formula, which reduces fees when volume goes up, was expected to cut doctors' Medicare income by 26 percent in six years. Recognizing at the time that Congress was determined to move to pay for performance, the AMA struck a deal with key congressional leaders: It promised that a group of specialty societies would develop 140 performance measures covering most medical fields. The pact also stated that, in 2007, "physicians would report voluntarily to CMS on at least 3 to 5 quality measures per physician." In return, the AMA obtained a vague promise that Congress would work with physician groups "to implement additional reforms to address payment and quality objectives." The lawmakers also postponed the scheduled reimbursement cut for 2006.[20]

Some specialty societies criticized the AMA for what they saw as "giving away the store." But Nancy Nielsen, MD, speaker of the AMA's House of Delegates, denies that the AMA has abandoned its goal of getting payment reform before committing to support Medicare P4P. In fact, she says, CMS's current payment formula is on a "collision course" with its desire to adopt P4P. "Pay for performance will increase the volume of services," she notes, "and the more that services increase, the more fees go down under the current system. So it just doesn't make any sense."

Evolution of P4P Programs   The roots of P4P go back to the managed-care backlash of the late 1990s. At that time, health plans began to scale back utilization review and preauthorization requirements for tests, referrals, and procedures.[21] Many began to rely more on persuading doctors to follow clinical guidelines to reduce inappropriate variations in care. But physician bonuses were still based mainly on efficiency in areas like test ordering and prescribing. To the extent that "quality" was factored in, it was usually measured through patient-satisfaction surveys.

In California and Minnesota, however, some plans were starting to measure the clinical quality of physician groups and put out comparative "report cards" on them. At first, this data, too, came from patient surveys: For example, the Pacific Business Group on Health, a California employer coalition, published group report cards based partly on what patients with diabetes, asthma, and other chronic conditions said their doctors had done for them.[22] But by the end of the decade, Health Partners, in Minneapolis, was posting on its Web site comparative data on blood-sugar control of diabetics in each group it contracted with. And West Coast–based plans like PacifiCare and Health Net were publishing report cards comparing groups on their adherence to clinical guidelines. While it was unclear how much effect these report cards had on consumers, they did prompt some California groups to step up quality-improvement efforts.[23]

California Takes the Lead   The next stage of the process began in 2002, when the Integrated Healthcare Association, a California health-policy group that includes providers, employers, health plans, and consumer groups, established a P4P program to reward the top-performing groups in the state. Among the association's current members are seven insurance companies that cover the majority of the state's commercially insured population.

The big achievement of the Integrated Healthcare Association program was to persuade the major health plans to use the same standardized performance measures. In 2004, six of these seven plans (the seventh joined in 2005) disbursed about $50 million in quality awards to California medical groups and independent practice associations (IPAs).[24]

Since the plans paid only top performers, some groups received little or nothing. Of the 215 organizations (representing 45,000 doctors) that participated in 2003, only 74 scored significantly high on most of the clinical measures, which determined 50 percent of the points needed for the rewards that were paid the following year. A consumer-satisfaction survey accounted for 40 percent of a group's score, and use of information technology contributed 10 percent. (The latter now accounts for 20 percent of the score, and the IHA plans to add efficiency measures.)[25]

The groups' quality data are posted on the Web site of the California Office of the Patient Advocate (www.opa.ca.gov/report_card). These scorecards include overall rankings in clinical quality and patient service, as well as drill-downs on how well each group does on each of the measures within those categories. Among the measures are childhood immunizations, breast and cervical cancer screening, and control of blood pressure and blood sugar.

Bridges to Excellence   The Integrated Healthcare Association program relies on competition among large groups and IPAs that have built an extensive infrastructure for managing care under prepaid HMO contracts. Since physicians in other parts of the country practice in a totally different environment, that approach is unlikely to work for them. So health plans and employers are looking for alternatives.

One alternative favored by some big corporations is called Bridges to Excellence. Launched by GE, Procter & Gamble, Raytheon, Verizon, United Parcel Service and Ford, Bridges to Excellence (BTE) measures doctors in three domains of performance: diabetes care, cardiovascular care, and office processes. For each patient with diabetes employed by a BTE member company, qualifying physicians get $80 a year; for each member patient with cardiac disease, they get $160. Physicians who qualify for bonuses based on office re-engineering, including the use of health information technology, receive $50 for each BTE patient.[26]

The BTE approach has some advantages over other P4P programs: It allows physicians to submit their own data, and the rewards clearly represent "new money," because they come directly from employers. But BTE has a serious defect: The participating companies initially provided the minimum number of patients required for a practice to qualify for rewards in only a few markets; even in those cities—Albany/Schenectady, Boston, Cincinnati, and Louisville—a small minority of practices have participated. During its first couple of years, in fact, BTE sponsors awarded only $4 million to physicians.[27]

BTE is expanding its reach. Employers in Arkansas, Colorado, Georgia, Illinois, and Minnesota are in the process of adopting its program. Also, CareFirst Blue Cross Blue Shield of Maryland, Blue Cross Blue Shield of North Carolina, CIGNA, and United Healthcare are supporting BTE.[28] CareFirst is paying physicians bonuses for acquiring electronic health records and improving office processes.[29] But CIGNA and United are only assisting employers that want to participate in BTE, rather than sponsoring the program themselves.[30]

Major Drawbacks of P4P

As mentioned earlier, physicians have serious reservations about P4P programs, and experts have pointed to deficiencies in them that may limit their effectiveness. In the following section, I describe some of the P4P drawbacks cited by doctors and other observers.

Inadequacy of Claims Data   While some of the California groups generate performance data from their own information systems, and BTE has doctors review their own records, most P4P programs rely on claims data (and lab values, if they're available) for performance measurement. Some plans supplement claims analysis with chart reviews in physician offices, but this approach is expensive and burdensome. That's one reason the government is pushing for adoption of standardized electronic health records.

Based on billing codes, claims data are severely limited. Not only do they fail to capture many important dimensions of performance, but they are full of errors and omissions. Some doctors talk about insurers sending them claims-based profiles that showed missing mammograms on men or that included patients who weren't in their practices. Robert Ostrander, a family physician in Rushville, New York, says one plan faulted him for not prescribing certain medications to patients. He did write the prescriptions; but the patients filled them at a local Veterans Affairs hospital to avoid co-payments, so they didn't show up in the plan's computer system. Claims-based measures also tend to be inflexible. Gregory Hood, an internist in Lexington, Kentucky, says, "I've received a number of reports criticizing me for not having every single one of my diabetic patients on ACE inhibitors. There's no allowance for the double-digit percentage of patients who are allergic to ACE inhibitors."

Insufficient Sample Size   While P4P started with large groups and IPAs that include hundreds of doctors, the majority of physicians are in small practices. So the plans are now measuring those doctors as well, and a few have begun to publish scorecards on individual physicians.[31]

The expansion of P4P to small offices raises the question of sample size. In a test of P4P in its PPO, for example, Blue Cross of California measured doctors who treated as few as thirty-five plan members with a variety of chronic conditions.[32] The East Coast division of Anthem Blue Cross and Blue Shield once set the cutoff at twenty-five total Anthem members per doctor, regardless of whether they had a health condition that required a measured service.[33]

To put this in perspective, Sheldon Greenfield, an internist and health care quality expert, says you must look at a minimum of twenty to thirty patients with diabetes to get valid data on diabetes measures for a single doctor. Greenfield, who is co-director of the Health Policy and Research Unit at the University of California at Irvine, adds that this minimum number works only under the right conditions. Those conditions include setting quality goals at a level that takes into account the severity of illness and patients' noncompliance with the doctor's orders. Few plans are doing the former and none, the latter.

The health plans could reduce the sample-size problem by collaborating with one another, as the California HMOs are doing. This move would also increase doctors' interest, since it has been shown that P4P programs don't have much impact until they affect 15 to 20 percent of a physician's patients.[34] But so far, there's little evidence that plans are interested in working together. "It's something employers would like to see, but it's hard for plans to get used to, because their natural instinct is to differentiate their programs for competitive advantage," says Beau Carter, former executive director of California's Integrated Healthcare Association.

Measurement Problems in PPOs   Compounding the sample-size problem, most P4P programs focused initially on HMOs, which require members to sign up with a primary-care physician. In a PPO, the other major type of health plan, patients can see any specialist without a referral, and they usually don't have to pick a primary-care physician. Since many people see multiple doctors, it's difficult for P4P programs to assign responsibility for providing preventive or chronic-care services to a particular PPO physician.

That hasn't stopped insurers from trying. The Hawaii Medical Service Association has used P4P in its PPO for several years, and many other carriers have recently expanded their programs to include PPOs.[35] But health-plan executives admit that it's a challenge. And since 60 percent of commercially insured people belong to PPOs, the difficulty of applying P4P to this kind of plan is bound to slow down the movement.

Lack of Standardization   One of the big achievements of the Integrated Healthcare Association is that it persuaded the California plans to use the same measures. Elsewhere, P4P programs use a variety of measures. While they're similar in many respects, physicians have a hard time dealing with multiple requirements from different plans. If too many different things are required of them, they're likely to ignore all of them.

Efforts are under way to standardize P4P measures, but they're far from unified. In 2005, the Ambulatory Care Quality Alliance, which includes two medical societies, the health insurers' association, and the Agency for Healthcare Research and Quality, announced a "starter set" of measures.[36] The National Quality Forum, an organization of 270 private and public health care stakeholders, later endorsed a list of 51 primary-care indicators.[37] Then CMS introduced still another set of P4P measures for a "voluntary" physician-quality reporting program.[38] Meanwhile the AMA-led consortium of specialty societies created the measures that Congress had demanded.

Noncompliance of Patients   One reason patients don't get all the care they need is that many don't comply with their doctors' orders or fill prescriptions. They might not come in for their regular check-ups or might not get necessary tests, such as an eye exam for diabetic retinopathy. Yet P4P rewards are based only on what the physician did for the patient. So if a patient doesn't come in or follow his advice, the doctor gets penalized.

This problem is especially acute with regard to P4P "outcomes" measures that show how well a chronic condition is being controlled. Patricia Roy, a family physician in Muskegon, Michigan, says that local plans measure "outcomes" such as the blood glucose and LDL cholesterol levels of her diabetic patients. Because they can't get that from claims data, the plans send auditors into Roy's office. They review six or eight of her patient charts, and if the clinical indicators aren't what they should be, she loses part of her bonus. That approach is already prompting some of her colleagues to encourage noncompliant patients to find other physicians, she says.

Kenneth Kizer, MD, former president of the National Quality Forum, says outcome measures of this kind are weak indicators of performance. "The caregiver should be judged primarily by things that are under his or her control. This may bias performance measurement toward process measures more than outcomes, because medical care may be only a small part of what determines the outcome for a lot of common conditions," he says.

Too Few Measures to Show Quality   Another problem with quality measures—no matter how well-validated and evidence-based they are—is that they examine only a small part of the picture. For example, internist Kenneth Kubitschek of Asheville, North Carolina, notes, the blood-sugar level of a diabetic patient (as measured by the hemoglobin A1c lab test) is just one indicator of his health. "The patient's HbA1c may be fine, but her blood pressure is 190 over 110. That's a higher risk factor than the hemoglobin in the setting of diabetes. So the doctor who doesn't score as well on the HbA1c may be taking much better care of the diabetic. I'm not negating the national guidelines. But there are so many potholes that it is a challenge."

Another example is the measure for LDL cholesterol, a common one in P4P programs. Physicians normally try to get patients to change their diet and exercise before putting them on an expensive, lifelong regimen of cholesterol-lowering drugs that have side effects. But they point out that their incentive under P4P programs is to put every patient on a drug like Lipitor or Crestor right away. Craig Wax, a family physician in Mullica Hill, New Jersey, says he normally tries diet and exercise first with people who seem motivated. "But if I'm being incentivized to get everybody to goal right now, I'm a pill machine. I dispense to everybody."

Practice Pattern Distortions   Most P4P programs use only a dozen or so measures, because physicians can focus on only so many things at once. On one hand, programs that measure groups on a multitude of services make it more difficult for physicians to comply and don't provide enough of an incentive for them to improve on any individual measure. On the other hand, concentrating on just a few measures may result in physicians' focusing on those areas to the detriment of other aspects of care. Moreover, no correlation exists between performance on those indicators and overall physician quality.[39]

What happens when a plan decides enough physicians have met its goals on particular measures and shifts its rewards to other measures? Would the doctors continue to do as good a job on the old measures? "Their performance would probably degrade, based on current evidence," David Nash of Jefferson Medical College says. "Everything degrades that doesn't get sufficient attention."

Improvement Isn't Rewarded   Many observers, including some who strongly support P4P, have criticized the plans for rewarding only groups or physicians that achieve excellence, not those that merely improve. Diane Laird, CEO of Greater Newport Physicians, a California IPA that's one of IHA's higher-scoring groups, says that paying only the top performers "makes it difficult for groups to keep investing in improvement."

Ronald Bangasser, MD, of Redlands, California, a former president of the California Medical Association, says some HMO executives in his state are content to let the lower-scoring groups "die off." He's especially concerned about the plans that are trying to steer patients to the top performers in tiered networks.

"If you paid only the top 20 to 40 percent [of groups] and said everybody's going to be steered to those doctors, obviously access is going to go to hell in a handbasket," Bangasser says. "That's not going to happen. So most people have come to the belief that you've got to raise all the boats, and improve access to care for every patient in California."

The plans in the Integrated Healthcare Association haven't done that yet, however, and neither have most other payers across the country. A 2004 Harvard study of P4P programs found that "the sponsor nearly always rewards good performance rather than improvement. This puts physicians or hospitals that have already figured out how to deliver good quality healthcare along the targeted dimensions at an advantage.... Physicians and hospitals that have a long way to go in terms of meeting absolute targets or are ranked low among their peers are less likely to find it worthwhile to strive for these bonuses."[40]

Not Enough Money   In 2005, P4P programs gave qualifying physicians rewards that ranged from 2 to 5 percent of their income from the health plan sponsoring the program.[41] Where most of the plans are involved, as in California, these percentages can amount to a fairly substantial sum. For example, some physicians in the Orange County (California) groups mentioned earlier received P4P bonuses of $5,000 to $10,000 in 2004.[42] But even this might not be enough to get doctors to change how they work. "The conventional wisdom," Beau Carter says, "is that you need to put 10 percent on the table to get doctors' attention."

Many California physicians wonder whether the HMOs' P4P rewards are really increasing their incomes or whether the plans are reducing their capitation rates to fund the incentives. They know that the money they're receiving from Blue Cross of California replaces bonuses they used to get for holding down the use of hospital services.[43] Elsewhere, as discussed earlier, physicians often view P4P as just another hoop they have to jump through to get the plans to return the "withholds" from their HMO payments.

Under a fee-for-service payment system, moreover, P4P adds less to income than simply speeding up visits would. One observer notes, "Physicians could increase their income more—with less additional work—by adding one or two patient visits each day than by meeting all the quality standards in current performance-based payment programs."[44]

Where Is P4P Leading Us?

There is evidence that P4P programs do improve care. The Roches-ter IPA, for example, has detected a significant rise in testing of LDL cholesterol in diabetic patients, reports Howard Beckman, MD, the IPA's medical director.[45] And a P4P program sponsored by the Hawaii Blues helped raise the percentage of heart-failure patients who were prescribed ACE inhibitors from 41 percent to 64 percent.[46]

In 2004, the second year of the Integrated Healthcare Association P4P program, average scores on some measures rose significantly among the 225 participating groups and IPAs. For example, the average rate of appropriate DTP immunizations jumped from 33 to 62 percent, and the mean rate of LDL cholesterol screening rose from 68 to 78 percent.[47] But Beau Carter and others say that some of the improvements can be attributed to better data collection.

The most dramatic improvement seen in a P4P program so far has been in the CMS Premier Hospital Quality Demonstration Project. On average, the 266 hospitals' scores on thirty quality measures improved by 11.8 percent in the first two years of the project, and Medicare paid the top-performing hospitals an additional $8.85 million in the first year and $8.7 million in the second.[48] But, since CMS published the grades of hospitals that scored in the top 50 percent, their improvement ef-forts were apparently aimed more at buffing their public images than at boosting their bottom lines.[49] "The bottom line impact to our hospi-tals is minimal," says Rick Hachten, president of Alegent Health, which includes 19 hospitals in Nebraska and Iowa. "But public reporting has been a huge incentive to focus on process improvement and produce the outcomes we've seen."[50]

The largest study to date on the quality impact of P4P programs shows mixed results. Performed by a team led by Meredith B. Rosen-thal of the Harvard School of Public Health, the study compared im-provements in clinical quality scores of California physician groups that participated in a P4P program with those of Pacific Northwest groups that did not. The California groups had the potential of receiving 5 per-cent quality bonuses from PacifiCare, which gave both sets of physicians quarterly feedback on their performance.[51]

The researchers found that the California groups improved signifi-cantly more than the Pacific Northwest groups did on cervical-cancer screening, but that there was little difference between the amounts by which the two cohorts raised their rates of mammography or hemoglobin A1c tests. In California, the bulk of the P4P rewards went to groups that already were performing above the program's goals when it began. The study's conclusion: "Paying clinicians to reach a common, fixed performance target may produce little gain in quality for the money spent and will largely reward those with higher performance at baseline."

The Prometheus Model   Dissatisfaction with the current P4P model has led some health care reformers to propose alternative methods of P4P. One group of experts led by the health care attorney Alice Gosfield and François DeBrantes, national coordinator of BTE, recently unveiled a new approach called "Prometheus payments." Their reimbursement model would require physicians, hospitals, and other providers to work together to provide care that conforms with "evidence-based" guidelines. Physicians would be paid on the basis of negotiated case rates that would cover all necessary care in a particular case. They would get 80–90 percent of the case rates in monthly payments instead of fee-for-service reimbursement. Depending on their efficiency and quality scores, physicians would receive additional payments from the pool of withheld money. Exceptional performers could earn even more.[52]

Doctors and hospitals would form a range of ad hoc associations to "bid" for case rates, and each provider would be paid for the portion of the practice guideline that they promised to deliver. But, although they'd cooperate clinically, their businesses could remain separate. To persuade unrelated providers to work together effectively, 30 percent of a provider's bonus would depend on whether other team members also delivered high-quality, efficient care.

Prometheus has some significant barriers to overcome, including the fragmentation of the delivery system and the limitations of evidence-based medicine (see Chapter 7). But because it seeks to knit providers together both clinically and financially, it's an experiment worth watching. And it has some heavyweights behind it. Among Prometheus's board members and designers are people from the Blue Cross and Blue Shield Association, the American Hospital Association, BTE, the Leapfrog Group, Partners Health Care, RAND Health, the Harvard School of Public Health, and the National Business Coalition on Health.

Pay for Results   The American Medical Group Association, which represents the largest groups in the country, favors an alternative to P4P that it calls a "results-based payment system." This approach would reorient the reimbursement system to pay doctors on the basis of the outcomes of care rather than slavish adherence to clinical guidelines. The association has assembled a blue-ribbon panel of experts to flesh out this concept.[53]

Donald Fisher, president and CEO of the association, says that P4P is a "terrific" step in the right direction, but that it does not go far enough. "If a patient comes to the ER with chest pain and you give him an aspirin within the first 30 minutes, you get an extra dollar in your pay envelope, because that's the protocol," he points out. "But if the patient had a hiatal hernia that was bleeding, the aspirin did more harm that good." So in his view, only outcomes matter.

Until now, outcomes of care have been excruciatingly difficult to measure. Not only do they often take a long time to become apparent, but some of them are gauged with patient-reported functional status measures that are hard to match with clinical data. Fisher is optimistic that these obstacles can be overcome with the help of the latest information technology. However, this is technology that only large groups like those in the American Medical Group Association currently possess.

Views of Physician Behavior   P4P and pay-for-results proponents regard the Institute of Medicine's 2001 report *Crossing the Quality Chasm* as a touchstone. They all want care that is safe, effective, patient-centered, timely, efficient, and equitable, and they agree with the book's conclusion that the reimbursement system needs to be changed to bring that about.[54] But Donald Berwick, a principal author of the report, rejects the idea of P4P, saying it runs counter to the philosophy of medicine: "At the individual [physician] level, I don't trust incentives at all," he told Robert Galvin, MD, in a published interview.[55] "I do not think it's true that the way to get better doctoring and better nursing is to put money on the table in front of doctors and nurses." The joy of doing a good job, in Berwick's view, is more important to most clinicians than financial incentives are.

Moreover, rewarding good performance on a few clinical measures won't fundamentally alter physician behavior, Berwick says. "The results we're after are more expansive than the adherence to a small set of criteria, which get them paid a little more. . . . We've got to support the culture, clinical care, and the underlying system that make healing, not scoring, the objective."

Ronald Bangasser, the former California Medical Association president, agrees with Berwick's premise but still supports P4P. "I think physicians just get up in the morning and try to do the right thing, and if you give physicians more information they'll do better," he says. "You don't need money to begin the process of change. However, there's only a certain amount of change you get without putting money into it."

Feedback to Doctors   While health-plan feedback to physicians on their performance has not been too successful, group practices—especially those with electronic health records—have been able to use data feedback to change physician behavior. And in many instances, they've done so without the lure of pay for performance.

Giving performance data to the physicians in the five-hundred-doctor Dean Health System of Madison, Wisconsin, for example, has helped them raise the number of the group's diabetic patients with their blood sugar under control from about 50 percent to more than 70 percent, Donald Logan, MD, Dean's chief medical officer, reports. The group has achieved similar results in lowering LDL cholesterol levels, he adds.

Posting Dean's quality numbers on a Web site alongside those of other groups in the Wisconsin Collaborative for Healthcare Quality has stimulated a certain amount of intragroup rivalry. But what has really motivated doctors to improve, Logan says, is the realization that they're not doing as well as they might on standard measures that Dean and the other groups helped develop. "What helped us more than anything was the recognition that when we measured their performance, it was not at the level they thought it was or should be," he says. "When you give physicians good data that they can accept and guidelines that are short, succinct and believable, they'll go along with it."

P4P wouldn't make much difference to Dean's physicians, Jack Bowhan, the group's administrator for clinical practice improvement, says. "I think professional pride in doing a good job is what motivates most people. Getting patted on the back and recognized for it is more important than the money. Because these doctors are making good money. All you can do is punish them by saying, 'We're going to take what we were paying you, and now you've got to do something else to get it. So jump through this hoop.' "

5   EHRs: Necessary but Not Sufficient

Many physician groups have made impressive strides in quality improvement without pay for performance. In some instances, the key to success has been health information technology.

Midwest Heart Specialists, a fifty-five-doctor cardiovascular group in the Chicago area, has had an electronic health record (EHR) system since 1997. A couple of years ago, the group decided to imbed national performance measures for coronary artery disease, heart failure, and hypertension into its EHR. The system prompts physicians to follow clinical guidelines, and, as they document patient visits, it automatically gathers data on how well they do.

As a result of the prompts and the feedback Midwest Heart Specialists gives the doctors on their performance, the group has produced startling improvements in some areas of cardiac care. In the first year after the measures were imbedded in the EHR, for example, the percentage of the group's patients who had their LDL cholesterol at goal increased from 22 to 78 percent. By extrapolating from studies of patients with coronary artery disease, Michael O'Toole, MD, the group's director of medical informatics, calculated that this one change has prevented 78 deaths, 158 heart attacks, and 38 strokes. It has also saved $3 million–$5 million in avoided hospitalizations, he says.[1]

Numbers like these have made many government officials and corporate leaders enthusiastic about the potential of health information technology. At a July 2004 conference in Washington, DC, to launch President Bush's initiative to make EHRs universal within ten years, Mark McClellan, who was then the administrator of CMS, said, "We have an opportunity to improve quality and reduce costs by driving our health care system into the new world of information technology." Tommy Thompson, former Secretary of the Department of Health and Human

Services, said, "Health IT is essential to improving care." And David Brailer, MD, then the administration's health information technology czar, declared, "This is about the transformation of health care."

The following February, Brailer explained his views more fully: "The important aspect of health IT is not software and computers—it is physicians making better treatment decisions, nurses and pharmacists delivering safer care, and consumers making better choices among treatment options. It is the way people connect together across a fragmented delivery system—from physician offices to hospitals to skilled nursing facilities and even to the consumer's home. It is putting consumers in control of their health status, and customizing care delivery to meet their needs."[2]

Some of this optimism about the power of information technology is warranted. By giving physicians and nurses instant access to patient information, EHRs can help avoid adverse drug interactions and can remind doctors to provide appropriate care for patients with chronic conditions. Hooking up physicians to regional data repositories can alert them to the allergies, medications, and diagnoses of new patients and avoid redundant tests. ER physicians can use information systems to find crucial data when saving time means saving lives. Finally, health information technology can give patients access to their own medical records and help them use the information to care for themselves.

But none of this means that superimposing information technology on a dysfunctional health care system will make it work properly. "It is insufficient to just automate the current culture and the current behavior," Donald Berwick of the Institute for Healthcare Improvement says. "It has to be part of a plan for a complete redesign of care processes. If we just automate the current environment without deciding that care is going to be safer and more effective, we'll get the current care."

Peter Basch, MD, a longtime EHR user and director of e-health for MedStar Health, a hospital system in the Washington, DC, area, agrees that health information technology is necessary but not sufficient to bring about systemic change. "Achieving value for our patients will take more than an affordable, adoptable computer system," he writes. "It will take intentional practice redesign supported by a sustainable business case for the activities that the optimal use of the EHR can enable: advanced information and care management and a heightened focus on quality."[3]

Why Most Doctors Don't Have EHRs

The Bush administration envisions a national health information network that will someday connect all health care providers and provide instantaneous access to information on any patient who needs care anywhere in the country. But before this grand vision can become reality, most doctors' offices, hospitals, nursing homes, and home health care agencies must have their own EHRs, and the data in them must be accessible to patients and their providers. Today, we're very far from that goal. Only about 30 percent of hospitals have EHRs,[4] for example, and even fewer physician practices do.

In 2005, 14 percent of physician practices of three or more doctors had electronic health records, according to a survey by the Medical Group Management Association (MGMA). The study also showed that large groups were more likely to have information systems. While just 12.5 percent of groups with three to five physicians had EHRs, 19.5 percent of groups of twenty or more had them.[5] Another study found that 9 percent of doctors in practices of one to four physicians were using EHRs, compared with 15 percent in groups of twenty or more.[6]

Why are EHRs spreading so slowly among physicians? A big reason is the upfront cost, which averages about $33,000 per doctor and is often much higher in small practices.[7] That tab breaks down to roughly a third for software, a third for computers, and a third for training and implementation. It does not include the annual software licensing fees and hardware maintenance costs, which total about 20 percent of the initial outlay,[8] and it does not take into account the doctor's loss of productivity during the six months or more that it takes to learn how to use the system. According to the MGMA survey, productivity typically drops 10–15 percent during this initial period.

Some physicians never really get the hang of their EHRs. For example, Jonathan Cheek, a pediatrician in Canton, Georgia, and his four colleagues have been using an EHR since 2001. Cheek still is seeing many fewer patients than he used to. While he concedes that his notes are more complete and more legible and that the EHR has raised the quality of care, he doesn't know whether the practice will ever break even on its investment.

The risk for a practice that considers sinking money into an EHR is even more acute than Cheek indicates: Around half of all EHR installations are unsuccessful,[9] either because of technical problems or because the doctors never learned how to use the system correctly. In many cases, only some of the doctors in a practice use the EHR, or the physicians use only a fraction of its features. When that happens, the practice usually retains its paper charts, so it doesn't get any of the increased efficiency that could justify its investment.

Return on Investment   According to a 2005 *Medical Economics* survey, most doctors who purchase EHRs believe they will see a return on investment.[10] Their decision to acquire health IT "has nothing to do with the quality of care," Jeffrey Hertzberg, MD, a medical informatics consultant in Minneapolis, explains. "It's about doing it a little faster, a little cheaper, with fewer employees."[11]

Rosemarie Nelson, an MGMA consultant based in Syracuse, New York, agrees. Having an EHR eliminates the cost of paper-chart handling, reduces time spent on prescription drug refills, and helps staff answer phone queries from patients, she points out. If physicians are currently dictating their notes, they can save $800 to $1,000 a month by eliminating transcription. Also, if an office has a link between its billing system and its EHR, she notes, it can cut the number of missing charges due to lost invoices.

EHRs also help physicians raise revenues by improving their documentation of what they did for patients during office visits. Primary-care physicians often "under-code" for visits—that is, they submit bills for a lower level of service than what they performed, because they're afraid that Medicare or health plans will audit them. The more complete their documentation is, the more likely they are to submit billing codes that carry higher reimbursement. Some EHRs even contain code checkers that suggest a code based on the services that are checked off.

A recent study of fourteen small practices across the country found that, on average, they recovered their investment in an EHR within two and a half years and that after that, their practices benefited financially. About half of the net financial gain of $23,000 per provider per year came from being able to justify higher office visit charges, and the rest stemmed from increased efficiency, including savings in personnel, supply, and transcription costs.

The authors also note, however, that "three practices experienced considerable financial risks," including EHR-related billing problems and a system crash that resulted in a total loss of patient data. "Moreover, this survey did not include practices that implemented an EHR and then returned to paper, thereby losing their total EHR investment."[12]

Payers Benefit, and Providers Pay   While health plans and CMS anticipate that EHRs will produce big savings for the health care system, the providers are expected to bear most of the cost. Even though they can profit down the road from going digital, physicians may have to sacrifice 10 percent or more of their income in the meantime.[13]

Neither the government nor private payers have yet made large-scale financial commitments to help physicians acquire EHRs. A few plans outside of California have followed the example of the Integrated Healthcare Association in rewarding physicians specifically for acquiring health information technology as part of pay-for-performance programs. But for the most part, insurers with P4P programs are paying for quality and efficiency only. And some insurance companies regard public reporting of quality and cost data as a better incentive than P4P to persuade physicians to adopt EHRs.

"We believe the best way to facilitate the diffusion of health IT is to promote transparency around different levels of clinical performance and efficiency," says Lewis Sandy, MD, executive vice president of clinical strategies and policy for United Healthcare. "We think that investments in IT will allow physicians to both deliver and to demonstrate higher levels of performance. As the marketplace evolves toward more of a consumer-oriented industry, efforts to promote transparency will accelerate the adoption and diffusion of this infrastructure."

Of course, if payers continue to award pay-for-performance bonuses in the 2 to 5 percent range, they won't have much impact on EHR adoption. The effect of the "transparency" that Sandy refers to—report cards that compare providers on cost and quality—will depend on how it's done and whether consumers pay attention. So far, most of them have not (see Chapter 6).

Medicare's Game Plan   CMS also wants to use pay for performance to accelerate EHR adoption. Although Congress has not yet spelled out how Medicare should proceed in this arena, CMS has considered giving physicians a small bonus when they acquire some form of information technology, such as an electronic registry or an EHR, and more when they use it to meet CMS's quality goals.[14]

Some observers, however, believe CMS will pay relatively little for information technology acquisition alone. If that award is only $2,000 per physician, say, and an EHR costs a doctor $33,000, "there's no way pay for performance will make a dent in that," says Molly Joel Coye, MD, president of HealthTech, a nonprofit research and education firm in San Francisco.

Coye's former colleague David Brailer agrees. "[Medicare] pay for performance might put 2 or 3 percent of practice revenue at stake," he says. "If a small share of that—maybe 20 percent at most—goes to health IT, that's a very small incentive for practices that face a pretty steep investment. And so a lot of them might say, 'Look, I'd rather get only 80 percent of the pay-for-performance maximum and not do the IT, rather than going the extra mile.' So pay-for-performance is helpful—it creates a milieu—but the question is whether it's really enough to bring small practices into the information age."[15]

How Do You Spell "Stark Relief"?   In another ploy to boost EHR adoption, CMS has created an exception to the Stark regulations (named after Representative Pete Stark, D-CA) that prohibit hospitals from providing anything of financial value to physicians who admit Medicare or Medicaid patients to them. This exception allows hospitals to pay up to 85 percent of the cost of EHR software for physicians on their staffs. (There is also a new "safe harbor" within the federal Anti-Kickback Act for the same purpose.)[16]

Despite this rule change, observers predict that some institutions won't provide any assistance to physicians, either because they can't afford it or because they have a long way to go in building their own information systems. Those facilities that do want to help doctors acquire EHRs may offer them the outpatient version of the hospital's information system or the EHR that a hospital-owned group uses. In that case, the program and the data—including practice management information—might be hosted on a hospital computer and served to individual practices over the Internet. But many physicians don't want a hospital to have access to their financial data; so some institutions are considering using outside computer hosting firms or going through IPAs or physician-hospital organizations to subsidize EHRs. Even in those scenarios, however, physicians probably wouldn't have a choice of EHRs—something that many of them won't like and that medical leaders oppose.[17]

Besides being practical—it's easier to support one EHR than many—the centrally hosted approach reflects the desire of some hospitals to bind physicians to them. Partly to counter that, CMS has designed the Stark exception so that it applies only to interoperable EHRs (systems that can communicate with one another).[18] But Dave Garets, who heads a health information technology research firm, doubts that this interoperability will emerge soon. In any case, Garets notes, the main reason for a hospital to offer cut-rate EHRs to doctors is to persuade them to work more closely with that institution, rather than its competitors.

Old Habits Die Hard   Money isn't the only obstacle to EHR adoption. It's also difficult for most physicians to learn how to use the software in their daily work and to customize the program to their individual practice styles.

Some physicians dodge the problem by dictating or typing some portions of the record. For example, Catherine Campion, a family physician who belongs to a nine-doctor primary-care group in Newport Beach, California, types all her notes, except for those concerning the physical exam, because she hates templates with drop-down "pick" boxes. A perfectionist, Campion decided to enter her old chart data into the record manually, instead of having it scanned in. This effort took eight months of evening work at home. Four to six weeks after starting on the EHR, she was seeing as many patients as before; but she was not able to complete all her documentation during office hours for a year.

Robert D. McCartney of Denver, an internist, combines typing with dictation, using voice-recognition software. He says he can't use the drop-down-box charting method that's characteristic of most EHRs, because he works exclusively in nursing homes. Most frail elderly patients have numerous problems, he notes, and it would take too long to navigate the templates for documentation. So he has his nurse enter vital signs and lab results, and he uses the automatic features of the EHR to generate drug and diagnosis lists.[19]

Why does it matter whether physicians take notes in a structured format? Because if they don't, the discrete data they need for quality improvement and disease management will not be available.

Limited Products Don't Stress Quality   Even if doctors were more willing to do data input, many of the products they use have a very limited palette of features. According to a *Medical Economics* survey of primary-care physicians, the only function that nearly all of their EHRs could perform was electronic charting. Beyond that, the most prevalent features were the ability to interface with a billing and scheduling system, electronic charge capture, electronic prescribing, and the ability to scan in paper documents. Only 59 percent of the EHRs allowed physicians to exchange structured e-mail messages with their staffs—a real workflow advantage to those who have it.[20]

Near the bottom of the list were drug reference and formulary data and the ability to call up lists of patients with specific diagnoses. Clinical alerts, including allergies, drug interactions, and reminders, were more widespread. (However, many doctors turn off these alerts if they pop up too often.)

Among the reasons more physicians don't buy advanced EHR programs is that they contain features they deem unnecessary. "The products that have a lot of functions related to data structuring, error checking and disease management tend to be expensive to buy and update," consultant Jeff Hertzberg says. "You just can't get the economies of scale in a small group to justify paying for that."

Consequently, most of the physicians who use high-end, sophisticated programs are in large groups. Even those EHRs can rarely help physicians do disease management. Few of them, for example, enable users to build registries that list patients with chronic diseases and what has been done for them.[21]

Lack of Connectivity · Another factor that limits the usefulness of many office-based EHRs is their inability to communicate with systems in hospitals, labs, pharmacies, and other health care facilities. In the *Medical Economics* survey, only half of the EHRs could exchange data with labs and hospitals, in most instances because interfaces are expensive. Physicians are eager to use free interfaces provided by some reference labs but don't want to pay thousands of dollars for them. Hospitals are even less likely than labs to offer free interfaces to specific EHRs, but they will do it for a large group or one that they're affiliated with.

Similarly, a study of thirty practices that have EHRs found that large practices are more likely than small offices to have electronic connectivity with other providers; many are also online with their internal labs. In contrast, the researchers said, "physicians in nine of the 18 solo/small group practices we studied could not view any electronic lab results within their EHR, seventeen could not view hospital data, and nine had EHRs that could not exchange any data with their practice management system."[22]

The Connectivity Conundrum

In April 2004, when President Bush proposed his plan to provide most Americans with EHRs within ten years, he focused on promoting on-line connectivity among all health care providers and patients. Every person, he said, should have a portable electronic file that consolidates his medical history, including every doctor he has seen and every test he has had.[23]

Shortly after announcing this ambitious plan, Bush appointed David Brailer as his national health information coordinator and charged him with leading the development of a nationwide, interoperable health information technology infrastructure. (Brailer quit that post in May 2006.)

"Among the features of such a system is the ability to store patient data securely and to share it with other systems, so the data can move around," Brailer explained in an interview with *Medical Economics*. "Clinical information should be able to move with the patient as they travel from site to site, and it should be available if they change clinicians or hospitals or move to a different area."[24]

Other experts agree that this type of data exchange capability is crucial to the goal of using health information technology to improve care. "Most health care data, whether on paper or electronic, are trapped in 'silos,'" notes William Hersh, MD, a professor of medical informatics at Oregon Health and Science University School of Medicine. "As a result, a patient may have a physician or a health system with an advanced EHR, yet if that patient requires care elsewhere, there is little likelihood the information from that advanced system will be accessible."[25]

National and Regional Networks   The government agenda for electronic connectivity is multifaceted. As set forth in Brailer's Strategic Framework, it contemplates a national health information network that would enable patients' records to move with them, facilitate the implementation of national quality measure, help consumers judge the quality of providers, enhance bio-surveillance to help authorities deal with epidemics and bioterrorism, and connect government information systems with those in the private sector.[26] This gigantic structure would rely on national standards for recording and transmitting data down to the level of the individual EHR. The national health information network would tie together a large number of regional health information organizations (RHIOs) that would provide access to local patient data.

Some of the groundwork for this national network has already been laid. In 2005, the government awarded contracts to private vendors and organizations to develop certification standards for EHRs and to test the components of a national health information network.[27] Another contractor was assigned to choose health information technology standards that will enable certified EHRs and other systems to exchange information online.[28] And government agencies are starting to interconnect their own health information systems.[29] All of this is going to be valuable as the national system develops, partly because standardization will break down the information "silos."

Except within agencies like the Departments of Defense and Veterans Affairs, however, the government is putting relatively little money into this gargantuan effort. Congress allocated just $61.7 million to the Office of the National Coordinator of Health Information Technology for fiscal 2006. In addition, the Agency for Healthcare Research and Quality handed out $166 million in grants and contracts for researching health information technology, including RHIOs.[30] Compared with the efforts of the United Kingdom, which has allocated 8 billion pounds to its health information technology infrastructure, and Canada, which has already invested $1.5 billion (Canadian),[31] the U.S. initiative seems puny.

Reliance on the Private Sector   Our government is relying on the private sector to carry the health care IT ball, but it's unclear whether or how that will happen. Take the hoped-for regional health information organizations: More than a hundred RHIO efforts are under way across the country, but only a couple of dozen RHIOs—nonprofit organizations that are supposed to enable connectivity among physicians, hospitals, labs, pharmacies, and other health care providers—are fully operational, and most are quite limited in scope.[32] This is a very new kind of enterprise, and one that's fraught with political, economic, and technical pitfalls. Dave Garets says it may be ten years or more before RHIOs exist in most parts of the United States. Many hospital executives agree, according to Mitch Morris, executive vice president for health at the First Consulting Group.

One obstacle is the lack of cooperation and trust among health plan systems, labs, and physician groups that have traditionally been rivals. For example, the Indiana Health Information Exchange has taken the first step toward building a RHIO by getting all of the hospitals in Indianapolis to send lab results and reports to doctors' offices through a common Web portal. But it took this organization and its predecessors many years just to get the hospitals to collaborate. "Nationally, the principal barrier to RHIOs isn't technology; it's the absence of trust and a shared sense that the effort is worth the cost," Molly Joel Coye of San Francisco's HealthTech says.

Wanted: An RHIO Business Model   HealthTech spearheaded the formation of CalRHIO, a nonprofit organization designed to support and unite the local networks springing up across California.[33] Kaiser Permanente, Wellpoint, and Sutter Healthcare, a big hospital system, have each put $1 million into CalRHIO. Similarly, Blue Cross Blue Shield of Tennessee supplied some of the startup funds for Care Spark, a RHIO in eastern Tennessee.[34] And Blue Cross Blue Shield of Massachusetts has given $50 million to launch the pilot RHIOs of the Massachusetts e-Health Collaborative, including funds to buy EHRs for about five hundred doctors.[35] But, except for these efforts, payers haven't yet committed major sums for RHIOs.

Mitch Morris of the First Consulting Group views the "immature business models" of RHIOs as the major stumbling block to their success. "We're involved in a number of discussions about RHIO formation," he says, "and they tend not to get very far because no one has a check book. They're all well meaning, but the checkbook isn't pulled out. So the business model is one of the biggest challenges, because nobody believes that the federal government is going to finance the creation of this national information network."

Blue-Sky Financial Projections   Some researchers have argued that a national health information network could have a real impact on reducing the growth of U.S. health care spending. According to a RAND paper, after a fifteen-year phase-in period, full EHR implementation and networking could save more than $81 billion annually by improving health care efficiency and safety.[36] Health information technology–related improvements in preventive and chronic care, RAND says, could cut another $40 billion a year.

But in a commentary on the study, Clifford Goodman, vice president of the Lewin Group, a Falls Church, Virginia, consulting firm, notes that the claimed savings would amount to only 1.6 percent of projected health spending in 2019, the year in which the building of the health IT infrastructure was expected to be complete. Overall health costs would not drop even that much, he added, because "the U.S. health system will find ways to reallocate the money."[37]

Another study, by the Center for Information Technology Leadership in Boston, states that standardized electronic information exchange between providers could save $77.8 billion a year.[38] The Government Accountability Office, however, cast doubt on the validity of the study's estimate in a February 2005 report, noting that it was based on "a number of assumptions and inhibited by limited data."[39]

Other critics agreed. Laurence Baker, a Stanford University professor, targeted the study's claim that connectivity with labs could save $32 billion.[40] This assumes, he points out, that the $40 average cost of a lab test could be halved by eliminating most labor costs involved in test-related paperwork. If office and lab workers earn an average of $15 an hour, he says, this means they'd be working an hour and a half to process a single lab test!

A 2006 paper by Jaan Sidorov, MD, a medical director at the Geisinger Health Plan in Danville, Pennsylvania, points out that the literature does not support claims that physicians' use of EHRs will reduce national health costs. Sidorov found little evidence that practices with EHRs significantly decrease labor costs. However, he notes, EHRs do enable physicians to justify higher charges with better documentation.[41]

Cost Estimates Vary Widely   According to the RAND paper, it would cost $98 billion for 90 percent of hospitals to adopt an EHR system, and $17.2 billion for physician adoption to reach the same level. Yearly maintenance bills would total $7.6 billion. In contrast, the Center for Health Information Technology study estimated that it would cost about $28 billion annually for ten years and $16 billion a year thereafter to construct and maintain a national health information network.

A third group of experts estimated that it would cost $156 billion in capital investment and $48 billion in annual operating costs to build a national health information network over five years. This estimate includes $51 billion for hospital systems, $31 billion for nursing homes, and $18 billion for physician offices.[42] The authors observed that the total investment would represent only 2 percent of national health spending in 2005. But, even if their cost estimate is accurate, it does not represent the full cost of using health information technology to obtain the predicted improvements in quality and efficiency. Referring to the RAND study, James Walker, the chief medical information officer at the Geisinger Health System, notes that the complexity of redesigning work processes to take advantage of EHRs is bound to reduce the financial benefits. He also observes that the human resources required to change how care is delivered far exceed the cost of implementing EHRs and systems of data exchange.[43]

Connecting with Patients: Why Not Now?

Even without EHRs, there is plenty physicians can do to reduce the amount of dysfunction in their own offices. As the Institute for Healthcare Improvement has shown, medical practices can be re-engineered to increase patient access, shorten waiting times, deliver more appropriate services, and provide nonvisit care when that is needed.[44] But the current reimbursement system discourages physicians from adopting these innovations. Because they don't get paid for phone or e-mail work, for example, most doctors avoid it and encourage patients to come into the office instead.

Joseph Scherger, MD, a professor of family and preventive medicine at the University of California, San Diego School of Medicine, pins much of the blame for poor quality on the visit-centered model of care. The typical primary-care physician, he notes, cares for between fifteen hundred and three thousand patients. If there are five thousand fifteen-minute visits a year, he points out, "a visit-dependent model of care allows a physician about an hour per year per patient! That is not enough time to provide good preventive care, let alone to treat illness. The first rule of a new model of quality care is not being dependent on visits."[45]

To provide the "continuous healing relationship" that the Institute of Medicine says is needed to handle the burden of chronic diseases, Scherger suggests that the system be restructured so that physicians can communicate easily with patients outside of office visits. This new system would also enable patients to take better care of themselves and to share more of the medical decision-making with physicians.[46]

Among the components of this multifaceted approach, he says, are e-mail communications between physicians and patients; physician Web sites that allow patients to see lab results and other parts of their health record, make appointments, request medication refills, and obtain educational materials; and Web-connected home monitoring devices, such as glucometers, digital scales, and peak-flow meters, that enable patients to track their chronic conditions and send data to caregivers.

Slow Uptake of Technology   The technology to do all of this has existed for several years, but relatively few physicians are using it so far. Home monitoring is costly because of the equipment required and the need for nurses to stay in close contact with patients; hence, disease-management firms do most of this.[47] But the direct costs for physicians to exchange secure messages with patients or to set up an interactive Web site are not high. What is expensive is the extra time doctors would have to devote to communicating with patients online. That, plus security and liability concerns, are the main reasons only about 10–15 percent of doctors exchange e-mail with patients.[48]

More and more doctors are doing this, however, now that they're starting to get paid for it. Some Blues plans, for example, as well as Aetna and CIGNA, have begun reimbursing doctors for e-mail consultations. Doctors in other plans have found that patients are willing to pay them directly for this service through secure messaging services such as Medem, RelayHealth, and ZixCorp.[49] And some doctors include e-mail among the extra services they provide to patients who pay them an annual fee.[50]

Among this last group is Charles Kilo, an internist who leads a five-doctor practice in Portland, Oregon. About 20 percent of the interactions that Kilo and his colleagues have with patients take place in face-to-face visits that typically last thirty minutes or longer. The rest of their work is about evenly divided between their e-mail and phone contacts with patients who don't need to be seen.[51] Patients pay about $350 a year to belong to the practice.[52]

Personal Health Records   Meanwhile, a growing number of patients are interacting with their doctors through something called a "personal health record" (PHR). While this is a diffuse concept that takes many forms, most PHRs are online medical records that consist of patient-entered data, payer-entered claims data, or data extracted from a physician's EHR and posted on a secure Web site. (In the latter case, patients may correct or add to the record.) Any of these kinds of PHRs may present patient information that, in some instances, doctors are not aware of. That capability is a big advantage for physicians, partly because it can alert them to medications that other doctors have prescribed for a patient.[53]

Bonnie Parten of Bellingham, Washington, recalls that her late father, Maurice Perrault, took twelve different medications for his ailments, which included congestive heart failure, diabetes, renal failure, and hypertension. By using a PHR that a local hospital system created and that family members filled out, Perrault made sure all of his doctors knew which drugs he was taking.

"I think it extended the life of my father because we avoided medication errors," Parten told *Medical Economics*. She and her siblings now have PHRs of their own, she added.[54]

Medem, a San Francisco-based company, has launched another PHR that contains only patient-entered health data. Aside from helping patients keep track of their own information, this PHR, which is usually attached to a physician Web site, replaces the medical history forms that patients must fill out for every new doctor they see.

Some large groups are starting to connect PHRs to their EHRs. For example, people who belong to Group Health Cooperative, a Seattle-based HMO, can view their health records and pick up lab results in a Web-based "shared record" that mirrors portions of the EHR used by medical groups that belong to the cooperative. About one hundred thousand Group Health Cooperative patients now have these PHRs. Matt Handley, MD, a medical director of the HMO and a practicing physician, says this is "the greatest lever we've ever had to work with patients."[55]

Several health plans, meanwhile, have launched PHRs based on claims and lab data. This type of record provides patients with an overview of their medications and what their doctors have done for them. It may also be combined with educational materials tailored to a particular patient's condition.

Among the plans that have recently launched claims-based PHRs are Tennessee Blue Cross and Blue Shield, Empire Blue Cross and Blue Shield, Aetna, and United Healthcare. In addition, America's Health Insurance Plans and the Blue Cross and Blue Shield Association have created a standardized PHR that will be portable when a patient moves from one plan to another.[56]

The Public Wants Doctors Involved   About 60 percent of Americans would like to have a secure PHR, according to a survey commissioned by the Markle Foundation.[57] While most people don't want either health plans or employers to have access to their PHRs, four of five Americans say they would want their primary-care physician to see the data. A majority also believe that other health care providers should be able to view the PHR.[58]

When consumers are asked what they'd use a PHR for, their answers show that they view it as an extension of the patient-physician relationship: They want to check and refill prescriptions, get lab results over the Internet, check for mistakes in their medical records, and conduct e-mail communications with their physicians.[59] They also believe that a PHR would help them clarify their doctor's instructions, prevent medical mistakes, change the way they manage their health, and improve the quality of care.[60]

If physicians got onboard and if most of them had EHRs, much of this could happen today. But even PHR proponents see several problems with the state of the art. Letting patients view portions of an EHR is fine, they observe, but current information is limited to what a particular physician or organization has done for the patient. Standalone PHRs like Medem's, they note, contain only data the patient has entered and usually cannot connect with their physician's EHR. And the Holy Grail to which President Bush and the Institute of Medicine aspire—a PHR that combines patient-entered information with comprehensive data from interoperable, community-wide EHRs—is still far in the future, these experts say.[61]

Nevertheless, that hasn't stopped supporters of "consumer-directed care" from stating that health information technology and quality report cards will empower patients to manage their own care and choose wisely among health care providers. "Technological empowerment and control by the informed citizen will be the cornerstone of our health care of the future," former Senate majority leader Bill Frist declared in a 2004 speech.[62]

In the next chapter, I examine this argument and consider whether it makes sense in the light of what we know about consumers and the limitations of health care–quality data.

6   Can Consumers Direct Their Own Care?

Caryn Tinn, a forty-one-year-old homemaker in Bridgewater, New Jersey, discovered a lump in her breast in 2003. Six months earlier, her obstetrician/gynecologist had given her a clean bill of health, but she hadn't had a mammogram in nearly five years. When she noticed the lump, she went back to the physician, who immediately sent her to get a mammogram and an ultrasound test. The test results indicated that she might have breast cancer. So Tinn went to see a surgeon that the ob/gyn had recommended. Neither Tinn nor her husband felt comfortable with the surgeon, who was incommunicative and wanted to do a biopsy in an ambulatory surgery center rather than a hospital. But they were going to use him, anyway, for lack of a better alternative.

Then they spoke with Tinn's uncle, who had a close friend who was a surgeon at Robert Wood Johnson University Hospital in New Brunswick. When they contacted this surgeon, he told them to come in right away. He did the biopsy, diagnosed cancer, and, after explaining the alternatives to Tinn, scheduled surgery for three weeks later.

While the surgeon mentioned the possibilities of lumpectomy and "watchful waiting," Tinn agreed that a mastectomy made sense because the cancer had spread to her lymph nodes. Later, after she'd had a breast removed, Tinn's doctors discovered that her cancer had metastasized. Because of the danger of its spreading to the other breast and also because she wanted her breast reconstruction to look natural, she had a second mastectomy.

Tinn is currently getting infusions of Herceptin, which slows the recurrence of the cancer. She has also joined a clinical trial in Seattle that's testing a cancer vaccine. Her husband found out about the trial on the Internet. Tinn doesn't think her doctors would have told her about it because, she says, "they usually only do that with patients who are expected to live for no longer than six months."

Reflecting on her experience, Tinn says that the only reason she received excellent care was that her uncle knew the surgeon at Robert Wood Johnson University Hospital. Not only did he recommend her oncologist, who proved superb, but he got her a fine reconstructive surgeon.

"When it came time to get a plastic surgeon, I said to him, 'Of these people on my insurance plan, who do you recommend?' And he said, 'None of them.' He recommended another surgeon and wrote a letter to my insurance company, saying that this was the surgeon he wanted to work with, and they approved it.

"I had a good experience with the health care system," Tinn concludes. "But the foundation was laid because of this family friend, who made sure I went to all the right people. I also think that as a patient, I don't sit idly by. I don't put all the power in the doctors. That helped me have a good experience as well. We're partners in this, and I think that's made a difference in how doctors deal with us, and how we deal with them."

What Everyone Should Know—and Doesn't   While Tinn's story illustrates the importance of being an informed consumer, it also shows that even well-educated people have a hard time navigating the health care system. Yet consumer-directed care, the latest stab at health care reform, asks ordinary people to shop for doctors and hospitals on the basis of quality and cost and to make detailed health care decisions on their own. As noted in Chapter 2, proponents of this approach claim that when consumers spend their own money (or a health spending account funded by their employer), they'll use fewer unnecessary services, thereby slowing overall cost growth. What this chain of cause-and-effect depends on, however, is the unproven assumption that consumers can make good health care choices.

Sheldon Greenfield is co-director of the health policy department at the University of California, Irvine, and an expert on coaching patients to ask doctors the right questions. He thinks it's foolish to suppose that most patients can understand complex medical issues. "My mother-in-law was told up at UCLA that she had something in her eye related to macular degeneration," he says. "Does she know the difference between macular degeneration and something else, and whether a procedure should be done at UCLA or in a community hospital and how much money to spend on it? How in the world would she know? I'm an internist, and I don't know."

Making Decisions in Survival Mode   Karen Davis, a health economist and president of the Commonwealth Fund, also questions whether most people can make good choices based on the information now available to them. "The consumer really should know what the total hospital bill should be—not just a fee for a service, but also all the costs related to surgery. That's the only way you can compare the cost at one hospital to that at another. Also, you have no idea of how the quality of care differs from one hospital to another. So it's impossible to make wise choices today. Even if you could, you might not be up to it. When you're in crisis mode, you don't sit around and think about what it will cost if the ambulance takes you to this hospital vs. that hospital. Even with cancer, where you may have a little more time to consider your options, you're a lot more focused on survival than on the bill."

Other experts are more optimistic about the ability of some consumers to direct their own care. David Lansky, director of the Markle Foundation's health care program and a pioneer in the field of patient experience surveys, for example, says that the foundation's data reveals that "about 30 percent of the public will be fairly active in managing their own care. That leaves about 70 percent who will not be nearly as active. Of that group, at least half will basically trust their doctors to do the right thing. But for those who want to be more active in managing their care, we should provide resources to let them be more involved."

The Birth of Consumerism   Consumerism has had a major impact on health care, but its reach has been more limited there than in most other industries. Among the barriers to greater consumer involvement in health care have been the paucity of relevant, reliable, high-quality information and doctors' reluctance to accept patient involvement in medical decisions.

Until about forty years ago, most doctors practiced in a paternalistic manner that left little room for patients to participate in managing their own care.[1] This paternalistic relationship led to travesties such as the performance of tonsillectomies long after they were known to be useless and of a large number of unnecessary hysterectomies.[2]

The tide began to turn in the 1960s with the emergence of the idea of "informed consent."[3] The concept was that patients had a right to participate in all medical decisions that affected them; therefore, doctors were bound to inform them of the risks of any procedure beforehand. Today, state laws require patients to sign informed-consent forms before any surgical operation.[4]

By the late 1980s, as health researchers discovered large variations in care across the country, the notion of informed consent broadened into the idea of "shared decision-making." Patients were now invited to collaborate with their physicians in deciding whether to have certain procedures, such as those involving breast and prostate cancer (see Chapter 8).[5]

Self-Care Movement   By the 1990s, when the Internet came along, a new generation of educated consumers were primed to search for health care information that could help them take better care of themselves and understand what their doctors were telling them. According to a 2005 study, about 52 million Americans—or 55 percent of those with Internet access—used the Web to get health or medical information, and nearly half of those said it influenced their health care choices.[6] It should be noted, however, that a high percentage of health care information on the Web is misleading or erroneous.[7]

While the Internet was fueling consumerism, both the positive and negative aspects of managed care were leading consumers to seek health care information from sources other than their doctors. On the plus side, many managed-care plans and employers implemented self-care initiatives to help people stay healthy. At the same time, the limitations placed on patient access to specialists and the decreasing amount of time primary-care physicians spent with patients induced many of them to find the information they sought on their own.[8]

Today, in contrast, health plans are actively promoting consumerism as an alternative to top-down restrictions on care. The insurers are providing an increasing amount of health care information intended to help patients take better care of themselves and engage their physicians more fully. In addition, public report cards on doctors and hospitals are proliferating. The latter trend raises two key questions: How helpful are these rankings, and are consumers willing or able to use them in selecting health care providers?

Provider Report Cards

Some plans, including Humana, Pacificare, Blue Cross of California, and United, publish their own report cards. Other insurers and employers contract with firms such as Health Grades and Subimo to provide the information to plan members and employees. (Those companies also make some data available to the general public.)[9] At least 30 percent of pay-for-performance programs include report cards, mostly on hospitals and physician groups.[10]

The Leapfrog Group, a consortium of large corporations and government agencies, publishes a report card that covers thirty measures of hospital safety. The group ranks hospitals on the volume of certain procedures, the presence of critical care specialists in their intensive care units, and the progress they've made in computerizing physician orders, among other things.[11]

Recently, the federal government has become directly involved in quality measurement. The Centers for Medicare and Medicaid Services (CMS) now publishes clinical quality comparisons among more than thirty-five hundred acute-care hospitals. Including data on nineteen indicators of quality of care for heart attacks, congestive heart failure, and pneumonia, as well as two measures of surgical infection prevention, this scorecard is the most extensive comparative report on the conditions that it covers.[12]

New York, Pennsylvania, and California all compare hospitals on the outcomes of coronary artery bypass graft surgery, and the first two states also publish data on individual cardiac surgeons.[13] Other states look at some other parameters of inpatient care. But in most state hospital reports, the measure of treatment effectiveness is mortality rates.[14] The reliance on mortality greatly limits the range of measured conditions and excludes other key quality factors.

In contrast, the Wisconsin Collaborative for Healthcare Quality, a consortium of employers, providers, and health plans, has started publishing data that allows consumers to compare nineteen hospitals and fourteen large multispecialty groups on forty-five quality measures.[15] New York's Alliance for Quality Healthcare, sponsored by employers and insurers, puts out hospital reports that combine procedure volume for seven conditions, mortality rates for fourteen procedures and medical conditions, and utilization rates for five overused procedures.[16] Health

Grades publishes complication and mortality rates for twenty-eight procedures, along with average costs and lengths of stay.[17]

About a dozen states, including California, North Carolina, and Wisconsin, have mandated the publication of hospital cost data.[18] In June 2006, CMS also began to post information on the Web about how much Medicare pays hospitals for two dozen procedures and inpatient stays for common conditions.[19] CMS disseminates cost data on physicians and ambulatory surgery centers, too.[20] But unlike the state data, the Medicare information consists of county-by-county averages.

The initial release of the hospital-specific price information drew a lot of media attention. The *Wall Street Journal*, for example, cited huge differentials between California hospitals' charges for services like chest X-rays and CT scans as well as drugs such as Tylenol and Percocet.[21] But consumers haven't shown much interest in comparative data on the costs of particular services.[22] And hospitals object that this information on charges is irrelevant to most consumers because actual payments are individually negotiated with each health plan.[23]

Physician Scorecards   Across the country, more public information is available on hospitals than on physicians. But in California, Minnesota, and Wisconsin, where large medical groups and independent practice associations (IPAs) are prevalent, scorecards comparing the quality and cost of physician organizations have emerged as well.

As mentioned earlier, the Integrated Healthcare Association in California collects quality data on more than two hundred groups and IPAs, and the results are posted on a state government Web site. Minnesota has created a "clearinghouse" site that provides links to combined health-plan report cards on hospitals and physician groups.[24]

Meanwhile, Aetna and United have begun publishing very basic quality data on individual doctors,[25] and a few medium-sized plans have posted more detailed physician information.[26] Aetna also tells its members how much it pays individual physicians in a dozen states and cities.[27] CIGNA has begun giving its members cost and quality information on specialists, using a star-based scoring system. The insurer also publishes comparative data on what it pays for ambulatory surgery procedures and high-end imaging tests.[28]

Validity of Report Card Measures   As noted in Chapter 2, cost comparisons are questionable when they're based mainly on each provider's negotiating ability. As for quality measures, most report cards today are based on claims data or patient satisfaction surveys or both. (An important exception is CMS's HospitalCompare, which also includes information culled from patient records.) Claims data, as explained earlier, contain a lot of errors and constitute a blunt instrument for measuring clinical performance.[29] Patient satisfaction has often been treated as a proxy for health care quality, but there is little evidence that patients' judgments of doctors' ability to communicate, their technical skills, and the length of time they spend with patients are related to clinical excellence, says Shoshanna Sofaer, a health-policy professor at Baruch College in New York.

Plans and providers agree that it would be better for practices to collect performance data from their own records. Large groups on the West Coast are already submitting their own clinical data for both pay for performance and report cards, and smaller practices in Maine are also beginning to submit electronically gathered data to an employer coalition. But until many more practices adopt health information technology, electronic submission of data will not become widespread.

Another problem with the validity of report cards is the small sample sizes: A study of seven surgical procedures discovered that, except for coronary artery bypass surgery, none of the operations was performed frequently enough to use mortality rates as a quality measure.[30] And, as discussed in Chapter 4, sample sizes limit the ability to measure physician performance on chronic-disease care.

Like pay for performance, report cards can also have unintended consequences, such as doctors' providing inappropriate care and avoiding noncompliant patients to reach "target" rates.[31] In western Michigan, for example, a major regional insurer named Priority Health has been publishing report cards on doctors since 2003. Frank Belsito, a family physician in Wyoming, Michigan, says he knows of colleagues who have "dumped" difficult patients—or patients who can't afford the copays to fill their prescriptions—in order to get their scores up. "It's a very slippery slope," he says, "if we start to go down that path without really understanding what we're trying to do."

Do Report Cards Describe Quality?   Physicians are also concerned about the fact that report cards represent only a small portion of what they do. "To look at only one or two diseases as a proxy for a patient's likelihood of good care in a particular physician's office is a bit shallow," Louis Hanson, a veteran family physician in Cumberland, Maine, observes.

Experts such as David Lansky agree that such scorecards can be misleading. "We have pretty good data showing that the performance of physicians with their diabetes patients is uncorrelated with their heart patients or asthma patients," Lansky says. Therefore, he notes, scorecard data on whether particular physicians provide appropriate diabetes care "is only relevant to people with diabetes."

Robert Brook, MD, vice president and director of RAND Health, slams the current efforts to depict an individual doctor's quality based on a handful of factors. Disease-specific scores, he says, don't tell you enough about a physician who sees patients with many different conditions—and they don't encourage physicians to improve the overall way they practice.

"The trick is not to say, 'I'm going to put all my discretionary resources into mammograms,' " he says. "You have to reorganize the way you do business. If you were trying to improve car quality and said, 'I'm just going to get the paint right, I don't give a damn if the transmission falls out, because I'm measuring quality on the basis of paint color,' we would not have the kinds of improvements in cars that we've had."

One-Dimensional Hospital Reports   Since hospital report cards are based largely on the volume of procedures, complication and mortality rates, and patient satisfaction, they represent only a small portion of hospital quality. And because a hospital is good at one type of care, experts say, that doesn't mean it handles a different procedure or condition equally well.

"You can have a hospital that does very well on one measure and badly on another measure," observes Shoshanna Sofaer of Baruch College. "So finding a pattern that allows you to make a choice is difficult."

A study of Medicare quality data buttresses her point. The researchers found that while performance on the quality indicators for heart attack, congestive heart failure, and pneumonia varied moderately among large hospitals in different metropolitan areas, there was no correlation between the quality of cardiac care in any given hospital and the same hospital's score on pneumonia care.[32]

Do Consumers Care about Quality?

Partly because of the inadequacies of report cards, relatively few consumers rely on them. In a 2000 article in the *Journal of the American Medical Association*, Brook and other researchers summarized evidence showing that this information "has only a limited impact on consumer decision making." For example, a survey of Pennsylvania consumers who had undergone heart surgery showed that only 12 percent of them were aware of the state's coronary artery bypass graft report-card at the time of their operation; of those, fewer than a quarter said that it had had a significant impact on their choice of surgeon. "The reasons for consumers' lack of interest in and use of performance data," the authors of the study say, "include difficulty in understanding the information, disinterest in the nature of the information available, lack of trust in the data, problems with timely access to the information, and lack of choice."[33]

The authors conclude that neither consumers nor employers "appear to search out, understand, or use the currently available information to any significant extent." But provider organizations, including hospitals and physician groups, were sensitive to the publication of quality data, which frequently spurred them to engage in quality-improvement projects.

This effect has been observed among medical groups in California[34] and among hospitals in Cleveland,[35] New Jersey,[36] and Wisconsin.[37] A study of Wisconsin report cards, for example, showed that hospitals that reported their data publicly improved their performance more than hospitals that didn't report. But, while many consumers were aware of the report cards, only 10 percent of survey respondents reported using them to recommend or choose a hospital in the two years after they appeared.[38]

Is the Glass Half Full or Half Empty?   Consumers are starting to become more aware of report cards. A 2004 survey sponsored by the Kaiser Family Foundation, the Agency for Healthcare Research and Quality, and the Harvard School of Public Health found that 35 percent of respondents had seen information comparing the quality of different health plans, hospitals, or doctors in the past year (up from 27 percent in 2000). Nineteen percent of respondents said they'd used the information to make a decision about their health care, compared with 10 percent in 2000.[39]

Another national survey, however, showed that, despite the proliferation of report cards, most people are still not tuning in. In a Harris Interactive poll, 22 percent of respondents said they'd looked at hospital quality information in 2005, and 13 percent had seen data on physicians. (Both figures were about the same as in a 2001 survey.) But only 4 percent and 2 percent, respectively, had considered changing hospitals or doctors as a result of the report cards, and fewer than half of those had done so.[40]

How to Make Report Cards Relevant   Some observers believe that consumer use of report-card data will spread if the quality of the data improves and the data are properly presented. The health-care-quality expert David Nash of Jefferson Medical College lists three factors that would stimulate more use of report cards: a pressing clinical need, the ability to distinguish adequately among providers, and data on the risk of being harmed in a particular institution.

Judy Hibbard, a health-policy professor at the University of Oregon who studies how people use quality data, agrees on the need to inform consumers about safety risks. But for that to happen, she observes, hospitals and physicians would have to reveal much more information than they do now. For example, she notes, it's very difficult to obtain hospital infection rates. (This is starting to change. Sixteen states now require hospitals to report these data,[41] several other states are considering legislation, and CMS's HospitalCompare reports compliance with infection prevention guidelines.)

Lansky and Brook also believe we need to add measures of appropriateness to report cards so that people will understand the extent to which some providers overuse or misuse particular services, sometimes to the detriment of patients. "That's a major patient safety issue," Brook says.

Health Literacy Obstacle   A huge obstacle to the use of quality data is that many consumers can't understand it. One reason is that the information is usually presented at a college reading-level, which excludes a large percentage of the population.[42] About 90 million adults have low health literacy, meaning they have difficulty understanding and using health information[43] So when a report card uses a term like "risk adjustment," Hibbard notes, it's likely to stop them in their tracks.

Some hospital report cards, including Health Grade's, use simple three-star systems that are easy for consumers to grasp. If they want to drill down to the data on mortality and complication rates, they can do that, says Sarah Loughran, executive vice president of Health Grades. It's doubtful, however, that most visitors to the HospitalCompare site understand the importance of the "percent of patients given ACE inhibitor or ARB for left ventricular systolic dysfunction" if they have congestive heart failure.

Shoshanna Sofaer questions how the rating services are presenting the information. "Are they presenting it in plain English? Are they using clear graphics? Are they helping people to interpret what they're seeing? Are they giving people advice on how to use what they're seeing?"

Sofaer and some other experts argue that it's easier for most consumers to get a handle on patient satisfaction data, which reflects the parameters they're most concerned about. "It's not clinical quality, it's people's experience of their care," Sofaer says. "That's across [medical] conditions, so it's easier to get enough data to be reliable. It resonates to people."

While there's no reason to doubt this conclusion, there are many people for whom the conventional notions of health care quality are irrelevant. Some consumers rate affordability, insurance coverage, and access as the most important components of quality. Others think that all physicians have equivalent clinical skills, or that more expensive providers are better. And a large percentage of the poor—especially immigrants who speak little or no English—don't even understand the question.

Gloria Mayer, whose Institute for Healthcare Advancement in Whittier, California, has put out a series of self-care books for the low-literacy population, says that their readers wouldn't understand treatment alternatives even if they were written in Spanish. These people, she says, want to know how close a doctor's office is, because many of them don't have cars. They also want to know about office hours, whether the staff speaks their language, and how well a doctor communicates. But clinical quality data is way above their heads, she adds. "I don't find the report cards are helpful to low-literacy people; they don't understand them. They don't see themselves as having a lot of options."

The Doctor-Patient Relationship

While consumers treat 80–90 percent of illness symptoms at home,[44] they usually rely on their physicians for advice on more serious (and sometimes not so serious) ailments. Today most physicians believe that patients should make the ultimate decisions, but many patients still want their doctors to tell them what to do. According to a recent New York Times/CBS News poll, "slightly more than half of the patients who received a diagnosis were given multiple treatment options. One-third made the decision on their own, with those between the ages of 45 and 64 most likely to do so."[45]

Forty-four percent of the respondents who received a diagnosis sought further information, either on the Web or from family and friends. Anecdotally, people seem to do this more often when they have a serious condition. "When a woman gets breast cancer, the first thing she does is speak to the ten other women she knows who've had it," says Ann Mond Johnson, president of Subimo.

Nevertheless, experts say that patients still usually go to the hospital or specialist that their doctor refers them to. And, despite the suggestion of a Solucient study that people would be willing to switch hospitals or doctors based on data,[46] they tend to trust their physicians more than Internet report cards.

"If personal experience (and positive emotional memories) with one's doctor contradict negative statistics about that doctor, consumers will probably stay with that doctor rather than change," the consultant Mark Hochhauser writes. "Consumers choose what they like and avoid what they don't like: Feelings trump data."[47]

Doctors' Experience   Primary-care physicians say that even if their patients brought them comparative quality information on hospitals or specialists, they'd be unlikely to give it much weight in their recommendations. Salvatore Volpe, an internist and pediatrician in Staten Island, New York, for example, says he sometimes sends patients who need parathyroid surgery to a surgeon he knows at New York University Hospital, and he sends cancer patients who want a second opinion to Sloan Kettering in New York. Otherwise, he usually relies on his local hospital, and he believes most doctors do the same, regardless of report cards.

Craig Wax, a family physician in southern New Jersey, is equidistant from three hospitals. While each has its strengths and weaknesses, he tries to make recommendations to patients "based on their needs and their expressed wants." He also tells them what to ask surgeons, whom he picks on the basis of their technical skill, medical knowledge, and ability to communicate. Although he learns these things from personal experience rather than data, he doubts that report cards on either doctors or hospitals would make much difference to him.

Wax doesn't believe that the current scorecards are reliable. Even if they were, he values the "warm, fuzzy" aspects of providers, because he wants his patients to be treated nicely. But most of all, he just doesn't trust any hospital or physician that he's not personally acquainted with. "I'm particularly culpable if I send a patient anywhere for anything and they have a bad outcome. So if I send a patient to a place I know, where I know what the plusses and minuses and limitations are, I can weigh the outcomes in that."

Lawrence Casalino of the University of Chicago does not believe that many people will use report cards to choose their hospitals or physicians in the near future. David Nash of Jefferson Medical College points out, however, that performance measurement has come a long way in the past decade, and that it's continuing to improve. So perhaps report cards will mean something to most consumers someday. In the meantime, public rankings are prompting some hospitals and physician groups to improve the safety and quality of care. As long as they do that, report cards are unlikely to go away.

Consumer Empowerment

Health plans have placed a big bet on consumer-directed care. So they're not relying only on provider report cards to support patient health care choices. They're also supplying information about the comparative costs of hospitals and physicians, guidelines for treating chronic conditions, preventive care reminders, and even coaching to help patients find out more from their physicians.

Humana, for example, has an online tool that estimates how much consumers would have to pay for certain procedures at different local hospitals, based on their insurance policies. It's also developing a Web-based method of comparing prescription prices at different pharmacies.

And it offers its own report card on hospitals that includes risk-adjusted mortality and complication rates as well as infection rates.

Humana tries to provide guidance to consumers on their current health status by having them fill out health-risk appraisal forms. It also sends out automated reminders to people who need preventive and chronic care.

According to Jonathan Lord, MD, senior vice president and chief innovation officer for Humana, the company now makes "in excess of 1 million automated outbound phone calls that are related either to reminders about getting preventive services like mammography, getting appropriate treatment for diabetics, like HbA1c tests, or people getting a brand-name prescription when they might have a less costly alternative, so they can ask their doctor about it."

Humana also has nurses call high-risk patients to intervene with them before they have a catastrophic illness or heart attack. The nurses try to motivate them to take better control of their health and understand the choices they need to make. Moreover, they help them ask doctors better questions. But Lord says this coaching is more related to the patients' concerns than to their medical needs. "Many times patients can think of a lot of things when they're in the waiting room. But they freeze up in the exam room, and then remember all the questions they didn't ask later on."

Different Approach to Coaching   If a patient doesn't understand his illness and what needs to be done for it, he won't, of course, be able to ask his doctor the right questions. Sheldon Greenfield of the University of California, Irvine, has done a lot of research on patient coaching, and his team has shown that, at least for diabetes, it can improve outcomes. But he doesn't believe that health plans will be able to do this well, and he predicts it will be fifteen to twenty years before proper coaching is available for most common conditions.

Sofaer holds out more hope for the health plans' efforts to inform consumers. But she wonders whether the public's distrust of insurers will sabotage their efforts. "For a long time now, consumers haven't believed their health plan has anything to do with the quality of their health care," she says. "And that's going to be the challenge for these plans: They're going to have to create trust in the consumer that they're an independent and reliable source of information. And it's not an easy sell."

Lord doesn't deny this difficulty. "When it comes to earning trust, it takes quite a while to build. And it can be frittered away fairly quickly." But Humana's experience with automated reminders, he says, shows that people will listen when the information is credible and important.

Humana maintains that patients should be given as much autonomy as possible to make their own health care choices, Lord notes. And he thinks that Humana's ability to give this autonomy has received a huge boost from "the democratization of information" on the Internet. While not every person is capable of making "the rational choice every time," he says, most people are, and they can probably make choices that are better than those that someone else would make for them.

The Proactive Patient   Many patients are becoming more proactive in their relationship with doctors. Research has shown that doctors don't mind patients' wanting to be more engaged in their own care, and some say they're quite comfortable with the idea of patients' bringing them information they've dug up on the Internet. In fact, says Kenneth Kubitschek, an internist in Asheville, North Carolina, patients sometimes mention things he didn't know about certain conditions.

"I have a patient with multiple sclerosis who definitely knows more about it than I do. She's in chat rooms with patients who have MS, and they tell her what their neurologists are doing. And she'll bring in information and say, 'What do you think about this?' It's very helpful for me."

Robert Hughes, a family physician in Murray, Kentucky, is less impressed by the quality of what his patients bring him off the Internet. "It's usually not something that's dramatically helpful or very profound. It's just background information for them about their condition. But it does enhance the conversation about their condition, and I appreciate that, because the more information you have about your condition, the more likely you are to have a favorable outcome."

Gullibility of Consumers   Unfortunately, people tend to be gullible, as marketers of prescription drugs and "alternative" therapies know quite well. The move to consumer-directed care will help these entrepreneurs part patients from even more of their money.

Take "direct-to-consumer" television ads for prescription drugs, which generate billions of dollars a year in advertising revenues. The pharmaceutical companies use Madison Avenue advertising techniques to create a desire or the perception of a need for drugs that consumers might not need or that could be harmful to them (see Chapter 11).[48] The kicker in these ads is always, "See your doctor to find out if this medication is right for you."

This caveat, of course, places a great deal of pressure on physicians—and just as when they prescribe antibiotics for colds, they often give patients what they want. In a study that used actors posing as patients with major depression, researchers found that when patients asked for Paxil, doctors prescribed some antidepressant in 53 percent of the cases and Paxil specifically in 27 percent of the cases.[49]

Alternative Medicine   More than 40 percent of patients use alternative medical treatments, and over 70 percent of those don't tell their physicians.[50] Some estimates indicate that patients spend as much or more out of pocket for visits to alternative practitioners than they do on doctor visits.

While alternative techniques such as chiropractic manipulation and acupuncture help some people, there's little scientific evidence to support most "complementary" medicine, and some herbs, such as ephedra and pennyroyal, can be quite harmful.[51]

Doctors find it difficult to advise patients about alternative medicine because they often do not know what treatments the patients are getting or what medicines they are using. One of the scariest aspects of consumer-directed care is the possibility that underinsured patients will seek care from poorly qualified practitioners or use herbs and supplements they don't understand and that aren't regulated by the federal government.[52] In addition, by seeking alternative treatments rather than seeing a doctor, they might prolong their acute illness or worsen their chronic disease.[53]

Bad Health Behavior   Our country's growing obesity problem generates an ever-growing burden of illness and health costs, despite doctors' telling patients repeatedly to lose weight. The percentage of the adult population that smokes has leveled off at just under 25 percent, and alcoholism and drug abuse remain health problems of epic proportions.[54]

While these facts present one of the strongest arguments against consumers' ability to make good health choices, they also underscore the need for consumers to take greater responsibility for their health—a major premise of consumer-directed care. Citing the self-destructive tendencies of many patients who overeat, smoke, and drink too much, Wax observes, "At some point it has to be incumbent upon the patient to make choices. I can't go home with them."

But Hughes doesn't believe that giving noncompliant patients more control over health spending will change their health behavior. "I think they'd decide they enjoyed their lifestyle as is and were unwilling to change it or couldn't change it," he says. In fact, he adds, being in a consumer-directed health plan "might encourage them to say, 'What the heck, I'm not going to bother doing anything, and I'll save some money in the process.' For those who are already irresponsible, I think you'll increase the likelihood that they'll be irresponsible, because now you've created a financial incentive for that. You've rewarded that behavior."

7   The Limits of Evidence

Consumer-driven care is not just about giving consumers incentives to use health care services more judiciously. Its proponents also seek to create a market in which consumer choices will force physicians to change how they practice. In this sense, it complements pay for performance, which is designed to influence physician and hospital behavior.

Both pay for performance and provider report cards rely on performance measures drawn from a set of "best practices." In the past, these "best practices" might have been based on expert opinion. But today, health plans, employers, and politicians expect physicians to practice in accordance with "evidence-based medicine," which they regard as a body of generally accepted scientific principles. If doctors followed "evidence-based guidelines" with the help of information technology, these parties maintain, practice variations and inappropriate care would vanish, and quality and efficiency would go through the roof.

Arnold Milstein, MD, medical director of the Pacific Business Group on Health, believes that someday, all physicians will follow step-by-step, computerized guidelines. In the regimented system he envisions, physicians would provide better, less expensive care by making fewer medical decisions.

"Think about a world in which treatment selection and application is prompted by structured, computerized workflow, where over time the doctor begins to play less and less of a role in these decisions," Milstein says. "You begin to have something more analogous to Big Blue playing chess. In the 1950s, when you said to a chess master, 'The computer's going to take over and outplay the chess masters,' he'd say, 'Get real, no way that's going to happen.' But by 1985, not even Bobby Fischer could beat Big Blue. That's my prediction as to what's going to happen in medicine."

Some large physician groups are already moving in this direction. At the Park Nicollet Clinic in Minneapolis, for example, the doctors depend on their electronic health record to help them adhere to guidelines created by the Institute for Clinical Systems Improvement, a consortium of the state's major groups and health plans. In an affiliated hospital, the physicians all order the same tests and drugs for each medical condition. "If a patient is admitted with acute myocardial infarction [AMI, heart attack], we create a standardized order set based on what patients with AMI should be receiving," David Abelson, MD, the group's vice president of strategic improvement, says. "So the patient automatically gets the best care."

To accelerate quality improvement and reduce waste, Abelson and other Park Nicollet executives have even attended Toyota "lean production" workshops. But Abelson admits that this industrial approach can be applied in health care only to a limited extent. "The Toyota lean production system doesn't help decision-making in the face of uncertainty," he says. "It doesn't help in understanding individual preferences."

Neither does evidence-based medicine. While it can be a powerful agent for change, it's no more of a silver bullet than electronic health records are. To harness evidence-based medicine properly as part of health care reform, we need to understand what it can and cannot do.

Three-Part Definition   According to the Centre for Evidence-Based Medicine at the University of Toronto, evidence-based medicine is "the conscientious, explicit and judicious use of current best evidence in making decisions about the care of individual patients. The practice of evidence-based medicine requires the integration of individual clinical expertise with the best available external clinical evidence from systematic research and our patient's unique values and circumstances."[1]

This approach represents a departure from the traditional concept of the physician as an omniscient expert who can be relied on to provide the best care. But it's also far from the interpretation of payers who view evidence-based medicine as the robotic application of rigid guidelines. Not only does it require physicians to pay more attention to patient preferences but it also retains a role for "clinical expertise"—the fruits of experience in treating many different patients with various diseases and co-morbidities.

We certainly should expect physicians to practice in conformity with the latest scientific knowledge. But even if they could always do so—and that's a big "if," considering the difficulty of keeping up with the ever-changing medical literature—adherence to the best evidence faces two problems: First, it's often difficult to apply these findings to particular patients; and second, the studies on a particular topic may be inconclusive or nonexistent. Evidence-based medicine cannot reach its full potential until there's more evidence that's relevant to clinical practice.

Large Areas of Ignorance   Solid, high-grade evidence justifies less than half and perhaps as little as 15 percent of what physicians do.[2] How can this be? The best evidence is the randomized controlled trial, but these trials are lacking in many clinical areas, either because nobody wants to underwrite the costs or because there are ethical problems in conducting trials that may withhold beneficial treatments from some patients.[3]

In the absence of randomized controlled trials, doctors have to rely on studies of lesser validity or on the opinions of experts in the field. Although current practice guidelines depend less on expert opinion than did those of twenty years ago, they're frequently based on chains of evidence of varying grades.

"It is difficult to produce clinical practice guidelines that are completely evidence-based," Earl Steinberg, MD, and Bryan Luce, MD, state in a 2005 *Health Affairs* article. "In fact, opinion often fills in gaps in the evidence base related to a chain of reasoning that underlies a clinical guideline."[4]

A comprehensive study of practice guidelines, most of which were developed by medical societies, shows that just 36 percent conformed to standards on evidence evaluation. Seventeen percent specified the methods used to identify the scientific evidence behind them, and only 7.5 percent of them reported or used formal methods to combine scientific data.[5]

The aggregation of data from multiple studies, also known as a meta-analysis, is a key ingredient in the "systematic research" that evidence-based-medicine advocates prefer: Researchers analyze many studies to see whether, taken together, they provide convincing proof that a particular test, treatment, or procedure works or is more effective or safer than the alternatives.

This evidence is often missing, especially in the pharmaceutical arena, where there are few comparative clinical trials (see Chapter 11). "Drug companies design their trials to make their drugs look good and give them some kind of market differentiation," notes Bruce Bagley, MD, medical director of quality improvement for the American Academy of Family Physicians. "If you have five different ACE inhibitors, doctors assume they work similarly, whereas the drug companies are trying to make them think that theirs works differently or better."

Clinical Trials Don't Fit All Patients   Even if a systematic review or a large, well-conducted randomized controlled trial shows that a certain medical technique or drug is superior to other ways of treating a particular condition, it often takes many years before most doctors apply that finding in their practices.[6] Among the reasons for this delay are inadequate dissemination of the data, poor educational methods, and a resistance to change among doctors who prize their clinical autonomy. But the slow diffusion of evidence-based medicine also reflects the difficulty of applying a particular piece of evidence to the care of an individual patient in many cases. If a randomized controlled trial shows, for example, that a certain medication reduces hypertension in people under sixty-five, a physician cannot necessarily assume it will work as well in a seventy-year-old. If the trial proves that a treatment for diabetes works well in patients who have no other major ailments, that does not tell a physician what to do about the woman in his office who has diabetes, heart disease, and arthritis and is taking medications for all three conditions.[7]

A recent study of nine clinical guidelines for common conditions found that only four (for diabetes, osteoarthritis, atrial fibrillation, and angina) considered the issues of older people with multiple co-morbidities. In addition, the researchers found that guidelines "rarely address treatment of patients with 3 or more chronic diseases—a group that includes half of the population older than 65 years." If such patients were treated in accordance with the guidelines for their diseases, the authors note, they'd be at high risk for medical errors, adverse drug interactions, and hospitalization.[8]

Long Lag Time   Some health care reformers brush such objections aside. For example, in Newt Gingrich's book *Saving Lives and Saving Money*, the former congressman decries the long lag time between the discovery and the widespread application of new technologies. Gingrich advocates a system "that rapidly diffuses new innovations and discoveries to the people who can use them."[9]

The Institute of Medicine has also said that this lag time is "unnecessarily long," and it clearly is when a new approach is highly beneficial. For example, three years after studies showed that heart-attack victims and those at high cardiac risk could benefit from taking a small dose of aspirin every day, this simple remedy was still not being prescribed for more than a quarter of heart-attack survivors. Similarly, by 1991 it was well-known that the H. pylori bacteria cause some kinds of stomach ulcer. Yet, five years later, only 10 percent of internists and family physicians were testing patients for H. pylori, partly because the tests were invasive and there was disagreement about the proper drug therapy.[10]

When there's money to be made on a particular technology, however, it tends to diffuse very rapidly. This rapid diffusion can occur where specialists stand to profit from the introduction of a new technique, such as the placement of stents in cardiac arteries, or where a pharmaceutical company is heavily promoting a new drug. But some innovations are no more beneficial than older, less expensive alternatives;[11] and sometimes, as with Vioxx and Rezulin, they may prove harmful to some patients. So rushing innovation into practice isn't always wise.

Searching for the Evidence   With 150,000 new studies being published each month,[12] practicing physicians can keep up with only a tiny fraction of the worldwide literature. And it's hard for them to evaluate the strength of the evidence in most studies. Some doctors use a rule of thumb—the corporate affiliations of the researchers—to assess whether a paper is even worth reading. But, aside from that, it's often difficult to put together the findings of one article with those in other studies and then decide how—or whether—to apply the results to patients.

When they don't know the answer to a clinical question, physicians can search the medical literature but seldom do. Until recently, searching the literature was too time-consuming for the average physician, especially during patient encounters. But today, specialized, Web-based services list the best evidence-based-medicine studies on various topics and distill their results. With a handheld computer and a little knowledge about how to search for the most relevant information, physicians can educate themselves while providing better care.[13] Unfortunately, relatively few doctors use this technology, partly because subscription costs are high.

Clinical Guidelines and Measures

In recent years, specialty societies, governmental agencies, hospitals, and health plans have issued a plethora of clinical guidelines. According to one estimate, more than a thousand new guidelines are created each year. Many of these are "overlapping, conflicting, and poorly constructed."[14] In Minnesota, physician groups and HMOs have agreed to use the same set of guidelines, which have been developed under the auspices of the Institute for Clinical Systems Improvement (ICSI). Similarly, groups in California and Wisconsin have adopted standardized performance measures based on guidelines, and there are ongoing efforts to build national measures. Other than that, there's little uniformity.

Where good evidence exists, why doesn't everyone use the same guidelines? One reason is that physicians have a hard time accepting protocols that come from outside their immediate circle of peers. In Minnesota, ICSI has solved this problem by having physicians from most groups participate in guideline committees. As a result, groups that include three-quarters of the doctors in Minnesota have adopted the guidelines, according to Gordon Mosser, MD, executive director of ICSI.

Ironically, he notes, the ICSI protocols all come from national specialty societies. The work of the committees consists largely of looking up studies that justify certain parts of the guidelines that committee members have doubts about. In the end, the physicians accept just about everything in the guidelines.

"All of this leads you to wonder why we do this over again," Mosser says. "The point isn't to do the scholarship even better than the American College of Cardiology did it. That would be arrogant, and it's unlikely we'd improve it. The point of doing the guidelines is to get the material in them to be familiar and accepted throughout Minnesota. So the purpose is organizational, not scholarly."

Complexity of Decision Making   Mosser admits that many guidelines have gaps in evidence. Nevertheless, he maintains that ICSI's guidelines are "supported by a lot of high-grade evidence. This isn't as odd or implausible as it might sound, because we stay away from topics on which there isn't much evidence."

ICSI has put out fifty-six guidelines over the past twelve years. While it is still creating one or two new guidelines a year, and updating around thirty, the existing guidelines already "touch on" about two-thirds of visits to physicians, Mosser says. "If a patient has diabetes and also has lupus, say, we'd be touching on the visit, because we have a diabetes guideline, but we don't have one on lupus."

ICSI guidelines cover every condition that accounts for more than 1 percent of patient visits, he notes. If that's true, and if there's solid evidence behind all the guidelines, how does it square with the fact that there's good evidence for only between 15 and 50 percent of what doctors do?

"We've got guidelines that will touch upon about two-thirds of visits, but there will be any number of decisions made in those visits that aren't covered by a guideline," Mosser explains. "Say the patient's there for diabetes, but they report this odd pain in the right side of their chest. We don't have a guideline for 'odd pains in the right side of the chest.' So the doctors and the nurses will be making any number of decisions that aren't based on evidence."

Another area where there's little evidence is the frequency of follow-up visits, notes Bruce Bagley of the American Academy of Family Physicians. Nobody knows how often patients with a particular condition should be called back in for follow-up care. Efforts to prescribe a particular frequency to doctors tend to run into resistance, as Howard Beckman of the Rochester (New York) Independent Practice Association discovered when his organization told doctors they'd be measured on whether they brought in diabetics four times a year.

"The doctors didn't like it. They said the patients thought they were trying to rip them off, and that there was no good evidence for this. And it turned out that the endocrinologists, when they made the community-wide guideline, wanted that frequency of follow-up; but the evidence was poor, so we took it out."

Even in large groups where physicians have agreed to follow certain guidelines, there's a limit to how closely the protocols can approximate their decision-making process. "Typically, a clinician will change about 5–15 percent of a protocol for a particular patient," writes Brent James, MD, vice president for medical research and executive director of the Institute for Health Care Delivery Research, a unit of Intermountain Health Care in Salt Lake City.

Nevertheless, he says, a guideline is useful if it covers more than 85 percent of the process. "That means that the most important tool in clinical care delivery—the trained human mind—can focus its attention on that small portion of a total care process that needs modification. Such an approach not only helps clinicians manage complexity, it also greatly increases clinical efficiency."[15]

Why Aren't Guidelines Followed?   Many experts have tried to figure out how to get doctors to follow guidelines, and their main conclusion is that a combination of techniques works best.[16] But, in the absence of a concerted campaign to persuade them, most doctors tend to ignore efforts to change how they practice.[17] This is especially true when the guidelines come from health plans, which the physicians regard as mainly interested in saving money.

"We've been putting out guidelines for thirty years and it's had very little effect," Bagley notes. "It does not work unless it can be condensed into a few measures that can be integrated into practice at the point of care."

When such measures are imbedded in electronic health records, as discussed earlier, they can be very effective. But, regardless of the technology employed, physicians won't necessarily follow guidelines if they don't believe in them.

For example, an expert panel called the Joint National Committee on Protection, Detection, Evaluation and Treatment of High Blood Pressure has been exhorting physicians for a decade to use inexpensive diuretics and beta blockers as first-line drugs in treating hypertension. A very large National Institutes of Health trial known as ALLHAT confirmed the Joint National Committee's position in 2002.[18] But many doctors continue to prescribe what they've been prescribing all along. While much of this is undoubtedly due to the influence of pharmaceutical salespeople, some physicians aren't convinced that a diuretic alone can control hypertension.

Doctors Go by Experience   Other guidelines also raise some doctors' eyebrows. Patricia Roy, a family physician in Muskegon, Michigan, says that it's "irrelevant" to require HbA1c tests for diabetic patients four times a year. Depending on the severity of their illness, "some diabetics need it once a month, some once a year," she notes.

Allen Wenner, who practices family medicine in Columbia, South Carolina, observes that "some guidelines recommend care that many patients can't afford. Others might tell you that you should be doing something that isn't part of your practice, like flexible sigmoidoscopy [for colorectal cancer screening]. Or they might say that you should refer patients with certain indications to specialists, even though you feel perfectly capable of caring for them."

In some instances, malpractice liability fears deter physicians from following guidelines. Charles Davant III, a family doctor in Blowing Rock, North Carolina, says, "A lot of us are practicing 'attorney-based medicine.' Sprained ankles are an example. There's a very well-documented algorithm called the Ottawa Ankle Rule that lets you examine an ankle, score it up, and say with a high degree of certainty that it's only sprained and you don't need an X-ray.

"Sometimes medical students ask me, 'Why are you X-raying this ankle? You know it's just a sprain.' I say, 'Davant's radiographic dictum is, "It's the patient's ankle, but it's my ass."' I would rather X-ray 100 sprained ankles than go through the hassle of defending a single missed fracture in a malpractice suit."[19]

Some physicians continue to insist on the superiority of their own experience and intuition. James Goodwin, a geriatrician, maintains, "Traditional science cannot predict complex systems. People are complex systems. Everything that makes an individual an individual, everything that importantly defines an individual's life, is outside the realm of science. The practice of medicine involves only individuals."[20]

This skepticism is understandable, considering what has already been said about the limits of evidence. Yet there is a well-accepted body of evidence supporting certain tests and treatments. The RAND study showing that patients receive only about half of recommended care looked at how treatment compared with guidelines for which the evidence is strong. Examples include prescribing long-acting drugs for asthma, lowering high cholesterol in patients with coronary artery disease, and giving flu shots to people who are sixty-five or older.[21] When doctors do these things, we know that patients have better outcomes.

National Performance Measures   Pay-for-performance programs, as discussed earlier, try to get doctors to follow guidelines by providing them with incentives to do well on particular measures, but the measures are all over the lot. In an effort to standardize them, the National Quality Forum, an organization of 270 private and public health care entities, released an initial set of fifty-one national performance measures in 2005.[22] These included primary-care-oriented metrics for treating conditions such as asthma, chronic obstructive pulmonary disease, depression, diabetes, heart disease, heart failure, hypertension, osteoporosis, and prenatal care.

But the measures endorsed by the National Quality Forum were not immediately accepted. The Ambulatory Care Quality Alliance, which includes the health insurance industry association, some medical societies, and the Agency for Healthcare Quality and Research, issued its own "starter set" of metrics.[23] And in October 2005, the Centers for Medicare and Medicaid Services (CMS) released thirty-six measures that included only a handful of the National Quality Forum criteria. The American Medical Association (AMA) criticized the measures for being too burdensome and too hospital-oriented.[24] Subsequently, CMS rescinded twenty of the measures but made it clear that it wanted metrics that would cover specialty areas as well as primary care.[25]

Meanwhile, as mentioned earlier, the AMA struck a deal with Congress to develop 140 quality measures covering thirty-four clinical areas by the end of 2006.[26] At the time, several specialty societies questioned whether the AMA's timeline was realistic, partly because relatively few of the existing measures had been field-tested.[27] Janet Corrigan, president of the National Quality Forum, said she expected the medical community to make substantial progress toward validating these and other quality metrics in the near future. But she predicted that it would take around five years to assemble a comprehensive set of physician measures.[28]

Field-tested or not, the AMA's consortium of specialty societies created 174 measures by April 2007. That month, CMS unveiled 74 measures for a new voluntary reporting program that would give physicians a 1.5 percent bonus if they reported some quality data. Most of CMS's measures came from the AMA set.[29]

Technology Generates Optimism   When national performance measures are available, and when more doctors have electronic health records, there's going to be a quantum leap forward in health care quality, some observers predict. Eventually, David Nash of Jefferson Medical College, notes, interconnected EHRs will provide a way to compare the outcomes of patients treated by different physicians.

Nevertheless, Nash does not believe that national guidelines should be rigidly applied. "It all has to be modified locally, because all medical practice is local," he says. "Jefferson College has three MRIs, and that's the number they have in all of Canada. What we do versus what a rural town can do are two very different things. So it all has to be modified."

If guidelines have to be tweaked locally, what good would it do to have electronic health records include reminders and alerts based on national guidelines? "These decision support tools are for very basic things like heart failure, asthma, hypertension, hyperlipidemia," Nash replies. "We're not talking about two-nodes-positive breast cancer; we're talking about bread and butter. For the bread-and-butter primary-care stuff on which we do a relatively poor job, sure, we could do it a lot better, even with cookie-cutter guidelines."

Limited Solutions   Evidence-based guidelines, disease management, pay for performance, and electronic health records can all play roles in quality improvement. But the fragmentation of U.S. health care and its perverse financial incentives will limit the impact of these innovations. Moreover, even a dramatic rise in quality won't save our system from economic disaster. While higher-quality care will eventually cut spending by reducing medical complications and waste, it's going to cost more in the short run.

There is evidence that better hospital treatment of patients with pneumonia and blocked coronary arteries can cut costs immediately,[30] and the same undoubtedly is true for other acute conditions. The common-sense improvements in hospital care that IHI president Donald Berwick champions have not only saved lives but also prevented complications that are expensive to treat. With chronic diseases generating 75 percent of health costs, however, the most Herculean efforts to improve inpatient care can have only a limited impact on spending growth.

The better-quality solution also ignores two other factors in the cost explosion: rapid advances in medical technology and the financial motivation to do more and to sell more. Until we address those issues, we will continue to see spending expand at a rate that will exclude more and more of us from high-quality health care. The next part explains how the profitability of health care has helped fuel this conflagration of spending.

Part III
The Money Machine

8   Supply-Induced Demand

Three years after having cardiac bypass surgery, Richard Knauer, a fifty-three-year-old computer services executive from Glen Rock, New Jersey, went to see his cardiologist because his blood pressure seemed unusually high. The cardiologist did the usual tests and told him his heart was fine. He then sent Knauer for an ultrasound test of his renal artery, which turned up what looked like a cyst attached to his abdominal wall. CT scans confirmed that it was, in fact, a cyst, and also revealed gallstones in his gall bladder.

Upon hearing about the cyst, the cardiologist referred his patient to a surgeon who specialized in minimally invasive abdominal surgery and who frequently operated on cancer patients. There was no indication that the cyst was cancerous; in fact, it seemed to be filled with liquid, a characteristic of benign cysts. Yet, Knauer recalled later, the surgeon did not lay out the options. "He looked at the CT scans and said, 'We'll make incisions here, here and here, and we'll pull out the cyst and also the gall bladder at the same time.' "

The surgeon then performed an endoscopic ultrasound—an invasive procedure—to get a better picture of the terrain before he operated. Assuming that he had no alternative, Knauer made an appointment for the surgery.

Why would a well-educated person like Knauer simply follow a doctor's orders without finding out whether he really needed this procedure? Knauer says he depended on his cardiologist, who had saved his life three years earlier. Since the cardiologist had told him he needed to see the surgeon, he felt that what the surgeon said must be correct. But after discussing it with his family and friends, Knauer decided to get a second opinion, and the cardiologist referred him to a gastroenterologist who was in his own medical group. That physician looked at the CT scans, said he didn't think the cyst looked cancerous, and referred him to another gastroenterologist in New York who specialized in this kind of case.

After the second specialist did an endoscopic ultrasound, he said that Knauer had a benign mesentery cyst. He recommended getting an MRI test in six to twelve months to reevaluate the cyst. As for the gallstones, he said they might not bother Knauer and that it made no sense to remove the gall bladder unless the cyst needed to come out.

Meanwhile, on the advice of his brother-in-law, Knauer had gone to see his general internist, who'd urged him to return after visiting the New York gastroenterologist. Knauer did come back to see him, and the primary-care physician said the New York specialist's advice was reasonable.

So what did Knauer learn? "One lesson I draw from this is that when a cardiologist wants to send me to a surgeon for something other than heart-related stuff, I'm going to go to the internist right away."

More Care Doesn't Mean Better Care   Lots of people go to specialists without consulting a primary-care physician. Perhaps they're afraid that the primary-care physician might miss something important, or they just assume that if anything is really wrong, their family physician or internist will just refer them to a specialist, anyway. But what these people don't realize is that their chances of receiving a test or procedure they don't need is greater if they consult the specialist first. Even if the specialist does the right thing, the quality of care they receive won't necessarily be better.

Proof of these statements comes from several recent studies about the large, striking variations in care across the United States. One study found that Medicare beneficiaries get lower-quality care in states where more is spent on each senior than in states where less is spent. The higher the percentage of specialists among all physicians in a state, the lower the quality of care is, and the more it costs. Conversely, the researchers write, "States where more physicians are general practitioners show greater use of high-quality care and lower cost per beneficiary." They estimate that this factor accounts for nearly half of the variation in Medicare spending from one state to another.[1]

Differences in Mortality   In another study, Barbara Starfield and her colleagues at Johns Hopkins University showed that a higher ratio of primary-care physicians to the population is associated with a lower mortality rate from all causes and from heart disease and cancer; in contrast, having more specialists in a particular locality does not decrease the overall mortality rate or deaths from cancer and heart disease.[2]

The ratio of generalists to the population, not the specialist ratio, affects death rates, the Hopkins team observed. One reason, they suggest, is that primary-care physicians tend to catch illnesses such as cancer at an earlier stage, when they're more treatable. Also, they note that when specialists provide care for conditions outside of their specialties, patients have higher mortality rates for such conditions as pneumonia, acute myocardial infarction, and congestive heart failure.

Edward Salsberg, director of the Center for Workforce Studies at the American Association of Medical Colleges, criticizes the Starfield paper for what he regards as its unfair treatment of specialists. "Increasing specialization has gone hand in hand with the advancement of medicine and science," he notes.[3] Lumping all specialists together on the basis of mortality alone, he says, does not represent the value of these physicians in improving the quality of life for many patients. Moreover, he states, "Numerous studies have documented that for specific conditions, care by a specialist leads to better outcomes."

Huge Cost Difference   Everything Salsberg says is true. But landmark studies by Elliott Fisher, MD, and David Wennberg, MD, of Dartmouth Medical School and other researchers show that nearly a third of Medicare spending pays for services that don't improve health, and that much of these are for specialty care. Independent of local prices, patient health status, and other variables, the researchers found, Medicare costs in the most expensive areas of the United States were about 60 percent higher than those in the least expensive areas.[4] Patients hospitalized in the low-cost areas for hip fracture, colorectal cancer, and acute myocardial infarction had outcomes that were just as good as those of similarly ill patients in the high-cost regions.[5]

While the overall rate of major surgery was "relatively constant" across the country, there were large differences in other services. In the highest-cost areas, for example, patients had more tests and more minor procedures.

"Regional differences in Medicare spending are due almost entirely to use of discretionary services that are sensitive to the local supply of physicians and hospital resources: more frequent physician visits, greater use of specialists, and greater use of the hospital and intensive care units as sites of care," concluded the researchers. "Policymakers and purchasers concerned with resurgent growth in health care spending will need to focus on these 'supply-sensitive services.' "[6]

Little Data on Causes of Variation   Managed-care plans have long tried to deny coverage of what they regard as unnecessary tests and procedures. But their data have been poor and their methods of control, ham-handed. Moreover, many of the variations in care occur in areas where little research has been done.

Take the proper frequency of follow-up visits, the number of specialists who should see a hospitalized patient with a certain condition, and when a patient should be transferred to the intensive care unit. "On most of those things, there's no evidence whatsoever," says Earl Steinberg, a clinical guideline expert and the president of Resolution Health Inc. "The bottom line on what type of doctor a patient should see in a particular circumstance and how often—that stuff is made up. By and large, it's influenced by turf battles and pocketbook issues," he adds, referring to the battles among different specialties for power and money.

What type of doctor a patient sees is also affected by regional practice patterns. For example, Medicare spends nearly two and a half times as much on the average beneficiary in Miami, Florida, as it does in Minnesota. This difference can't be explained on the basis of how sick the Medicare populations are in the two states, and other explanations have also fallen short of the mark.[7]

Mark Sprangers, a family physician who used to practice in Minnesota and now works for a managed-care company in Florida, says there's a vast difference between doctors' practice patterns in these states. In Minnesota, he notes, primary-care physicians have a close relationship with their patients. But in Florida, "the patient and the primary-care doctor have no real connection." When he reviews medical records, he says, he often notices that a doctor has seen a patient only a couple of times, and before that, he or she had a different physician. "I don't know whether they change because of insurance or convenience or some other reason—but there's no real continuity of care."

In Minnesota, he observes, doctors normally followed their own patients in the hospital. Now that they have begun referring patients to inpatient physicians known as hospitalists (see Chapter 20), the communication is usually good, because the hospitalists are members of their own group practices. But in Florida, he says, there seems to be little or no communication between outpatient physicians and inpatient physicians, who are often part of hospitalist groups that contract with hospitals.

What often happens, he says, is that a patient goes to the emergency room, and the ER doctor has the hospitalist admit him without informing the patient's primary-care physician. "The hospitalist orders up a bunch of consultations and then kind of drops the patient," Sprangers says. "The specialists march through, and each one takes a piece of the patient and puts in the charges, and in the next day or so, someone may or may not look to see what the specialists have said. Eventually, people run out of tests to do, and the patient gets discharged."

Variations within Local Areas   Practice patterns vary not only from state to state but also from one local area to another. In 1998, for example, a senior living in Fort Myers, Florida, was nearly four times more likely to have back surgery than a Medicare patient living in nearby Miami. An operation to reduce the size of swollen prostate glands was performed in Columbus, Georgia, at three times the rate it was done in Augusta, Georgia.[8]

These examples come from the *Dartmouth Atlas of Health Care*. A compilation of practice variations across the nation, the *Atlas* grew out of a thirty-year body of research spearheaded by John Wennberg, MD, of Dartmouth Medical School. Wennberg and his colleagues have established that most practice variations are unrelated to medical necessity or the health status of different populations.

In a 1989 study, for example, Wennberg's team discovered that "for reasons that had nothing to do with illness rates, the number of staffed beds per capita in Boston is about 60 percent greater than in New Haven, Connecticut. And Bostonians' rates of hospitalization for high-variation medical conditions are also 60 percent higher."[9] Nevertheless, the study found that Medicare enrollees hospitalized in both cities had about the same mortality rates.

"Bostonians aren't sicker than people in New Haven," Wennberg told *Medical Economics*. "In fact, the pattern of initial hospitalization for certain conditions is similar. For instance, our group published one paper comparing patients with hip fractures in Boston and New Haven.

The hospitalization rates were the same in both places. But over a three-year period, the Boston patients had a 60 percent higher readmission rate."[10]

When a patient needs surgery for an emergent condition such as a hip fracture, a physician will normally admit him to a hospital. But when a physician has to decide whether to admit a patient who has a medical condition such as heart failure or pneumonia, Wennberg says, the supply of beds in local hospitals seems to influence his decision. He attributes this to the complexity of medical decision-making: If a physician is uncertain about what to do, it's easy to use an available hospital bed.

According to Wennberg, there's also a correlation between the availability of diagnostic procedures and the amount of surgery done. "For example, there's a strong linear relationship between the capacity to diagnose coronary artery disease through angiography and combined rates of angiography and coronary artery bypass surgery," he says. "The numbers of surgeons and operating rooms also matter. But the variations in utilization associated with bed supply are mostly related to medical, not surgical, hospitalizations."

Inappropriate Care   While Wennberg was analyzing variations in care, other researchers, notably Robert Brook and his colleagues at RAND, were trying to measure the extent of inappropriate care.

A 1989 RAND review of the literature found that "as much as one-fifth to one quarter of acute care services were felt to be used for equivocal or inappropriate reasons."[11] While there were wide differences among experts in what they deemed appropriate, the studies of hospital admissions, procedures, and medications examined by the RAND team showed at least double-digit rates of inappropriate care in nearly every category.

In another study, Brook and his team found that the use of three procedures—coronary angiography, carotid endarterectomy, and endoscopy of the upper gastrointestinal tract—was inappropriate in 17 percent, 32 percent, and 17 percent of the cases, respectively. They defined an operation as appropriate if its expected health benefits exceeded its expected negative consequences "by a sufficiently wide margin that the procedure is worth doing."[12]

As shocking as these findings were—and continue to be—the researchers picked up something else that was even more surprising: While there were more instances of inappropriate procedures in areas where overall utilization of services was higher, they said, "in no case can differences in appropriateness explain the large differences in overall [use] rates."

Supply-Induced Demand   Since then, Wennberg and his followers have demonstrated that "supply-induced demand"—the tendency of physicians to create demand for their own services—is implicated in both inappropriate services and overutilization.

In one study, researchers followed for seven years about 159,000 Medicare patients who'd been hospitalized for acute myocardial infarction. They found that younger and healthier patients were more likely to receive invasive treatment and medical therapy, even though those strategies "primarily benefit elderly or high-risk patients and may not be warranted in lower-risk patients."[13] Where cardiac catheterization labs were more numerous, patients were more likely to receive that procedure, regardless of age or health status. In those areas, patients were also less likely to receive beta-blocker medications, which have been shown to reduce the chance of a second heart attack.

Another study looked at rates of back surgery and knee and hip replacement among eight contiguous areas in south Florida. It found marked differences in practice patterns, and patient preference was deemed to have little impact on the relative rates of surgery. "It seems improbable, for example, that Medicare retirees living in Fort Myers prefer back surgery 2.4 times more often than residents of Miami," the researchers note.[14] What did matter were the practice patterns of surgeons working in each area, and their recommendations to patients. The study found that these "surgical signatures" varied just as much from area to area in 2000 as they had in 1992, despite a big jump in the volume of those procedures, both in Florida and across the nation.

Logic might suggest that the way to reduce these unwarranted variations would be to do clinical trials comparing the outcomes of different interventions for particular types of patients and disseminate the results to surgeons. But an act of Congress ten years ago blocked that avenue of inquiry.

A Political Football

When Wennberg began publishing his variations studies in the 1970s, they had little impact at first. But as Congress groped for ways to limit the explosion of Medicare costs in the 1980s, the legislators began listening to the arguments of Wennberg and his colleagues in favor of finding out what works best in medicine. The upshot was that in 1989, Congress created the Agency for Health Care Policy and Research (AHCPR). Among other things, AHCPR was charged with conducting comparative outcomes studies and formulating clinical guidelines to reduce the variations in care.[15]

The AHCPR's investigations into conditions such as angina, peripheral vascular disease, arthritis, and low-back pain were based only partly on epidemiological analyses—the kind of studies that Wennberg had done. They also involved literature searches, focus groups of physicians and patients, the development of standardized measures of patients' preferences and outcomes, and the organization of practice-based clinical trial networks to test the outcomes of new medical techniques (see Chapter 22). The use of these networks was less costly than randomized controlled trials, and the practice-based studies looked at groups of patients more representative of those encountered in real practices.[16]

Nevertheless, some critics regarded these outcomes studies as simple database analyses rather than valid clinical research. They also questioned whether outcomes studies could have any impact on clinical practice. "The particular reasons that lead doctors to choose a particular treatment make most nonrandomized outcomes analysis untrustworthy," Richard Peto, an Oxford University epidemiologist, maintained.[17]

Meanwhile, 1995 reports by the U.S. General Accounting Office and the Physician Payment Review Commission questioned the effectiveness of the AHCPR's clinical guideline program. And an Office of Technology Assessment report concluded that the agency's research comparing the effectiveness of different treatments probably would not save money.[18]

Counterattack from Surgeons   What almost killed the ACHPR in 1995, however, was the finding of one of its patient outcomes research teams (PORTs) that spinal-fusion surgery was unproven and potentially harmful. A group of politically-connected back surgeons added fuel to Republican complaints that the ACHPR was wasting taxpayers' money. The fact that the agency had been involved in the development of the Clinton administration's ill-fated health plan also did not endear it to the new Republican majority.[19]

While the agency was saved at the last minute, it soon ended its comparative outcomes research. Under its current moniker, the Agency for Healthcare Research and Quality (AHRQ), it now funds systematic literature reviews. In addition, it houses the National Guidelines Clearinghouse and supports the U.S Preventive Services Task Force. In recent years, it has also delved into medical error prevention and health information technology. And it has begun publishing consumer-oriented comparisons among different treatments, based on the available studies.[20]

That's a lot for an agency with a relatively small budget ($318 million in 2005).[21] But the PORTs created AHRQ's most notable achievements when it was still the AHCPR. For example, the PORTs helped establish anticoagulation drug therapy as the treatment of choice for stroke prevention for patients with atrial fibrillation. They also helped clarify the risks and benefits of prostate surgery for cancer and for noncancerous enlargement of the prostate. Over 60 percent of urologists now use a PORT-developed prostate symptom score.

The low-back-pain guidelines that angered the spine surgeons are now used as a teaching tool in medical schools. After Washington State's disability program asked the PORT to develop a guideline for elective lumbar-fusion operations, spinal-fusion rates fell by 33 percent without any changes in outcomes.[22]

Shared Decision-Making   By the time outcomes research began running into trouble, Wennberg had decided that the best way to mitigate supplier-induced demand was to have physicians provide patients with more information about their treatment options. To start the ball rolling, he and some like-minded colleagues created the Foundation for Informed Medical Decision Making in the early 1990s.

The not-for-profit foundation produced and disseminated a series of videos that explained the risks and benefits of treatment alternatives and included interviews with patients who'd made various choices. Among the early topics were benign prostate disease, early-stage prostate cancer, early-stage breast cancer, low back pain, high blood pressure, stable angina, hysterectomy, and hormone replacement therapy. The idea was to have patients view these programs before conferring with their physicians.

The scenarios in the videos were based on patients' actual concerns. "With prostate surgery, for example, we look at objective measures like incontinence and impotence, and subjective measures like worries about sexuality," Wennberg told *Medical Economics* in 1993. "Those factors are rarely discussed when patients consider prostate surgery. But we feel that doctors should discuss them with patients before deciding on surgery."[23]

This "shared decision making" had a dramatic impact on patient choices. At Kaiser Permanente in Denver, the rate of prostate surgery dropped 44 percent in the first year after offices started showing the video; the surgery rate fell 60 percent at the Group Health Cooperative HMO in Washington State.[24]

Wennberg was cautiously optimistic that this approach could reduce overall health costs. "Informing patients about the risks and benefits of surgery vs. watchful waiting will probably lead to a decline in surgery, because most patients are naturally risk-averse," he said.

His approach to shared decision-making, however, did not catch on widely, partly because in the early 1990s, the laserdisc equipment and software were too expensive for the average physician office. But Wennberg also admitted, "With private practitioners, there's often a real question whether they want to use a video, particularly if it may reduce the demand for their services."[25]

More Decision Aids, No More Use   Fast-forward to 2007. The Foundation for Informed Medical Decision Making, through its for-profit partner Health Dialog, has put out about twenty of what are now called "patient decision aids."[26] Other organizations around the world are also releasing patient decision aids on about five hundred different conditions. These are now delivered on DVDs, in print and audio media, and over the Internet. Thirty-four clinical trials have examined the impact of patient decision aids, and some have shown a significant impact on patient choices.[27]

Among women with breast cancer who used a decision aid in one study, for example, only 23 percent chose a mastectomy rather than a lumpectomy or some other option, compared with 40 percent who did not receive the extra information. In another study, the uninformed patients who chose a cardiac operation for angina outnumbered the informed patients by nearly two to one.

Yet despite the obvious benefit to patients, the use of patient decision aids is still not widespread. In the United States, Health Dialog sells most of its programs directly to patients whom the company has identified as being in need of outreach and "health coaching."[28] (Health Dialog does this work on behalf of its employer and health plan clients.) Physicians have not generally accepted these tools. They may be unaware of them, have difficulty obtaining them, or be unable to fit them into their workflow. It's also apparent that neither doctors nor hospitals devote much effort to nonreimbursed activities, especially when those activities might result in a diminution of income.[29]

"Until incentives are realigned and providers have an incentive to help patients make informed medical choices that are consistent with their values toward benefits and risks, things are unlikely to change much," observes John Billings, an associate professor in the Robert F. Wagner School of Public Service at New York University.[30]

Follow the Money   This is an understatement. Allen Wenner, a family physician in Columbia, South Carolina, tells a story about a surgeon who wanted to do a new kind of operation on one of Wenner's patients. The surgeon told the patient that the success rate on this operation, to unclog the carotid artery, is 94 percent. Wenner had never heard of the procedure before, so he looked it up. He could find only one study on it, involving eighteen patients. The Food and Drug Administration had approved the procedure just six months earlier, and the surgeon himself had done it on only a few patients. So Wenner had the patient ask the surgeon where he'd found his data; after the doctor confessed it came from a small study, the patient decided not to go ahead with the operation.

This is not to say that all physicians are greedy. Based on my fourteen years of reporting for *Medical Economics*, I believe that most doctors want to provide top-notch care, save lives, and relieve suffering. Yet they also want to make money, like everyone else, and new technology gives them a way to do that. In 2004, for example, spending on physicians grew 9 percent, more than drug or hospital costs. Actuaries at the Centers for Medicare and Medicaid Services attributed this cost rise largely to technological advances and increased use of services, both old and new.[31]

When new technologies are truly beneficial, they quickly become the standard of care. Moreover, as Jonathan Weiner, of Johns Hopkins University, notes, there's a public demand for specialists who can wield these powerful new tools. So supply-induced demand is not the only reason for cost growth. But, as I've explained, there is a significant correlation between the supply of physicians, equipment, and facilities and the amount of care ordered by those same clinicians, especially when doctors own the means of production. The next chapter shows how physician ownership of imaging and surgical centers and other facilities has become a major cost driver.

9   Physicians Go for the Gold

The Imaging Explosion

In recent years, medical imaging services have been growing rapidly. The total cost of CT, MRI, and PET scans, X-rays, ultrasound, and other imaging tests was roughly $100 billion in 2005, compared with about $75 billion in 2000.[1] Between 1999 and 2002, the use of CT and MRI tests by Medicare patients increased 15 to 20 percent a year, and the cost of those tests shot up 10 percent annually.[2]

Beneficial medical advances accounted for some of this cost growth. For example, MRIs are used to detect brain tumors. CT scanners using "multi-slice" technology allow better imaging of soft-tissue organs.[3] And image-guided biopsies to diagnose bone cancer produce fewer complications and faster wound healing than open surgical biopsies.[4]

The new imaging technologies, however, are often overused or misused. For example, many primary-care physicians order X-rays for chronic back pain or CT scans for stomach pain;[5] MRIs for persistent headaches are not unknown, either.[6] Much of this inappropriate use of imaging technologies is, of course, driven by doctors' constant fear of malpractice suits.[7] Recall the physician who said that he'd rather X-ray a hundred ankles unnecessarily than have to defend himself against a single suit because he missed a broken ankle.

Consumer demand is also a big factor: Americans feel they deserve to have every test under the sun and that someone else should pay for it. When noninvasive imaging studies replace invasive tests or exploratory surgery, the demand rises even further.[8] But current market dynamics explain much of the current explosion in imaging work.

Proliferation of Technology   Once upon a time, doctors would order tests, and radiologists would perform them in hospitals or imaging centers. That still happens, but radiologists performed only about half of the 543 million diagnostic imaging tests done in 2003.[9] Most of the rest were conducted by other doctors in their offices or in imaging facilities that they owned.

Why did this occur? Partly because, in certain fields, advances in imaging techniques and related procedures obligated physicians to learn how to use the new technology. Cardiology is a good example. From 1999 to 2004, the number of cardiac nuclear imaging procedures, including echocardiagrams and electrophysiology studies, jumped from 3 million to 5 million a year.[10]

Orthopedists have also found new uses for imaging tests: At one time, for example, they might have just splinted a sprained wrist. Now if a group can afford an MRI machine, they might perform the $800 test to see whether there are any torn ligaments that need repair.[11]

More and more specialty groups can afford the $1.2 million for a CT scanner or the $1.35 million for an MRI unit, and even primary-care groups can pony up the $250,000 for an ultrasound machine.[12] One reason is that single-specialty groups have grown larger—and conversely, physicians have formed bigger groups partly in order to invest in imaging equipment.

In some instances, new technology can ignite an "arms race" among specialists, just as it does among hospitals (see Chapter 10). Take the new sixty-four-slice CT scanners that some physicians say can pinpoint blockages in the coronary arteries as well as invasive cardiac catheterization does.[13] Even though Medicare hasn't yet approved routine coverage of this technique, and commercial insurers are paying for it only case by case, cardiologists expect a boom in this area as patients demand to know whether they're at risk for a heart attack.[14] So, like the hospitals that their imaging facilities compete with, many cardiology groups are buying the $1.7 million machines. If they don't, they risk losing business to other practices or hospitals.

Retreat of Managed Care   The imaging explosion has coincided with the retreat of tightly managed care and the restoration of fee-for-service.[15] When HMOs moved away from prepayment and reduced preauthorization rules for imaging tests, specialists such as cardiologists and orthopedists stood to benefit from investing in equipment and imaging facilities. These physicians also did better in single-specialty groups where they didn't have to share any of the profits with primary-care physicians.

Meanwhile, primary-care groups began to buy "ancillary" equipment that could be used for tests their doctors frequently ordered, such as X-rays, ultrasound, bone density scans, and mammography. Larger multi-specialty groups also invested in imaging centers that had CT and MRI units, sometimes contracting with radiologists to read the studies.[16]

Insurers' reimbursement cuts have made these ancillary investments essential for many groups. For some primary-care practices, especially, the profit from imaging tests spells the difference between rising and declining income.[17] Specialists also complain about the deep discounts they have to give health plans; but to judge by the recent increases in their compensation,[18] they've reaped handsome rewards from their investments in technology.

Self-Referral of Imaging Tests   Regardless of the formula for compensating physicians in a group, those who own in-office machines or imaging facilities tend to order more tests than those who do not. A 1992 study published in the *Journal of the American Medical Association*, for example, found that self-referring physicians perform between two and eight times as many imaging tests as those who refer their patients to radiologists.[19] The U.S. General Accountability Office reported similar findings in a later study.[20]

The Ethics in Patient Referrals Act (generally known as the Stark law) was supposed to restrict this kind of self-aggrandizement. The statute prohibits physicians from referring Medicare or Medicaid patients for certain services to providers with whom the referring doctor has a financial relationship. But the Stark law exempts nuclear medicine (including MRI and PET scans) from the list of covered services and allows physicians to own entities that furnish services and equipment to providers of covered services. According to a government report on medical imaging, "Physicians can lease an MRI to an [imaging] center for a fixed amount per use. Every time the physicians refer a patient to the center for an MRI, they receive a fee. This allows physicians to increase the return on their investment by referring additional patients."[21]

Unintended Consequences   While spending on newer tests such as MRI, CT, and PET scanning is increasing the fastest, more and more X-ray and ultrasound tests are also being done; together, these two kinds of studies consumed about half of the imaging dollar in 2001.[22] This trend illustrates a basic principle of new medical technology: it tends to be used in addition to older technology, rather than replacing it or reducing its use.

A 2005 report from the Medicare Payment Advisory Commission (MedPAC) suggests that the increased use of some imaging techniques, such as mammography, may improve outcomes. "However," the report states, "using imaging to detect disease may present risks, particularly when patients have minor or no symptoms. Imaging technology can identify trace amounts of disease (e.g., cancer) or abnormalities (e.g., of the back and knee) that frequently never affect the health of the patient. Detection often causes patient anxiety and leads to follow-up testing and treatment, and may have only a limited chance of improving patient outcomes. In these circumstances, the costs of imaging services may outweigh the potential benefits. . . .

"Equally disturbing is evidence of misuse of imaging services. For example, some providers have been found to produce relatively high numbers of inaccurate carotid ultrasound tests, which could lead to inappropriate surgical interventions. . . . The experience of imaging benefit managers and health plans also suggests that faulty equipment or poor imaging techniques harm the quality of images and may result in repeat studies."[23]

Does Imaging Save Money?   Naturally, associations representing physician groups have not taken criticism of their imaging business lightly. In a June 2005 article in *Group Practice Journal*, Susan J. Mertes, a lobbyist for the American Medical Group Association, attributes much of the growth in imaging tests to the aging of the population. She also notes that technology itself creates demand. "With the availability of less invasive, more comfortable, and more convenient diagnostic screening, more patients will be screened and, of course, more problems will be found."

Finally, she asserts that calculations of imaging costs under-represent the degree to which they offset other expenses: "Costly hospital-based procedures are being supplanted by non-invasive diagnosis and treatments that have likely curtailed the number of invasive, expensive procedures thought necessary and performed in a higher cost setting."[24]

There is some truth in this. For example, the abovementioned sixty-four-slice CT scans cost only about $550, compared with $1,000 for a diagnostic cardiac catheterization.[25] But if this noninvasive test becomes widely accepted, it's likely that many more tests will be done on healthy people, driving total costs higher.

According to the Blue Cross and Blue Shield Association, imaging tests are often used inappropriately to determine the stage of prostate cancer: Nearly a quarter of patients with low-risk disease and half of those with intermediate-risk disease receive MRIs and CT scans not indicated by current recommendations, while almost 20 percent of those who have high-risk disease receive therapy without being tested.[26]

Moreover, MedPAC points out, there's a three-fold variation in the use of imaging tests across the country. Yet, according to unpublished research by Elliott Fisher and his colleagues, the MedPAC report says, "increased use of imaging services was not associated with improved survival" among Medicare patients who had heart attacks, colon cancer, or hip fractures.[27]

Private-Sector Solutions   Many HMOs and PPOs have brought back preauthorization of expensive tests, which is the most common cost containment technique today. Depending on how aggressively they pursue it, plans may deny as much as 20 percent of requests for high-end imaging studies.[28] But this approach carries high administrative costs and can antagonize doctors and patients.[29]

MedPAC suggested that the Centers for Medicare and Medicaid Services (CMS) use some of the other techniques that private insurers have employed to get a handle on imaging costs. In the 2006 budget bill, Congress went along with this suggestion, cutting in half Medicare's payments for multiple scans on contiguous body parts, for example. The same legislation authorized CMS to cap payments for most kinds of imaging tests, starting in 2007.[30]

Ambulatory Surgery Centers

While imaging centers have mushroomed, there has also been a tremendous boom in freestanding ambulatory surgery centers (ASCs). Between 1997 and 2003, the number of Medicare-certified ASCs jumped 50 percent to nearly four thousand.[31] Just two years later, the American Association of Ambulatory Surgery Centers (AAASC) placed the number of facilities at between four and five thousand.[32] While hospitals, local investors, and national, publicly traded companies invest in ASCs, physicians usually have an ownership interest in them as well.[33]

More than half of high-volume ASCs specialized in a narrow range of procedures in 2002, according to MedPAC. A third of them offered ophthalmology services, particularly cataract removal, and nearly 20 percent performed only gastroenterology services. Most of the rest were general surgical facilities.[34]

Physicians profit in two ways from investing in ASCs: They get professional fees for performing procedures, and they share in the facility fees. Not surprisingly, physician-owners send plenty of business to their ASCs. "From 1998 to 2002," MedPAC notes, "the number of procedures generated by ASCs increased by 75 percent." This figure refers only to services provided to Medicare patients, which accounted for about 40 percent of ASCs' unit volume and 25–30 percent of their revenues.[35]

The number of surgical services provided to Medicare patients has increased faster in ASCs than in hospital outpatient departments. During 1998–2002, when ASC services were increasing at 15 percent a year, the same procedures rose only 1.7 percent annually in the outpatient departments. And the huge growth in ASC business occurred despite the fact that Medicare payments to ASCs for each unit of care rose less than 1 percent a year during that period.[36] While MedPAC doesn't speculate on the reason for this growth, the business activity suggests that physician-owners and investors in ASCs made good profits at Medicare rates.

Which Is More Cost Effective?   According to the AAASC, ambulatory surgery centers bring "healthy competition" to the market and save Medicare a bundle: "In most instances where a Medicare beneficiary undergoes surgery in an ASC instead of a hospital, the Medicare program saves money. In fact, ASCs save the Medicare program hundreds of millions of dollars each year, because Medicare payments to ASCs for outpatient surgical procedures are substantially lower than payments to hospitals (both on an inpatient and outpatient basis)."[37]

There is no doubt that it's cheaper to perform surgery in an ASC than in a hospital operating room. But ASCs aren't necessarily paid less than hospital outpatient departments. In 2004, MedPAC reports, CMS paid ASCs more than outpatient departments for only 13 percent of the surgical procedures it covered in ASCs, but that included four of the ten highest-volume ASC services.[38] In 2005, CMS paid the ASCs more for nine of the top twenty services.[39] Those services included a cataract procedure (35 percent difference) and biopsy of the prostate (47 percent difference). So, while some procedures cost much less in ASCs, it's hard to say how much the ambulatory facilities save Medicare. What is certain is that, because of ASCs' growth, Medicare payments to these facilities more than tripled from 1992 to 2002.[40]

In 2006, CMS proposed changes in the ASC payment system. While the list of Medicare-approved ASC procedures would be expanded, the agency also proposed to pay ASCs on the same basis as hospital out-patient departments, starting in 2008. Although the payments could not be higher than those allotted to outpatient departments, they could be lower, because they'd be based on the actual costs of doing procedures in ambulatory surgery centers.[41]

Hospitals versus ASCs   Some hospitals have threatened phy-sicians who founded ASCs with loss of staff privileges.[42] But many others have found it more prudent to partner with the doctors. In fact, says Craig Jeffries, president of the AAASC, hospitals own an interest in 44 percent of ASCs. Why have hospitals done this? According to an article in *Hospitals & Health Networks*, they're "fearful of losing profitable business to upstart ambulatory surgery centers." Since that business is bound to move away from the hospitals, they've concluded that "half of something is better than 100 percent of nothing."[43]

The article cites Genesis Health System in Davenport, Iowa, which has joint ventures with ASCs providing urology, ophthalmology, and gas-troenterology services. Genesis also collaborated with a big cardiology group to create a "heart institute" on the hospital campus.

Wherever possible, however, physicians prefer to own ASCs and other ancillary facilities outright "to maximize autonomy and revenue," according to one study. "Respondents perceived that investments in ancillary services proved largely successful for physicians and medical groups, despite the large capital outlay sometimes required. Medical group respondents claimed that [the ancillary services] usually generated profits and operated at or near capacity and in some cases were critical to medical groups' financial standing."[44]

One unintended consequence of the ASC boom is that, in combina-tion with fear of malpractice suits and other factors, it has led to special-ists' refusing to take call in emergency departments unless hospitals pay them extra for their time. In fact, some surgeons have dropped hospital privileges so they can spend more time in their ASCs.[45] These developments have made it more difficult for hospitals to provide high-quality care. Along with an insufficiency of critical-care beds and overcrowded emergency departments, specialist shortages are partly to blame for wide-scale "diversions" of patients from one hospital to another.[46]

Specialty Hospitals

Some surgical and multispecialty groups are also investing in specialty hospitals. Since 1990, more than a hundred of these hospitals have been built across the country. While the bulk of these are heart hospitals, they include a number of orthopedic and general surgical hospitals as well.[47] Traditional hospitals have protested this invasion of their turf, claiming that the specialty facilities drain off their most lucrative business without having to provide emergency services or care for the uninsured.[48] Moreover, physicians are sending their less complex cases to specialty hospitals and admitting sicker patients to the traditional institutions. Since Medicare pays the same for procedures on both groups of patients, the specialty facilities are raking off the more profitable cases.[49]

Hearing the hospital industry's cries of woe, Congress in 2003 placed an eighteen-month moratorium on the construction of new specialty facilities.[50] CMS extended this ban twice before ending the moratorium in August 2006.[51] When it did so, the agency attempted to level the playing field between general and specialty hospitals by changing how Medicare paid hospitals for procedures (see Chapter 19). CMS also established disclosure requirements for physician investors.[52]

Physicians are the driving force behind the construction of specialty hospitals. According to a CMS report, doctors own 34 percent of cardiac hospitals and 80 percent of general surgery and orthopedic hospitals. These physician-owners refer or admit the majority of Medicare patients in these hospitals.[53]

Now that physicians and other investors are being allowed to build more specialty hospitals, observers believe they will, because these hospitals are very profitable.[54] Not only can physicians benefit from referring patients to a facility in which they have an interest, but they can also perform more procedures there because of shorter turnaround times.

Because of the increased productivity at one specialty hospital, for example, physicians raised their incomes by 30 percent.[55]

Medical Arms Races   Before the CMS moratorium, the advent of specialty hospitals ignited medical arms races in some markets. In Indianapolis, for example, specialist groups have grown in size and strength since the late 1990s. In 2002, cardiovascular groups at two of the city's four private hospital systems threatened to partner with Med-Cath, a company that invests in heart hospitals, unless the health care systems agreed to join with them in the construction of specialty hospitals. The health care systems caved in, and soon each of the four hospital systems was building or operating a freestanding heart facility. Physicians were allowed to invest up to 30 percent and 50 percent in two of these specialty hospitals.[56]

Meanwhile, the Indianapolis hospital systems were busy building new wings and even new hospitals to serve well-insured patients who were moving out to the suburbs. By 2005, the hospital systems had committed more than $1 billion to current and planned projects.[57]

Throughout all of this, no one suggested that there had been a sudden outbreak of heart attacks or a spike in the overall disease burden or that the population of Indianapolis was growing. In fact, the city's population remained nearly constant from 2000 to 2004.[58] The only epidemic was the fever of construction.

"The array of expensive capital expansion projects underway in Indianapolis threatens to push the already high cost of health care even higher," researchers at the Center for Studying Health System Change note. "According to health plan respondents, hospitals already are demanding large payment rate increases to help finance expansions, and some observers feared that costs will accelerate further because of increased utilization stimulated by physician-owned facilities."[59]

Quality Conundrum   The AMA and other defenders of specialty hospitals argue that they provide better, more cost-effective care than full-line hospitals do.[60] They cite a 2005 CMS study that found that, after case-mix adjustment, selected specialty hospitals had significantly lower mortality rates and complication rates than traditional hospitals did.[61] However, about the same number of moderately ill patients were readmitted to the specialty and community hospitals, and far more se-

verely ill patients were readmitted to specialty cardiac facilities. (Orthopedic specialty hospitals had a lower readmission rate.)

While it's been established that surgeons who do a higher volume of
procedures have better outcomes,[62] it's unclear why those same doctors
should produce better results in a specialty hospital than in a traditional
hospital. CMS researchers were told that the experienced staff and the
low nurse-to-patient ratio were part of the formula for success. In addition, physicians believed that "the amenities offered to patients improved quality of care. They particularly cited the use of private rooms,
which they said helped patients rest and recover better."[63]

What this evidence indicates is that if traditional hospitals improved
their facilities and services, they could provide care as good as that of
specialty hospitals. But hospital representatives note that upgrading their
facilities is difficult to do with the drag on their bottom line of serving
indigent and poorly insured patients—which specialty hospitals don't
have to do—and of offering a full array of services.[64] So, while specialty
hospitals might challenge conventional institutions to improve their quality, they could also be draining away some of the resources the hospitals
need to do that.

The Bottom Line   Physician investment in ancillary services
is not limited to specialists. Many primary-care physicians, trying to
counteract reimbursement cuts, have added a wide range of income-
producing ancillaries. Among these are dermatological services, bone
densitometry, audiology, spirometry, botox injections, nutritional counseling, X-ray tests, and in-house labs.[65] Some primary-care groups, in
fact, receive up to a third of their income from ancillaries.

But the specialists are the ones who are making the big money from
imaging facilities, ASCs, and specialty hospitals. While the portion of
their revenues these activities generate is a matter of conjecture, there's
no doubt that the bigger groups are doing particularly well. For example,
the Medical Group Management Association notes that, in 2004, the median net income of orthopedic surgeons leveled off at around $535,000.
But the larger orthopedic groups—the ones most likely to invest in facilities—saw increases ranging from 4.83 percent (practices of thirteen or
more doctors) to 7.88 percent (practices of seven to twelve doctors).[66]

Government regulations have not been effective at dealing with the
incentives of specialists to invest in and steer patients to self-owned
facilities. Part of the answer lies in creating regional health planning

agencies—a blocked thrust of earlier reform efforts—that would decide whether their communities need new facilities (see Chapter 21). But it's equally important for physicians themselves to agree on guidelines for the use of imaging technology. For that to happen nationwide, we'd have to restructure health care delivery in a way that would change physician incentives and the relationship between primary-care physicians and specialists.

Meanwhile, expenditures on traditional hospital care are rising nearly as fast as physician costs. The next chapter will explain why hospital spending is out of hand, despite decades of efforts to contain it.

10 Hospitals Flex Their Muscles

Spending on hospitals is rising much faster than the number of patients they take care of. The number of beds and the length of stay in community hospitals dropped slightly from 1999 to 2003, and the annual number of admissions rose a modest 8.2 percent over those four years. Yet during that period, total net revenue (including that of outpatient departments) jumped 35 percent.[1] U.S. hospitals as a whole posted a net profit margin of 5.2 percent in 2004—an all-time high—and aggregate profits leaped 16.4 percent.[2]

Overall, the nation's hospital costs increased 8.2 percent to $571 billion in 2004.[3] If hospital-cost growth continues at that level, we'll spend roughly a *trillion* dollars on hospital care in 2014.[4]

While new technology, more intensive care, aging population growth, and labor shortages all contribute to hospital cost increases,[5] so does the consolidation of hospitals into ever larger and more powerful systems. The mid-1990s saw a tremendous wave of hospital mergers, which was largely a reaction to the threat of managed-care plans that were selectively contracting with hospitals that met their price.[6] As that danger receded because of employers' demands for broad networks, the number of mergers fell sharply. But, as hospitals have sought to increase their market power and generate more capital for expansion and information systems, mergers are again on the rise. In 2004, 130 hospitals were acquired or merged in transactions totaling $9 billion. This value was three times greater than the annual average in the previous four years.[7]

In the past, the Federal Trade Commission has been unable to prevent mergers that result in monopolies or near-monopolies in individual markets. The agency lost a string of seven antitrust cases challenging hospital combinations in the 1990s.[8] But the FTC won a recent suit that sought to undo a merger between Evanston Northwestern Healthcare in Evanston, Illinois, and a nearby hospital. If that decision is upheld on appeal, observers say, it could allow the Federal Trade Commission and perhaps even individual states to retroactively challenge hospital mergers if they result in higher prices.[9]

Mergers drive up costs to the extent that they reduce competition. For example, it was reported in 2000 that hospital consolidation in North Carolina had resulted in monopolies that made it impossible for health plans to negotiate prices.[10] Also, there have been allegations of price-fixing by an eleven-hospital system on Long Island, New York.[11] And in 2004, the twenty-eight-hospital Sutter Health System in northern California raised prices so high that the state retirement system, known as CalPERS, dropped thirteen Sutter hospitals from its network.[12]

Passing the Buck   Few self-insured employers or health plans are powerful enough in any particular market to take such a strong stance. And with consumers and employers demanding that plans include most hospitals in their networks, it has become increasingly difficult for insurers in some markets to walk away from hospitals that won't compromise with them. It's much easier to pass on the price increase to employers—and that's what many plans have done.

"The general thrust of recent findings is that hospitals have picked up a lot more leverage over plans in recent years," Robert Berenson of the Urban Institute says, citing research by the Center for Studying Health System Change. "And so plans are paying more than they did because they can't negotiate prices. But what they figured out, in the aftermath of the managed-care backlash, is that they can pass it on to the employers and, ultimately, the employees."

How much is this costing all of us? According to one study, while mergers did not improve quality and increased efficiency only a little, they raised prices an average of 7.7 percent for managed-care patients and 4.1 percent for patients covered by indemnity plans.[13] Every 1 percent increase in hospital market share due to consolidation leads to an approximate 2 percent increase in inpatient expenditures, according to Maureen Sullivan, vice president of the Blue Cross and Blue Shield Association.[14]

Build It and They Will Come

Meanwhile, a building boom is going on among the nation's hospitals. It started around 1999 and accelerated after hospitals recovered from earlier Medicare reimbursement cuts, forced private plans to pay them more, and shed money-losing physician practices. Many hospitals have expanded or renovated existing facilities; but much more is being spent on new hospital construction than on additions or alterations to existing facilities.[15] New hospitals and outpatient clinics under construction in late 2005 were valued at $22 billion.[16]

As of 2004, about 20 percent of the eight hundred new hospitals planned in the United States were concentrated in six southern and western states: California, Colorado, Florida, Georgia, Texas, and Virginia.[17] But a year later, Illinois led in new hospital construction, and Ohio, in renovations.[18] According to the health care consultant Michael LaPenna, there's also a "fever" of new construction in the East. "Go to New Jersey, Connecticut, other East Coast states," he says. "They're going like gangbusters. They have money, real money."

Quite often, the hospitals follow their better-insured customers as they move from the cities into affluent suburbs, notes David Scroggins, a practice management consultant in Cincinnati. In his area, he says, three hospitals are being built fairly close together in the suburbs. "Within a ten-mile radius, we're going to have a lot of doctors and facilities, because all those people are chasing the better insurance and will eventually try to minimize their facilities in the inner city." For example, he notes, the owners of one downtown hospital have closed the facility and opened another in a middle-class area. The old hospital was excluded from the local insurance networks, but the plans have picked up the new facility because of its favorable location.

While some of the new construction is replacing aging facilities, a majority of hospital executives say they've simply run out of space for patients.[19] That statement may be hard to square with community hospitals' average occupancy rate of 66 percent[20] or with the trend to replace semi-private rooms with the private rooms that many consumers are demanding.[21] But some experts make a strong argument that we're going to need the extra hospital capacity soon.

The Boomers Are Coming   Noting that the United States lost about a hundred thousand hospital beds in the 1990s, Stuart Altman, a health economist at Brandeis University, says hospitals may have to add twice that number of beds by 2012.[22] In 2003, Altman and several colleagues observed that hospital use and spending had increased substantially in 2001 and 2002, reversing a decade-long decline in the inflation-adjusted rate of spending growth. They argued that if this trend continued, "real hospital spending per capita will increase 75 percent between 2002 and 2012, and the demand for hospital beds will increase considerably."[23]

Altman and his colleagues predicted that aging and population growth would account for less than a third of this growth. The rest would come from two other factors: "the excess of hospital inflation over the amount of inflation in the general economy," much of it related to labor costs; and the use of new technology and the greater use of hospital care in general.

The authors argued that baby boomers have a greater propensity to spend money on health care and more disposable income than the previous generation did. Consequently, they expected the need for hospitals to grow, adding that even if hospitals could absorb 10–20 percent more patients, they'd need 136,000 to 211,000 additional beds to accommodate this demand.

Where the Action Really Is   Other experts disagree. Jeff Goldsmith, a health care consultant and futurist, says: "Stuart Altman is basing a straight-line forecast for 10 years on the 1998–2001 run-up in hospital days, and I think that's nuts. There were very specific reasons why bed days increased, and they certainly weren't the reasons that Stuart and his colleagues alluded to. The people who are out there building that capacity in anticipation of this huge wave of demand for inpatient care are going to get their heads handed to them. . . .

"Boomers are going to demand more health care, but it's going to be all outpatient. I don't see a reversal of the two-decade trend of a continued increase in the intensity of ambulatory care. We've got the very real prospect of overnight laminectomies and overnight joint replacements for knees and hips. So the idea that the boomers produced this big increase in hospital demand is bogus."

In Goldsmith's view, the rise in admissions in the late 1990s had nothing to do with technology or a rise in boomers' disposable income. During that period, he says, "physicians shed a lot of their unstable cases onto hospitals. . . . There was a huge increase in emergency room volume and admissions that wasn't necessarily intensity-driven."

What this means, he explains, is that physicians are using the emergency room [ER] to manage their own malpractice risk. In other words, rather than trying to treat patients with certain acute conditions, they're sending them to the ER. That way, they avoid the chance that the patients will experience an adverse event at home and sue them later.

Other Viewpoints   Mark Pauly, a health economist at the Wharton School, agrees that the trends indicate a continuation of the shift to outpatient care. In Philadelphia, he sees mainly construction of ambulatory facilities, not new hospitals. And those new hospitals that are going up, he says, are replacing older buildings, so they aren't adding any net capacity.

"Altman may be entirely right; the population is getting older," he says. "But I'm more inclined to bet on the trend to keep people out of the hospital as much as possible."

Gloria Bazzoli, a health economist at Virginia Commonwealth University in Richmond, also doubts there will be a need to build many more hospitals. "When I look at the trends, I see growth in technology and more and more care outside the traditional hospital. I also see new technology coming into the hospital, but a lot of it is supporting a lower length of stay." For example, she says, the stents used to keep arteries open after angioplasties have enabled "quicker movement of patients from surgery to recovery outside the hospital. Also, due to some of the new robotic surgery, incisions for CABG [coronary artery bypass graft] or angioplasty are so small that patients are often up and about in a couple of days. That's the kind of innovation that reduces lengths of stay."

"We'll always need hospitals, but all the trends are toward other settings of care, with hospitals becoming the institutions that provide really intensive care for certain types of patients."

Rise in Disease Prevalence   Kenneth Thorpe, an Emory University health economist who coauthored the hospital paper with Altman, agrees that the rise in outpatient spending will continue. But he also believes that inpatient costs will soar as a result of the increasing burden of disease. "If you look at the rise in treatment for type 2 diabetes, back problems, asthma—the whole range of chronic illnesses—we're seeing the population prominence of those things skyrocketing. That's resulted in somewhat higher hospitalization rates than we'd anticipated."

While physicians treat these chronic conditions in their offices, "the bad consequences of something like diabetes are treated in the hospital," Thorpe says, citing amputations and kidney failures.

Are we short of hospital capacity today? "On a typical day on the inpatient side, perhaps not," he replies. "The problem is the relationship between what's going on in the ER and the outpatient side of the hospital, which is drawing a huge amount of resources. And certainly at peak periods on some types of floors—particularly the surgical floors—there's a major problem. So we've had this explosion in outpatient utilization in the hospital by many people who will ultimately be hospitalized. During peak periods, a lot of hospitals I know do have capacity problems."

Capacity Management　　Gloria Bazzoli and her colleagues at the Center for Studying Health System Change examined hospital capacity in twelve markets.[24] While most facilities had problems handling demand for emergency services, the hospital leaders surveyed expressed less concern about the adequacy of their general medical or surgical beds or their intensive care units. Since only a few institutions had problems in these areas, the researchers concluded that hospital capacity was poorly distributed rather than insufficient.

Most respondents in the 2003 study cited a lack of nurses as one of the major reasons for capacity constraints. While the nursing shortage diminished somewhat,[25] 72 percent of hospital chief executives in a 2004 survey said their facilities still lacked sufficient nurses.[26] Most of the new nurses lured by higher pay are foreign-trained or middle-aged,[27] and nurses' average age is now over fifty, which points to greater shortfalls as they retire. Goldsmith wonders where the new hospitals will get the staff they need and whether they'll start bidding wars for personnel. If so, hospital costs may rise even faster.

It's Hard to Close a Hospital

When Beryl Gardner spoke at a public hearing of the New Jersey State Health Planning Board in Orange, New Jersey, in January 2004, the elderly woman seemed close to despair. The 130-year-old Hospital Center at Orange (HCO) was about to shut down, and she was about to lose her job.

"I am a dietary worker, representative of about 25 or 30 concerned workers," she said. "Poor workers. Black workers. Every one of us is black in the department of dietary. I am old. I don't know how to fill out a resume anymore. This is it for me. I have two more years until retirement. . . . I don't need unemployment for six months. I am not qualified for Social Security. I need a job. All of us need a job."

Many others testified at the hearing in support of the 270-bed hospital, including town council members, physicians, ministers, a local union representative, a firefighter, and an assistant to Mayor Hackett Mims, who read a letter from the singer Dionne Warwick. Born in East Orange, Warwick said her mother and her sister had been cared for at HCO. "It is our right to have a facility that actively cares for our elderly and all in this community," she concluded.[28]

Despite the storm of controversy, HCO closed later that month, laying off about eight hundred people. Only its emergency department stayed open until the state gave permission to close it. The state also required HCO to put up $1 million for the operation of a temporary primary-care clinic and to contribute $500,000 to the building of a permanent clinic—something that was sorely needed in this inner-city community, with its many indigent and Medicaid patients.[29]

Within a short time, local doctors switched to some of the ten other hospitals in the area. For the most part, their patients have received good care in those facilities, and none is more than a twenty-minute drive away. Yet doctors note that it's difficult for poor people who don't own cars to get to these other hospitals. Moreover, the disappearance of an old, familiar institution shocked many. To Curtis Johnson, a pediatrician, "It was like a family member being stabbed in the heart."

No Alternative to Closure   Some physicians and politicians accused the Newark-based Cathedral Healthcare, which controlled HCO, of closing the hospital to benefit its other local facilities. But the biggest beneficiary was the nearby East Orange General Hospital, which is not owned by Cathedral.

Terrence French, executive vice president of Cathedral, notes that HCO was plagued by an antiquated, poorly maintained physical plant. Prior to its closing, he says, HCO was trying to raise funds to build a new hospital on the campus of a nearby nursing home. What made that plan infeasible, he says, were cutbacks in federal and state aid.

The first blow came in June 2003, when CMS changed how it paid hospitals with high Medicare volume and a long average length of stay. As a result of this change, the hospital received $14 million less from Medicare in 2003 than it had the year before. Meanwhile, the state of New Jersey cut its reimbursement to hospitals for charity care. Together, the federal and state cuts added up to more than $17 million, or about 25 percent of HCO's annual operating budget.

Before HCO shut down, its annual number of admissions had plummeted from sixty-four hundred in 1996 to below five thousand in 2003.[30] The average length of stay of its Medicare patients, who provided 70 percent of its business, was far above the state and national averages—a testimonial to its inefficiency. At one point, state regulators closed its operating rooms, citing unsafe conditions.[31] HCO simply could not compete with the area's newer, more efficient hospitals, which themselves were running at only half to two-thirds of capacity.[32] Yet HCO, which was on the verge of bankruptcy back in 1998, didn't finally collapse until 2004.

Fewer Hospitals Are Closing   If it was so difficult to close a hospital as feeble as HCO, how about all the other underperforming hospitals in the country? Over the long run, many of the weaker ones have gone under. From 1990 to 1999—a period when managed-care plans were cutting hospital utilization and much inpatient care was migrating to ambulatory clinics—the number of community hospitals dropped by 11 percent. But from 1999 to 2003, that figure leveled off at around forty-nine hundred.[33]

Why is it so hard to close a hospital? One reason is that area residents often feel an emotional attachment to their community hospital; they may have been born there or been treated there. They may be reluctant to travel farther to another hospital. And in rural areas, consultant Michael LaPenna notes, hospitals are often community centers. "It's where the Boy Scouts meet, where people have church socials. It's also the only source of jobs outside of agriculture. It's the only thing that keeps the local stores and gas stations going. If you have a little hospital in Iowa closing, it's really a catastrophe for the entire town."

Jobs are also the key in metropolitan areas. Overall, U.S. hospitals employed nearly 5 million people in 2004. The hospital industry ranked second as a source of private sector employment. Directly or indirectly, it supported one of every nine jobs in the United States.[34] Closing a large hospital is like shutting down a military base: It has a major impact on the local economy.

"We generally don't shut down hospitals, any more than we're willing to talk about rationing care," Robert Homchick, a health care attorney with Davis, Wright, and Tremaine in Seattle, says. "There are stakeholders involved, and it's a complicated enough regulatory area that they can usually find some political leverage to keep a hospital open. We'd be better off if hospitals could close more easily, but I don't see that changing very quickly."

Inefficiency Means Higher Costs   Although hospitals mean jobs, keeping underused hospitals open is not good for the employers, employees, and taxpayers who fund health care: Regardless of how low a hospital's occupancy rate is, it will still have the same fixed costs, and it will try to pass on some of those costs to payers through higher prices. Inefficiency also means longer lengths of stay, which can cost more. Yet it is very difficult to shrink local hospital capacity to match demand.

Buffalo, New York, which has lost half of its population in the past fifty years, still has eight hospitals with a total of 2,425 beds. The occupancy rate of Buffalo hospitals is 61 percent, several points below the national average. But it's difficult to talk about closing facilities in a city where the official unemployment rate is 7.3 percent. While recognizing the need for downsizing, local health care leaders all claim their own institutions deserve to survive.[35]

Near the end of his tenure, former New York Governor George Pataki formed a commission to close unneeded hospitals across the state as part of a plan to restrain soaring Medicaid costs.[36] In November 2006, the commission delivered its report, which called for closing or merging twenty or more hospitals and consolidating service lines in other institutions to avoid duplication.[37] While the federal government has agreed to give New York $1.5 billion to carry out this mission,[38] and Eliot Spitzer, the currrent Democratic governor, supports the idea, it was unclear at press time whether or not the affected hospitals, unions, and communities would prevent it from being implemented.[39]

Services Promote Competition The New York hospital commission's report addresses the duplication of services in areas such as maternity care and mental health. But it doesn't tackle the pervasive redundancy in service lines such as cardiac care and orthopedic care, even though this is what generates a lot of hospital construction and renovation. Letting every institution offer all of these services often creates a supply that exceeds community needs. It also intensifies competition. And, for reasons unique to health care, this increased competition leads to higher, not lower costs.

As George Halvorson points out in his 1993 book *Strong Medicine*, hospitals compete not for patients but for physicians, who usually determine where patients are admitted.[40] Hospitals especially need the surgeons and the specialists who do the lucrative procedures that keep the cash registers ringing. So they have to offer the new technology that these doctors use and build the surgical wings or outpatient facilities that will attract the right doctors. This kind of competition drives up costs as more and more hospitals add the capacity to do open-heart surgery or hip and knee replacements. Why? Because there are only so many patients who need these procedures. So, to get a return on investment and cover their fixed costs, the hospitals have to charge more for each case.

When hospitals merge, they tend to preserve redundancies between their service lines. "If two hospitals have hip surgery programs, they'll generally keep both open," LaPenna notes. "Sometimes when hospitals merge, it throws more costs into the system. You have to have true consolidation—with programs closed and people taking advantage of economies of scale—to save money."

So far, we've looked at the duplication of services created by competition among specialists, ambulatory-care facilities, and hospitals. But there's another type of redundancy that's responsible for some of the waste in the system: the competition among pharmaceutical companies to market "me-too" drugs that have very similar effects. This, and the perverse effects of profit-driven medical research on patient care, are among the subjects of the next chapter.

11 Why Do Drugs Cost So Much?

Have insomnia, restless leg syndrome, adult attention deficit disorder, heartburn, arthritis pain, or erectile dysfunction? There's a prescription drug for your condition, and you've probably seen it advertised on television or in a magazine. Of course, the medication usually has a host of potential side effects, and the ads always tell you to discuss it with your doctor to see if it's "right for you." But what that really means is that the drug companies want you to urge your doctor to prescribe it. And in a lot of cases, that's exactly what he does. Because when a physician is asked for a justifiable prescription, and he has only ten or fifteen minutes to spend with the patient, he's not disposed to argue. He reaches for his Rx pad.

Most of the widely advertised drugs have a few things in common: They're supposed to treat or prevent a widespread chronic condition; there are other drugs just like them; and they have to be taken long-term or forever. Among these are medications used to lower cholesterol or blood pressure or to treat depression or arthritis.

Sometimes the pharmaceutical firms medicalize a condition that most people have learned to live with. Take insomnia. Since the dawn of time, people have had trouble getting to sleep or sleeping through the night. But now, with the help of advertising, the drug makers have convinced consumers that there's no need to put up with even mild insomnia. As a result, the use of sleeping pills—mainly Ambien—doubled from 2000 to 2004 among adults aged twenty to forty-four, and rose by 85 percent among children aged ten to nineteen. In 2004, Americans filled more than 35 million prescriptions for these drugs at a cost of $2.1 billion.[1]

All that prevented this market from growing even bigger was that Ambien, made by Sanofi-Aventis, could be prescribed for only short periods. But then along came Lunesta, which had been approved for long-term use. Sepracor, Lunesta's maker, poured $185 million into advertising the drug when it was launched, triggering 3.3 million pre-scriptions in 2005. In response, Sanofi-Aventis increased advertising of Ambien and Ambien NR, the new controlled-release version that would take over after the original Ambien patent expired in 2006. And several other companies are developing drugs for this burgeoning market. By 2008, it's estimated, it will cost around $3 billion a year to help Americans sleep.[2]

Volume and Price Determine Cost   For decades, drug advertising on television was limited, because the Food and Drug Administration (FDA) required pharmaceutical companies to include a great deal of information about a product's risks and side effects. Then in 1997, the government loosened the restrictions, and a flood of drug ads followed. The results were predictable: Television advertising ignited a "raging demand for prescription drugs among consumers, often putting physicians on the defensive," one observer noted.[3] Now worth about $4 billion a year,[4] direct-to-consumer advertising was one of several factors that helped drive up U.S. prescription-drug spending from $81 billion in 1997 to $252 billion in 2005.[5]

The pharmaceutical companies also raised their prices substantially during this period. From 2000 to 2003, for example, prices of the most common drugs rose 28 percent.[6] Just in the first quarter of 2006—the first three months after the new Medicare drug benefit went into effect—prices of brand-name prescription drugs jumped 3.9 percent, four times the general inflation rate.[7] For many brand-name products, U.S. prices are now 30 percent to 100 percent higher than prices in Europe and Canada.[8]

Yet higher prices explain only part of the rapid growth in U.S. drug costs. According to the consulting arm of IMS Health, which tracks pharmaceutical sales, the rising volume of prescriptions accounted for 65 percent of sales growth from 1994 to 2004; price increases generated just 25 percent of the expansion.[9] Express Scripts, a leading pharmaceutical benefit manager, attributed about half of the 17.4 percent increase in drug spending in 2000 to higher prices. The rest, it said, was the result of higher utilization and the introduction of new drugs.[10]

Advertising is not the only force that has helped create demand for these new products. Doctors, patients, and even health plans have also contributed to rising drug costs. Changes in the agreed-upon indications for treating conditions such as hypertension and high cholesterol have encouraged doctors to prescribe certain drugs for more patients. So have pay-for-performance programs that reward physicians for better preventive and chronic care. And the rising prevalence of conditions such as obesity and diabetes, linked partly to bad health behavior, has also fueled the increasing use of ever-more expensive drugs.[11]

So it's unfair to blame the explosion in prescription drug costs—which in 2005 accounted for 11 percent of total health spending[12]—entirely on the drug companies. But even though they've fed a market that was poised to grow, the pharmaceutical firms do generate about two-thirds of their worldwide profits in the United States,[13] which is the only advanced country that does not control drug prices.

Research and Drug Costs   The drug makers maintain that they have to keep prices high in the United States because they need to invest in new "life-saving" medications. According to the Pharmaceutical Research and Manufacturers of America, the industry trade association, only one in ten thousand "potential medicines" makes it through the R&D process—which takes an average of fifteen years—and is approved by the FDA.[14] Citing a 2003 Tufts University study, the association claims that it costs an average of $802 million to develop and test a new drug.[15]

But Marcia Angell, MD, a former editor of the *New England Journal of Medicine*, contends that the $802 million figure has nothing to do with the average cost of drug R&D. The Tufts study, she says in a book about the drug industry, looked at just sixty-eight drugs developed at ten companies, and these were all novel products. In contrast, she points out, most new drugs aren't significantly different from medications already on the market. Of the innovative drugs, she adds, "only a fraction are developed entirely by the drug companies themselves. Most of the rest are simply licensed or otherwise acquired from university or government laboratories or biotechnology companies."[16] Since the Tufts researchers looked only at novel products created by the drug firms themselves, she concludes, they vastly overstated the typical cost of new drug development.

Angell notes two other problems with the industry's estimate. First, it includes the "opportunity cost" of investing in drug research, or the amount that could have been earned if the money had been invested in something else, such as stocks and bonds. That opportunity cost equaled nearly half of the $802 million figure. Second, she observes, the estimate is in pre-tax dollars, but R&D expenses are fully deductible.

The real facts, Angell says, are these: "In 2002, when the ten U.S. drug companies in the Fortune 500 list had combined worldwide sales of about $217 billion and spent just over 14 percent of that on R&D (about $31 billion), they had a profit margin of 17 percent ($36 billion). *Thus, profits were substantially more than R&D costs*" (emphasis added).[17]

Families USA supports Angell's thesis. The national consumer organization analyzed financial reports submitted to the SEC by nine of the largest U.S. drug makers. It found that of the $168 billion in revenues that these companies reported for 2001, 27 percent went for marketing, advertising, and administration; 11 percent was invested in R&D; and 18 percent was declared as profits.[18]

According to Pharmaceutical Research and Manufacturers of America, its member companies devoted 18 percent of their combined domestic sales to R&D in 2002.[19] If their margins were similar to those of the companies analyzed by Angell and Families USA, however, that would still mean their total profits were roughly equivalent to their research investment.

"Me-too" Drugs Proliferate   What do consumers get for all of those R&D costs that are passed onto them in the form of higher prices? They get many fine medications that save lives, cure or slow diseases, and improve the quality of life. But they also get a host of drugs that are not very different from one other. For example, there are several patent-protected prescription drugs in the statin class that lower high cholesterol, including Lipitor, Vytorin and Crestor. Your physician can also choose among several antidepressants (e.g., Paxil, Zoloft, Effexor) that work basically the same way. While these drugs are all useful, there's little scientific evidence that any of them is superior to others in the same class.[20] (Doctors do, however, report some variations in their effectiveness and side effects in different patients.)

According to Angell, of the 415 drugs that the FDA approved from 1998 to 2002, only 14 percent were truly innovative, 9 percent were updated versions of older drugs, and the other 77 percent were "me-too" drugs. While each is chemically distinct from other medications, the FDA classified these drugs as being no better than the products already out on the market.[21] Again, other observers have made similar estimates of the percentage of me-too medications.[22]

Why would the FDA approve new drugs that simply jam an already overcrowded medicine cabinet? It does so because the law states that, to be approved for sale, a drug need only be proved safe and effective. And under the FDA's rules, "effective" means that the medication must simply work better than a placebo, or sham pill. It doesn't have to work better than an older drug. So naturally, pharmaceutical companies place many of their R&D bets on "me-too" drugs that they can sell into an already established market.

Taxpayers Get the Crumbs   Rather than spend money on finding new drugs, the pharmaceutical firms have shifted much of their R&D investment to late-stage clinical trials geared to getting FDA approval.[23] Consequently, research supported by the National Institutes of Health (NIH) is responsible for most of the breakthrough discoveries, says Angell.[24]

This public/private nexus grew out of the Bayh-Dole Act of 1980, which allows NIH-funded universities and small businesses to patent discoveries and license them to pharmaceutical firms. Some drug companies have exploited those licenses to make huge profits on breakthroughs that were achieved at public expense. One example is the AIDS drug Fuzeon, which was discovered at Duke University, developed by a local biotech company, and then licensed to Roche. The drug maker now charges $20,000 a year for Fuzeon.[25]

The Bayh-Dole Act requires drug companies that license taxpayer-supported research to make the resulting drugs available to the public "on reasonable terms," which could be interpreted as "reasonable prices," Angell points out. If profits are very large, she adds, part of the money is supposed to be returned to the government. However, she avers, NIH has not enforced the reasonable pricing requirement.[26] According to Jerry Avorn of Harvard Medical School, the pharmaceutical industry persuaded NIH that it's more important to encourage the introduction of new drugs than to police pricing.[27]

In another book about the industry, Avorn supports Angell's contention that drug companies have not compensated NIH fairly for the research that they've exploited. He relates the story of Taxol, the top-selling oncology drug. The NIH paid for most of the clinical trials to develop Taxol at a cost of $484 million, he says. Bristol-Myers Squibb then marketed the drug, reaping $9 billion in sales through 2002. Under a 1996 licensing agreement with NIH, the drug company was supposed to pay the government one-half of 1 percent in royalties on that money, or $35 million, but its payments fell short of even that paltry sum.[28]

Commercialization of Research   While NIH and private foundations fund most basic research, the drug and biotech industries sponsor 80–90 percent of clinical trials.[29] That's why the combined domestic R&D budgets of the drug companies—which totaled an estimated $30.6 billion in the United States in 2004—exceed the amount that NIH spends on biomedical research.[30] All of this private money pouring into the research enterprise has had a major impact on both universities and physicians.

As the commercial support of drug studies increased in the 1980s and 1990s, universities became progressively more dependent on the pharmaceutical firms, John Abramson, MD, of Harvard Medical School notes in his book *Overdosed America: The Broken Promise of American Medicine*. Meanwhile, the drug companies started to outsource many trials to organizations known as clinical research organizations (CROs). These companies gained access to patients through community-based doctors, whom they paid thousands of dollars for each patient they recruited. The CROs began to exert an increasing amount of control over the research design, the data analysis, and even the writing of articles. At the same time, the number of trials done in academic medical centers declined, and the universities showed a greater willingness to accede to the drug companies' demands so they could compete for the remaining funds.[31]

The results of these shifts have been far-reaching. First, Abramson notes, "the odds are 3.6 to 4 times greater that commercially sponsored studies will favor the sponsor's product than studies without commercial funding." Also, as editors of several leading medical journals warned in an unprecedented joint statement in 2001, researchers "may have little or no input into trial design, no access to the raw data, and limited participation in data interpretation."[32]

Patient Safety Compromised   The commercial dominance of clinical trials has, in some instances, led to the concealment of data related to patient safety. For example, a 2000 study of Vioxx, the arthritis pain medication that was later withdrawn from the market, excluded three subjects who had suffered heart attacks. That fact elicited an indignant editorial from the *New England Journal of Medicine*, which had published the study, after the missing data were revealed in 2005.[33]

In the wake of the Vioxx withdrawal, Pfizer denied that it knew of studies of either Celebrex or Bextra—drugs in the same class as Vioxx—indicating that they caused cardiac problems. But the company later admitted that studies it had sponsored showed that both drugs could hurt the heart. It withdrew Bextra and put a warning label on Celebrex, which continues to be a top-selling medication.[34]

While most prescription drugs are beneficial, there's a lengthening list of those that have caused more harm than benefit. Among these drugs—each of which netted billions of dollars in sales before being withdrawn—are Rezulin for diabetes, Redux for weight loss, and Propulsid for heartburn. These medications, respectively, caused liver failure, heart-valve damage, and other cardiac problems.[35]

Physicians also prescribe many medications for purposes not approved by the FDA, often at the urging of drug company reps or on the basis of questionable research. For example, doctors give patients epilepsy drugs for depression and weight reduction; anti-psychotic medicines for insomnia and attention deficit disorder; and blood pressure drugs for headaches and anxiety.[36] In some instances, these "off-label" prescriptions—which comprise about one in five of all drugs prescribed[37]—have hurt patients, and the government has sued some pharmaceutical companies for fraudulent marketing. But that hasn't stopped them from profiting on these drugs.

In 2004 Warner Lambert, a unit of Pfizer, paid $430 million to settle government charges that it had hired doctors to prescribe Neurontin, an epilepsy drug, for everything from restless leg syndrome to manic depression. It was also alleged that the company hired ghostwriters to draft articles promoting the off-label uses and then found doctors willing to put their names on these articles. Despite the large fine, however, Warner-Lambert still came out ahead: In 2003, it sold $2.7 billion worth of Neurontin, 90 percent of it for off-label uses.[38]

Where's the FDA?   While doctors are allowed to prescribe medications for any purpose, the Food and Drug Administration is supposed to protect the public against harmful drugs. Yet some observers believe that the agency is failing in this mission.

Among these critics is David Graham, an official in the FDA's Office of Drug Safety. In congressional testimony in November 2004, Graham, a twenty-year FDA veteran, raised questions about the safety of Crestor, an anticholesterol drug that has caused kidney failure in some patients; Bextra, the pain medication that was later withdrawn because of its heart effects; Meridia, an obesity pill that sometimes raises blood pressure; Accutane, an acne medication that can cause birth defects; and Severent, an anti-asthma medication that has raised the incidence of asthma-related deaths. The companies that make these drugs have all denied that they pose a threat to the public.[39]

Other critics asked why the FDA was so slow to act in the case of Vioxx, which was withdrawn in 2004. They noted that studies going back to 2000 showed that Vioxx increased cardiac risk. Yet, until a trial of the drug's effect on precancerous growths in the colon accidentally showed that Vioxx increased the risk of heart attacks, the medication was being prescribed to millions of patients.[40]

Representative Henry Waxman (D-CA) recently released a report that said the FDA was falling down on the job. From 2000 to 2005, he charged, the number of warning letters issued by the agency for violations of federal requirements plummeted by more than 50 percent.[41] (The FDA responded that enforcement cannot be measured by the number of actions taken.) Similarly, a third of nearly a thousand FDA scientists surveyed by the Union of Concerned Scientists said that outside political and industry influences had impeded their work.[42]

Client of the Drug Companies?   Some observers think the problems at the FDA are partly related to how the agency is funded. In 1992, Congress enacted the Prescription Drug Fee User Act, which requires the pharmaceutical companies to pay user fees to the FDA. Today, the $260 million a year that the industry gives the FDA funds about half the cost of drug approval. So in essence, say these critics, the agency has become a client of the drug firms that it regulates.[43] Recent revelations about conflicts of interest among outside experts who advise the FDA show further evidence of drug company influence on the agency.[44] (At press time, the FDA announced new rules to deal with these conflicts of interest.)[45]

The Bush administration has pushed the FDA to expedite approvals of new drugs. The acceleration of regulatory action has been accompanied by an increase in the number of hastily approved drugs being pulled off the market.[46] And after companies receive expedited permission to market new drugs, only a third of them perform the postmarketing studies that the FDA requests but doesn't have the regulatory authority to require.[47] The "Phase IV" trials that they do conduct are often little more than flimsy attempts to support off-label uses of their drugs.[48] Recent legislative efforts to give the FDA additional authority over these trials have run into a stone wall.[49]

As safety concerns have risen, the FDA has been under pressure to more strictly regulate direct-to-consumer pharmaceutical advertising. Some critics have called for a ban on direct-to-consumer ads,[50] and former Senate majority leader Bill Frist suggested a two-year wait before new drugs could be advertised to consumers.[51] (The American Medical Association later requested a temporary moratorium on the advertising of newly approved drugs and medical devices.)[52] With congressional action brewing and the FDA announcing a review of its advertising policy,[53] the industry association released new advertising guidelines in 2005.[54] While these were considered weak, the association did urge member firms to submit ads to the FDA before they ran, and most are doing so.[55]

Marketing to Physicians   While advertising to consumers continues to grow, 90 percent of the $21 billion that the drug firms spent on marketing in 2004 went to influence physician prescribing.[56] The two main avenues for this vast promotional enterprise are pharmaceutical companies' support of continuing medical education and visits to doctors' offices by drug salespeople.

The pharmaceutical companies employ nearly ninety thousand sales reps, about one for every five doctors in practice.[57] When these "detailers" visit doctors' offices, they bring drug samples and sometimes little gifts for the doctors and their staff members. Sometimes they take doctors out to lunch or bring in lunch for the whole staff—all in the interests of getting some time alone with a doctor to make their pitch.[58]

Most physicians are willing to give the detailers some time. For one thing, they want the free drug samples, which they dispense to patients who can't afford prescription drugs or to other patients as a favor. (Of course, these samples aren't really "free," because they're designed to get patients used to a particular medication.) Also, physicians are often too busy to keep up with the medical literature. So they tend to get the bulk of their "education" from the drug reps, who are only too happy to give their companies' one-sided view of the research.[59] While the majority of physicians say that detailers don't influence their prescribing decisions, there's an abundance of evidence indicating that they do.[60]

Tainted Education   Physicians must receive a certain amount of continuing medical education in order to keep their medical licenses. There are many ways to meet this requirement, including various self-learning methods. But physicians like to travel and congregate with their peers, so they frequently attend continuing medical education conferences that are sponsored wholly or partially by drug companies. A prominent feature of these conferences are dinner "symposia" that focus on the sponsors' drugs.

The pharmaceutical firms or their proxies—known as medical education communication companies—also invite many "high-prescribing" physicians to dinner meetings where they can hear experts talk about the latest techniques for treating particular diseases. Some physicians get a "consulting fee" for attending these meetings.[61] Among the drugs discussed, of course, will always be the one that the sponsor is trying to promote, and there's evidence that speakers tend to slant their talks in favor of those drugs. As a result, physicians who attend the meetings often prescribe more of the promoted medications afterward.[62]

Jerry Avorn describes the combined impact of detailers and industry-sponsored continuing medical education on the treatment of high blood pressure. While a very large, NIH-funded study showed in 2002 that diuretics should be the first-line drug for treating this disease, patented calcium-channel blockers and ACE inhibitors are still widely prescribed for hypertension. One reason, he says, is that detailers have convinced doctors that the new drugs are better. In addition, the manufacturers have sponsored hundreds of seminars and symposia to promote these products. So millions of patients are taking calcium channel blockers, which cost $900 a year, rather than diuretics, which cost $60.[63]

Medical Leaders Protest   While many academic experts and physician opinion leaders are glad to accept the industry's gifts and to spout its line, others have taken an increasingly strong stand against what they see as the corruption of scientific research and physician integrity. In 2006, ten leading academicians, along with the head of the Association of American Medical Colleges, criticized the conflicts of interest that have led to this situation. In a widely discussed article in the *Journal* *of the American Medical Association*, they called for "the elimination or modification of common practices related to small gifts, pharmaceutical samples, continuing medical education, funds for physician travel, speakers bureaus, ghostwriting, and consulting and research contracts."[64]

The report's authors say that the recommendations by medical and pharmaceutical associations to curb these practices have not gone far enough. First, they say, limitations on drug company gifts have not produced the desired results, because even small gifts create positive attitudes toward drug reps. And they decry the practice of medical school faculty members serving as speakers for drug companies that use them as part of their marketing apparatus. They would replace drug samples with "vouchers for low-income patients or other arrangements that distance the company and its products from physicians." And they favor a similar arm's length system for pharmaceutical company support of continuing medical education events. The article calls for teaching hospitals to lead these reforms.

Tellingly, academic medical centers contacted by one publication declined to comment on the report.[65] While a few institutions, including Stanford, Yale, and the University of Pennsylvania, have since taken action to reduce industry influence,[66] most universities are not going to bite the hand that feeds them.

Generic Drugs   If you've ever turned on a television set, you've seen the ubiquitous ads for the "purple pill," aka Nexium. This heartburn drug, which costs $200 a month, is essentially the same as an older drug, Prilosec, which is now available both as a generic prescription drug and as an over-the-counter nostrum for a small fraction of Nexium's cost. AstraZeneca, which makes both drugs, introduced the purple pill in 2001, just as Prilosec's patent was about to expire. It then launched an unprecedented advertising blitz that cost $257 million in 2003 alone. That helped boost Nexium sales to blockbuster status.[67]

Protected by over-the-counter exclusivity from the FDA,[68] AstraZeneca has repromoted Prilosec OTC, which contains a limited dose of the drug. But nobody is advertising generics like Mevacor, the first of the big-selling statin drugs for high cholesterol, or Prozac, the initial wonder drug for depression. Nobody is interested in them anymore because, as generics, they can be manufactured by any company. When multiple firms put out generic versions of a drug, they normally sell for about 20 percent of the price they fetched while under patent.[69]

These generics have effects similar to those of other drugs in the same class, however, and some older generic drugs are even better than patented pills. A recent NIH-sponsored study, for example, compared four new schizophrenia drugs known as "atypical antipsychotics" and one older drug called perphenazine. It found that the generic medication was just as effective as three of the atypicals. Patients didn't stick with it as long as they did with Zyprexa, a bestselling atypical, but Zyprexa caused more weight gain and increased cholesterol levels more than the other drugs did. A month's supply of perphenazine costs $60, compared with $520 for Zyprexa.[70]

Because of persistent efforts by health plans and state Medicaid programs, generic drugs account for an increasing percentage of drug sales. Generic revenues grew 21 percent in 2004, and six of the ten most prescribed drugs that year were generic.[71] But an Express Scripts study showed that consumers could have saved $20 billion in 2004 by using more generic medications. For example, only 7 percent of the prescriptions for cholesterol-lowering drugs were generic.[72] There are signs that the tide is turning in favor of generics. Mevacor sales are growing, and generic and brand-name versions of Zocor now hold 20 percent of the market.[73] The recent move by Wal-Mart to sell nearly three hundred generic drugs for only $4 a prescription should give a further boost to no-name medications.[74] But brand-name drug sales are also soaring.

Medicare Part D   Partly because Medicare drug plans emphasize the use of generic drugs, the pharmaceutical firms initially claimed that they would not make much from the new Medicare Part D drug benefit.[75] This was a curious argument. While much of the $593 billion cost of the drug benefit over ten years[76] will represent a shift of private-sector and Medicaid drug outlays to Medicare,[77] nine million Medicare beneficiaries lacked any drug coverage before the new law took effect.[78] Those who have signed up for Part D are bound to use more prescription drugs. Moreover, drug makers are receiving 25 to 30 percent more under Part D than they received from state Medicaid programs that formerly bought drugs for low-income seniors.[79] Not surprisingly, pharmaceutical firms are reporting higher profits and are making a larger percentage of their sales in the United States.[80]

The pharmaceutical companies played a major role in writing the Medicare Modernization Act of 2003, and they received pretty much what they wanted. The law prohibits the Centers for Medicare and

Medicaid Services (CMS) from negotiating prices with the drug firms. Instead, the Part D drug plans bargain with companies known as pharmaceutical benefit managers that also administer drug benefits for most large, self-insured corporations.[81]

The health insurers also helped shape the law, and it shows. Not only do they get a piece of the Part D drug action, but they also have the opportunity to lure seniors into Medicare HMOs that are now much more lucrative than they used to be—again as a result of the Medicare drug statute.[82]

The legislation turned out this way because President George W. Bush and the Republican majority in Congress wanted to provide a Medicare drug benefit without impinging on the prerogatives of free enterprise. So, instead of a big government program in the mold of the original Medicare, Part D was envisioned as an innovative use of the free market to carry out social objectives. By competing with one other, the drug plans were supposed to hold down prices—and in fact, the average monthly premiums have been significantly lower than expected. But liberals argue that it would be simpler and cheaper to just let CMS buy the drugs.[83]

The privatization of the drug benefit has proved to be more difficult and complex than anticipated. Medicare beneficiaries in many areas can choose among forty or more different drug plans, each with its own lists of approved drugs, copayments, and premiums.[84] This huge amount of choice proved too confusing for many seniors when the program was launched in January 2006, and enrollment went slowly at first. But by May 15, after the enrollment deadline for the year, nearly 39 million elderly and disabled beneficiaries—90 percent of those eligible—had drug coverage. Of these people, 22 million had insurance through former employers, other government programs, or Medicare HMOs, and about 6 million low-income seniors were automatically enrolled in Part D.[85] Approximately 11.5 million people signed up voluntarily, leaving 4 million to 5 million beneficiaries without drug coverage.

Polls show a majority of seniors with drug insurance are satisfied and that about half are saving money.[86] But in 2006 about 35 percent of Medicare beneficiaries were in danger of falling into the infamous "doughnut hole"—the gap between drug costs of $2,250 and $5,100 a year that the government doesn't cover.[87] While most of those people could find drug plans that provided some coverage in the doughnut hole, some of these plans covered only generic drugs; far fewer are expected to pay for brand-name drugs in 2007; and those that do will jack up their premiums significantly, according to Families USA.[88] The consumer organization's report also notes that, of the top twenty-five drugs prescribed to seniors, eighteen are unavailable in generic form.

The data on drug savings under the Part D program show mixed results. According to CMS, Medicare beneficiaries are getting a 27 percent discount on drugs, compared with the 15 percent that had been predicted.[89] But according to a government report, drug-plan prices are higher than those paid by holders of the interim Medicare drug cards before Part D took effect.[90] Families USA also notes that the Veterans Administration pays only about half as much as Medicare beneficiaries and taxpayers spend for seniors' twenty most widely used drugs.[91] But the industry responds that the Veterans Administration's prices exclude the costs of drug distribution.[92]

Caveats on Price Controls   Critics, including the Democratic leaders in Congress, argue that Medicare could save far more if it negotiated drug prices directly. That begs the question of price controls and whether they would be limited to Medicare. If so, asserts the association of pharmaceutical benefit managers, the private sector would pay more for medicines, because drug companies would charge higher prices to health plans and people under sixty-five.[93] Universal price controls would solve that problem; but they'd also stifle innovation, argue the drug manufacturers.

Moreover, price controls alone would not address the problem of rising prescription volume. Although the growth in U.S. drug spending has slowed, partly because of rising copayments and deductibles, CMS actuaries expect national drug costs to expand 8.2 percent a year, on average, from 2007 through 2015. The effect on drug costs of the increased use of generics, they predict, will be offset by the growth in utilization.[94]

Reform Proposals   Part IV of this book explains how a restructured health care system could contain drug costs. Before moving on, however, I'd like to suggest a few ways to address the issues examined in this chapter.[95]

Free the FDA. To make prescription drugs safer and more effective, we have to insulate the FDA from industry pressure. An essential step is to sunset the Prescription Drug User Fee Act rather than renew it in

2007. That way, the FDA will not be dependent on the industry for a big chunk of its budget. Instead, the government should allocate sufficient funds to the FDA to perform its regulatory function. Also, let's give the FDA authority to mandate the completion of postapproval studies of drug safety in the broader population, as the Institute of Medicine has urged.[96]

Conduct comparative studies. The pharmaceutical firms have no incentive to conduct studies that compare their products with other medications for the same disease, leaving physicians and patients guessing about which are the most effective.

Like Jerry Avorn of Harvard,[97] I favor "practical" clinical trials—stripped-down studies in typical physician practices—to test comparative effectiveness at a reasonable cost (see Chapter 22). Some of this money could come from the NIH.

Discourage the production of me-too drugs. Some observers would like the FDA to require evidence that a new drug is more effective than older medicines before approving it. But that would deter companies from developing any new product that is not a medical breakthrough. A less onerous solution would be to tell the companies that their pills might be included in comparative trials after going on the market. In that scenario, they'd be less likely to put out me-too drugs that didn't offer any advantage over other medicines.

Reduce advertising. The FDA should restore the requirements for television drug advertising that it had before 1997. While this action wouldn't ban all such ads, it would keep them to a very dull roar—which should limit the production of me-too products. There is also merit in the AMA's proposal that the agency prohibit television ads for new drugs for some period after they're approved, to prevent situations where dangerous side effects are discovered only after millions of people are taking a medication.[98]

Promote integrity of research. To combat the drug firms' deleterious effect on scientific independence, let's put legal teeth into the leading medical journals' rule that all studies be registered at their inception.[99] That's the only way to make sure that studies with negative results are reported. The pharmaceutical firms and their contractors must also give researchers access to all trial data and allow them to publish what they've found. If the free exchange of ideas is protected, research tainted by corporate influence will not go undetected for long.

Separate medical education from commercial interests. Finally, let's get the pharmaceutical firms out of medical education. The companies influence the prescribing decisions of doctors from the time they enter medical school until they're out in practice and attending CME conferences. This is not the way to keep physicians up-to-date on medical advances. Instead, physicians should be taught how to use evidence-based-medicine resources on the Web and encouraged to get their CME credits the same way. Medical societies could support meetings out of membership dues and attendance fees. While fewer conferences would be held, the information that physicians got there would be less biased and more useful.

The pharmaceutical companies are not the enemy. These companies perform an important function, and we must be careful not to impede them too much in their pursuit of profits. But their financial motivation must be channeled in a way that helps produce better care at lower cost for people who can really benefit from their products.

Part IV
Rx for Health Care Reform

12 This Market Needs Regulation

Supporters of the current paradigm of health care reform argue that more competition and less regulation will reduce costs. But as explained in Part III, greater competition in health care does not lead to lower prices or less use of services. The more doctors there are, the more work they create for themselves; the more hospitals there are, the more services they offer; and the more drugs of a particular type there are, the more the pharmaceutical companies are able to expand the market. The conservative reformers' last hope, consumer-directed care, is another mirage: They can publish as many provider report cards as they like, but the vast majority of consumers won't be able to make head or tail of the information.

The tendency of health care players to merge in order to become dominant in local markets is another reason health care defies all attempts to make it competitive. As the health insurance market shrinks, insurance companies gobble each other up, reducing the choices of employers, individuals, and health care providers. As hospitals consolidate into larger systems to extract more revenue from the health plans, there are fewer choices for doctors and patients and higher costs for employers. As specialists form ever larger groups, they jack up their rates to payers and invest in imaging and surgical facilities that suck more money out of local economies.

A number of observers have commented on the tendency of health spending to expand at a far faster rate than inflation or GDP in a free market. Some of these commentators blame the free-enterprise system and favor a single-payer, government-run system.

Free enterprise *is* partly responsible for runaway health spending. But countries with national health insurance, although they spend less than we do, have not solved this problem, either. Their health costs are also rising faster than inflation or GDP because of factors such as aging, population growth, technology, national wealth, and consumerism. Some nations, recognizing that government cannot counter these forces alone, have introduced various market-based elements to restrain cost increases. Most countries with national health insurance also allow some private practice or private insurance.

In the United States, any reformer who tries to build a model for comprehensive, universal health care must reckon with the core ethos of this society, which revolves around market competition. The chapters that follow explain how we can blend that ethos with some structural elements of a single-payer system to provide universal coverage at a price we can afford. In general, this means taking some—but not all—of the profit out of health care. It means imbuing health care with more of a social consciousness than it has today. And it means government intervention to ensure that the market works.

There can be no real market for health care unless the government sets the rules for one. This is well understood—although rarely enforced—in the antitrust field. If insurance companies, hospital systems, or physician groups are allowed to keep growing, they will raise prices in markets where they acquire monopoly or near-monopoly power. Similarly, if there are no restraints on how many new cardiac surgery programs or imaging facilities can be introduced in a region, supply-induced care will raise the amount of health care spending.

If it were possible, however, to construct a limited form of free enterprise, strictly regulated by the government, and if everyone had insurance, competition could lead to lower costs and higher quality. This was the central insight of Alain Enthoven and the other advocates of managed competition, and it led to Bill and Hillary Clinton's bold but flawed attempt to achieve universal coverage. What if there were another way to negotiate the same passage, avoiding the Clintons' mistakes and engaging health care reform on today's terms?

The central premise of this book is that a different form of managed competition could succeed if it changed the equation in two ways: First, all primary-care physicians would have to join groups of a certain size that would be financially accountable for all professional services. And second, competition among these physician groups, rather than among insurance companies, would create the health care market. By incorporating a strong yet flexible regulatory framework that delegated power to regional authorities, this approach could prevent the federal government from gaining too much control over health care.

Naysayers will object that such radical reforms could never be adopted, given the determined opposition of the insurance and drug industries and the small-business lobby. Perhaps they're right. But forces are building up to support fundamental change. Employers are getting mad, and they're not going to take it much longer. Unless the ever-growing cost of health care is contained, many large companies might just drop coverage. And if enough voters eventually conclude that their choice is between lack of health care access and a government-run system, they might choose the latter. At that point, an approach like the one described here could suddenly look very appealing to those who'd prefer not to have decisions about their health care made in Washington.

13 Putting Doctors Together

In his book *From Chaos to Care*, David Lawrence, MD, a pediatrician and chairman emeritus of Kaiser Permanente, describes the odyssey of a fictional asthma patient named Rebecca.[1] Between the ages of two and six, Rebecca was a regular visitor to the emergency room (ER), because neither her pediatrician nor any of the specialists to whom he referred her could figure out how to control her asthma. Her doctors communicated poorly with one another and often disagreed about her treatment. She was hospitalized a few times, and during one hospital stay, almost died from an allergic reaction to an antibiotic. The next time she went to the ER, a doctor was about to prescribe the same antibiotic for a cold, because he didn't have access to her inpatient medical record; she avoided harm only because her father had written down the name of the drug she was allergic to.

When she was six, Rebecca's parents switched to a group-model HMO similar to Kaiser. While Lawrence doesn't minimize the problems they had at first in dealing with a large, seemingly impersonal clinic, he sketches out a scenario for improving this little girl's care: After placing Rebecca on a drug regimen recommended by the latest studies and giving her written instructions for self-care, her new primary-care physician sent her to a specialized nurse who took time to explain in detail what she and her parents had to do. The HMO also offered a twenty-four-hour call center, a support group for parents of asthmatic children, and a visiting nurse who would make sure there were no asthmatic "triggers" in Rebecca's house, such as dust or cat hair.

When Rebecca got sick again and had to go to the ER, the ER nurse and the doctor who saw her had immediate access to all her records on their computers. Her medication was adjusted, and her parents were instructed to pay closer attention to the readings on her peak-flow meter. With extra help from a call-center nurse and a pharmacist whom they met at their daughter's next office visit, Rebecca's parents eventually became adept at caring for her. They no longer had to rush her to the ER, because she was able to control her asthma.

Most Americans are not in group-model HMOs, and that form of health care delivery is not likely to grow. But Lawrence's story—a composite of many actual cases—demonstrates the huge difference between what an organized care delivery system can do and the care that a physician in a small practice can provide.

Inefficiency and Waste   According to the Institute of Medicine (IOM), the fragmentation of health care is a prime reason for medical errors, waste, and inefficiency.

"The health care system as currently structured does not, as a whole, make the best use of its resources," the IOM reports in *Crossing the Quality Chasm*. "There is little doubt that the aging population and increased patient demand for new services, technologies and drugs are contributing to the steady increase in health care expenditures, but so, too, is waste. Many types of medical errors result in the subsequent need for additional health care services to treat patients who have been harmed. *A highly fragmented delivery system that lacks even rudimentary clinical information capabilities results in poorly designed care processes characterized by unnecessary duplication of services and long waiting times and delays*" (emphasis added).[2]

The IOM advocates a vast reorganization of health care delivery centered on the leading chronic diseases, such as cancer, diabetes, heart disease, hypertension, and emphysema. Among the components of this reorganization are improved coordination of care, better information systems, new financial incentives, the use of guidelines based on scientific evidence, disease management, team-based care, performance measurement, and the availability to consumers of reliable, useful quality data.[3]

If physicians, hospitals, and other providers could pull this off, patients would receive high-quality care far more often than they do today. Lives and money would be saved, and health care would be more affordable.

But it's impossible to accomplish these goals without organizing health care providers into larger, more tightly knit units. Today, the only health care organizations in most communities are hospitals; in a few areas, there are also physician groups large enough to serve as hubs for the local medical community. Most physicians belong to health-plan networks, but these are mainly financial arrangements. Apart from the insurers' use of financial incentives to steer patients to particular physicians and hospitals, they have had little impact on clinical organization. (California is an exception that is explored later in this chapter and in the next chapter.)

Marcus Welby Lives   The biggest obstacle to a better-organized delivery system is the prevalence of small physician practices. In 2001, 47 percent of U.S. physicians in private practice were either soloists or had one partner; in contrast, only 9 percent were in groups of 20 or more.[4] These percentages haven't changed much since then.

Why haven't more physicians joined groups? According to a recent survey of medical community leaders, "physicians' desire for autonomy and difficulty in cooperating with each other" are the biggest barriers.[5] Reflecting on why many physicians have left groups to strike out on their own, Gary Matthews, an Atlanta-based health care consultant, observes, "Every single one of them says, 'I want to practice the way I want to practice medicine.' "

David Lawrence views this independent, self-reliant attitude—reminiscent of the 1970s television show *Marcus Welby, MD*—as a dangerous anachronism. In *From Chaos to Care*, he writes, "Now at the beginning of the 21st Century, medicine faces unprecedented challenges. Shifting expectations among those who require care, accelerating advances in medical science and technology, and the rapid growth in the number of people with chronic illnesses have changed the nature of medicine itself. . . . Continuing to rely on this timeworn approach in the future carries unacceptable risks to patients and costs to our society. Medical care as organized today is obsolete."[6]

Prepaid Groups Have Led the Way   Other observers agree that large, prepaid groups have a lot of advantages over the traditional cottage industry of small practices. Donald Berwick, president of the Institute for Healthcare Improvement, and his colleague Sachin Jain, for example, say that because of their incentive to keep people healthy, "prepaid group practices seem . . . to be better positioned to learn and improve continuously and to focus those efforts, especially on the needs of the chronically ill." [7] Compared with doctors in small, fee-for-service practices, they observe, physicians in those groups are much more involved with disease management. Prepaid group practices have also led the way in implementing evidence-based guidelines.

No improvement is possible without measurement, and here big groups are also ahead of the pack, Berwick and Jain say. Many large groups, whether prepaid or not, profile individual physicians and provide data to each doctor so that they can see how they compare with their peers within the group. The leading groups have been automating clinical data for decades, and the majority of them now have electronic health records.

While about 10 percent of small practices have EHRs,[8] most solo and small-group physicians don't have the infrastructure, the time, or the financial incentive to do any care coordination. That's one reason disease management falls far short of its potential, as discussed in Chapter 3.

Physicians cannot meet the IOM's quality goals unless they practice together in sizable groups, says Lawrence Casalino of the University of Chicago. Stephen Shortell, dean of the School of Public Health at the University of California at Berkeley, agrees. Citing the need for care management processes and expensive information systems, he says, "The fact that most U.S. doctors continue to practice in small groups is a major challenge to improving care."

The Market Doesn't Favor Big Groups   Besides the many doctors who do not want to join large groups, consumer preferences are another impediment to more organized health care delivery. Except in a few areas of the country, big group practices—whether prepaid like those of Kaiser or fee-for-service like the Mayo Clinic—have failed to build a critical mass of either doctors or patients.

This failure to grow is not an indication that they offer poor-quality care. Studies comparing prepaid group practices with fee-for-service plans show that prepaid group practices "seem to deliver preventive services more often and have lower patient satisfaction" but otherwise offer quality comparable to that of fee-for-service medicine.[9] In the 2006 ranking of health plans by the National Committee on Quality Assurance, Kaiser's northern and southern California plans were rated "excellent" in nearly every category.[10] And two recent studies, one in California[11] and the other based on national data,[12] show that large, organized groups tend to deliver better care than small, unrelated practices do.

Limited evidence suggests that group-model HMOs' cost of delivering health care is about 25 percent lower than that of other health plan types, including PPOs and HMOs that principally contract with small practices.[13] However, Kaiser's lack of success outside of California, Colorado, and Hawaii is one indication that many people prefer small, independent practices to large clinics.

As the market has repudiated capitation and moved to broad provider networks over the past several years, some group-model HMOs have gone under or been forced to shift their emphasis away from group practice. Even the venerable Harvard Community Health Plan, Berwick's own alma mater, went bankrupt. Under the name Harvard Pilgrim, it spun off its core group and was revived as a plan that contracts with many small practices.

Surveying the wreckage of the past decade, James C. Robinson, a health economist at the University of California at Berkeley, writes, "Vertical integration [of health care] survived only where the staff- and group-model HMOs constituted a large portion of the local market and hence offered sufficient physician choice and enjoyed economies of scale comparable to those of non-integrated competitors."[14]

Obstacles to Large Groups   Even large multispecialty groups that are not prepaid or exclusive to any one insurer have had trouble. Since the late 1990s, dozens of big group practices have broken up, gone bankrupt, or been sold. Among them are such well-known groups as the Nalle Clinic in Charlotte, North Carolina, the Burns Clinic in Petoskey, Michigan, the Thomas-Davis Medical Centers in Tucson, Arizona, and the Mullikin Clinic in Los Angeles.

What afflicted these groups? Some of them made the mistake of selling out to the physician practice management companies that swept across the United States in the late 1990s, offering investors visions of fantastic returns. When these firms were unable to deliver on their promise, they self-destructed. Doctors often didn't get paid, and some left their groups; others took on mountains of debt to buy back their practices. In some instances, the groups just sank in a sea of economic turmoil.[15]

Even well-run multispecialty groups tend to have higher costs per doctor than single-specialty groups do, so doctors can expect to earn less in them.[16] Also, specialists and primary-care physicians are constantly at loggerheads in multispecialty practices, because the primary doctors generate less income and have higher overhead costs. While groups have tried many methods to make income distribution equitable, the specialists tend to feel they're subsidizing the generalists and that they could do better on their own.[17]

According to a study of physician groups in twelve large markets, some multispecialty practices were formed in the 1990s "to gain negotiating leverage with HMOs and to spread the financial risk of risk contracting [i.e., prepaid care]." However, when it became clear that prepaid care was not the wave of the future, these efforts faltered. By 2001, "attempts to create large multi-specialty groups had ceased at all 12 sites, as groups' continued financial problems plus the growing backlash against managed care led HMOs to pull back from narrow provider networks and risk contracting."[18]

Specialists Feel Their Oats   During much of the 1990s, specialists were on the defensive. HMOs tried to limit the use of expensive tests and procedures, and they rewarded primary-care physicians who did as much as possible for patients before referring them to specialists. As a result, specialists' incomes sank, and an increasing number of young physicians entered primary care.

Today, because of the retreat of managed care, the pendulum has swung the other way. "Gatekeeper"-style HMOs are fading out; direct access to specialists is widespread; and primary-care physicians tend to do less for patients before referring them out.

"We pay them so little for their evaluation and management services that in many cases, if a primary-care physician can't figure right away what's wrong with a patient, he's not going to sit there and take the time," says health-policy expert Marilyn Moon. "He's going to send the patient to a specialist. Because he's not getting compensated to do more."

By working harder, primary-care physicians generated 31 percent more revenue in 2002 than in 1998, but their net incomes increased less than 10 percent.[19] That's partly because their overhead costs grew much faster than revenue: The average physician had to add an extra employee just to handle the additional paperwork generated by health plans and the government. Also, government and private payers weren't increasing their reimbursement enough to keep up with inflation. In real dollars, primary-care physicians earned 10 percent less in 2003 than in 1995.[20]

Meanwhile, the wide gap between the incomes of primary-care physicians and specialists has kept growing. Generalists earned an average of 2.4 percent more in 2003 than in 2002, while specialists' income rose by 8 percent.[21] In 2005, invasive cardiologists earned a median $400,200 and gastroenterologists, $300,000; general internists, in contrast, made $157,000, and family doctors, $150,000.[22]

Considering the difference in income expectations, it's not surprising that so many young physicians are flocking to the specialties and avoiding primary care. The number of U.S. medical school graduates who choose residency training in family medicine has been steadily sinking in recent years. The only reason this isn't true for internal medicine is that many internists subspecialize in high-paying fields like cardiology, gastroenterology, and pulmonology. In fact, three-quarters of internal-medicine residency graduates go on to fellowships in subspecialties rather than into primary-care practice.[23]

Not surprisingly, only about a third of U.S. physicians work in primary-care fields.[24] In countries such as Canada, Germany, and France, which spend far less than we do on health care, about half of the doctors provide primary care.[25] And as we've discovered, the regions of our country that have the fewest primary-care physicians receive the poorest care at the highest cost. That situation can only worsen as the percentage of specialists in the workforce increases.

One hopeful sign is that the Centers for Medicare and Medicaid Services has finally recognized that it's paying too little for cognitive services, which are the bread and butter of primary care. Recently, the agency proposed changes in its fee schedule that would raise Medicare payments to family physicians and general internists by about 5 percent, while chopping reimbursements of medical specialists and surgeons. But if the planned cuts in overall Medicare payments to physicians are implemented (see Chapter 4), primary-care physicians won't see any of this increase.[26]

Primary-Care Coordination   While effective care management requires the cooperation of many specialties and the integration of services across many different settings of care, good care coordination does not require multispecialty groups. But it does require a method of ensuring that providers work together.

"There are several mechanisms for coordinating care across priority [health] conditions," the IOM report states. "First, coordination could be performed by a health professional acting as a liaison across patients' multiple needs, ensuring the exchange of information and any necessary follow-up. This individual could be a physician, nurse, case manager, or other type of professional working in the care delivery system. . . . Primary-care models offer one approach to coordination, in which the primary-care practitioner is both provider and coordinator of care."[27]

Primary-care coordination of professional services makes sense because only primary-care physicians—defined as family physicians, general practitioners, general internists, and pediatricians—have a comprehensive view of a patient's needs, and because they're the best-equipped to oversee the work of specialists, at least on the outpatient side. (As I show in Chapter 20, a particular kind of primary-care physician who does only hospital work is best-suited for supervision of inpatient care.)

Need to Form Groups   Primary-care physicians can coordinate care effectively and provide systematic disease management, however, only when they work together in groups. Primary-care physicians in groups can implement electronic health records, reduce practice variations, measure performance, and improve the quality of care much more easily than they can in small practices. And if these groups are big enough, they can safely take financial responsibility for all professional services—a key component of the reform model proposed in this book.

Must doctors be in commonly owned groups or could they remain in separate practices that belong to independent practice associations? Most independent practice associations (IPAs) that have achieved a significant degree of clinical integration (meaning that doctors collaborate to improve care) are in California, where the HMOs have delegated financial accountability and medical management to both IPAs and physician groups. In the rest of the country, it's doubtful that most doctors would be able to work together effectively in IPAs. Most of these organizations are simply too weak and, up to now, have contributed too little of physicians' income to get their attention.

However, it would be difficult to assemble sizable physician groups in most rural areas. In those regions, clinically integrated IPAs with common information systems would serve the need better. While these IPAs might never overcome the inherent obstacles to cooperation, they could at least help physicians practice in a more uniform manner and find the resources they would need for their patients.

Parameters of Group Size   Except in rural areas far away from cities, primary-care groups of sufficient size to take financial risk and improve care could be built almost everywhere. This means that primary-care practices could be the basis for competitive markets across the country.

How big is a group of "sufficient size"? Stephen Shortell says his research shows that doctors don't start using care management processes extensively until they're in groups of at least a hundred physicians. Lawrence Casalino cautions, however, that very large groups tend to be bureaucratic and lose the "warm intangibles" in the patient-doctor relationship. Yet he admits that small groups may not be able to afford the information systems and infrastructure required to do disease management and measure performance. Under a system in which doctors were financially rewarded for meeting quality goals, a medium-sized group—say, one of ten to thirty doctors—might be able to do this, he says.

Some groups of this size have taken financial responsibility for primary and specialty care. For example, PacifiCare, an HMO based in Cypress, California, has delegated full professional risk to many groups that range in size from twenty to eighty doctors.[28] And about ten years ago, a firm called North American Medical Management succeeded in organizing dozens of small, multispecialty networks that were financially accountable for all professional services.[29] On the average, these IPAs included only about twenty primary-care physicians and thirty to sixty specialists

Geographical Considerations   When calculating the optimal size for primary-care groups, one must also consider how many doctors practice in each market where these groups would compete with one another in a reformed health care system. In 2002, the population of the one hundred largest cities in the United States ranged from about 8 million (New York) down to about 200,000 (Spokane, Washington).[30] In New York, there were about 30,100 primary-care physicians; in Spokane, only 430.[31] In cities that are half of Spokane's size, there might be as few as 200 primary-care physicians.

Allowing for the inclusion of doctors in outlying areas, enough groups of twenty to fifty primary-care physicians could be formed to offer real competition in these less populated regions. However, they'd need some outside administrative support to provide effective care management. Larger metropolitan areas could host competing groups of fifty to a hundred physicians. Those organizations could build most of the requisite infrastructure by themselves.

To summarize, primary-care groups could coordinate all patient care in cooperation with hospitalists, and enough of them could be formed in most nonrural areas to create a competitive market for health care services. But if we want these groups to coordinate care and practice cost-efficiently, they also have to take financial responsibility for professional services, which is the subject of the next chapter.

14 Why Groups Should Take Financial Risk

Sarah, a resident of Oklahoma City, was eighty-seven when she suffered a stroke in 2002. The stroke paralyzed her on one side and affected her speech. Until then, she'd been living at home and taking care of herself with some help from her family. She was mentally sharp and physically healthy for someone of her age. Her physician, an internist named Mary Ann Bauman, thought Sarah would be an excellent candidate for inpatient rehabilitation therapy. But the patient's health plan declined to pay for rehab, which can take two to six weeks. So she went to a nursing home, where she died a short time later.

"Sometimes when you just warehouse older people, they die," Bauman notes. "She would have had a better shot at survival if she'd gotten rehab. My relationship with the managed-care company deteriorated after that, because I felt they were not trusting my judgment."

None of this would have happened a year earlier, when Bauman's medical group, Integris Physicians, was taking financial responsibility for patient care. That meant that, in return for a fixed sum each month, Integris and its affiliated hospital were providing all care that each patient needed. Under that financial arrangement, known as "global capitation," Bauman could have done whatever she thought was best for Sarah, she notes.

"The difference under our old contracts was that we took the financial risk. I knew that I was spending the group's dollars, but that was my decision. If the rehab people said she could go, then she could go. The managed care company didn't care; they had already paid us a set sum, and they had their profit."

The number of physician groups taking financial responsibility for care has declined radically in most parts of the nation since the 1990s.

The most important reason is that, outside of California and a few other areas, most physicians simply didn't understand how to practice cost-efficiently without sacrificing quality. Consequently, they didn't do well under prepaid care, and they resented it. Coupled with the public back-lash against managed care, physicians' resistance eventually persuaded many insurers to end this form of contracting.[1]

By the time Integris Physicians' capitation contracts were rescinded, however, the fifty primary-care physicians in the group had fully embraced prepaid care, Bauman says. One reason was that it benefited them economically. The typical Integris physician was earning 40 percent more per unit of service for taking care of HMO patients than traditional, fee-for-service Medicare paid him or her for the same unit of service. Today, after the deep discounts that plans extract from them, the doctors are reimbursed just slightly more than Medicare pays them for doing the same work.

High Quality Equals Good Outcomes The rap on capitation is that it encourages physicians to stint on care. But that wasn't true at Integris, Bauman maintains. While it took most of the physicians some time to learn how to deliver care efficiently, she says, they never cut corners, and patient outcomes were excellent.

"You don't have good outcomes if you don't have good quality," Bauman says. "There's no sense in saving a bunch of money and then having a catastrophic case that costs you a million dollars. And if your patients are unhappy because they always feel they're being denied stuff, they're going to complain and they're not going to stay with you."

Shared financial accountability also gave the group's doctors a strong incentive to improve their quality of care and to make sure their colleagues did the same. "If someone had a deficit in a given year, we all made it up for them," notes Bauman. "So it was important for me to know that Dr. X on the north side of town was practicing the same style of medicine and with the same cost effectiveness as I was. That's how we really became a group. We started making decisions as a group, formed our quality committee and so on. Yes, we had a financial interaction, but we also had a quality interaction."

Although Bauman's group is trying its best to preserve the care guidelines that served them well under capitation, the physicians have had to adjust their approach to maintain their incomes. All of them are seeing more patients and ordering more tests from the group's labs than they used to, and they're not practicing as cost effectively as before, because they have no incentive to.

"Under our former system, when a person was ready to leave the hospital at eight o'clock at night, I discharged them," Bauman recalls. "I told them, 'You can stay another day, but you'll have to pay for it, because you're ready to go home.' I was making the medical decision, just as I do now. But I was also going over to the hospital to discharge them at eight o'clock at night. Now, there's no incentive to do that, so I'll wait until the next morning. That's a $1,500 hotel bill. And this is happening all over the country."

Taking It to the Max   The new paradigm of primary care is what doctors call "eat what you kill." Under this productivity-driven, fee-for-service approach, primary-care physicians run like hamsters on a treadmill, trying to jam as many patients as they can into their office schedule. If they're in group practices, physicians add ancillary services and order as many tests as they can from their own labs.[2]

You can't blame primary-care physicians for trying to maintain their incomes. Even while overall health spending shoots up, their revenues are barely keeping pace with inflation, and their overhead—including malpractice insurance premiums—continues to escalate.[3]

Nevertheless, a growing number of doctors are using questionable tactics to keep their earnings up. Some physicians have resorted to scheduling follow-up visits for minor matters, like prescription refills or normal test results that could have been dealt with over the phone or by mail. Some practices even charge "access" fees that give patients the right to have after-hours phone consultations with doctors, call in refill requests, exchange e-mail with physicians, and so on.[4]

The Bad Old Days   Despite the perverse incentives of fee-for-service, most physicians prefer it to capitation, partly because it's what they're used to. Some medical societies also oppose prepaid care on the grounds that it motivates doctors to undertreat patients and undermines the doctor-patient relationship. Underlying both attitudes is the conviction that, even if fee-for-service doesn't pay well, doctors would do even worse with a monthly budget. These fears aren't entirely misplaced: Physicians do earn less on the West Coast, where HMO penetration is high, than they do in the southeast, where fee-for-service has always held sway.[5] But in California, fee-for-service PPOs pay less than doctors can make under capitation contracts.[6]

Across most of the country, neither physicians nor patients had had much experience with managed care until the early 1990s. Then, all of a sudden, they had a profit-driven version of the California managed-care formula crammed down their throats. A phalanx of insurers, vying for the business of employers who wanted to cut their health costs, set up physician networks, contracting either with independent practice associations (IPAs) or with individual practices. These HMOs had their own requirements for referrals, authorizations, and permissible drugs, but they all demanded deep discounts from doctors and hospitals in return for business.

Primary-care physicians often received capitation payments for their own services, with the promise of a bonus or return of a "withhold" if they kept down the number of costly tests and referrals to specialists. All this meant to many doctors was that they'd be paid less if they didn't limit care. Many confused the monthly payment they received for each patient with the amount that fee-for-service plans paid them for office visits, not realizing they were getting paid for patients who did not come in.

Many HMOs also required primary-care physicians to act as "gate-keepers," meaning that they had to provide referrals for HMO members to see specialists. Health plans also had to approve the referrals. In reality, few were denied, but both doctors and patients resented having to jump through these hoops.

The Rise and Fall of "Risk" Contracts   Some primary-care and multispecialty groups signed "professional risk" contracts, under which they received a monthly sum to cover all physician services and diagnostic tests for each patient. These agreements usually allowed doctors to share some of the money saved by reducing the use of specialists, tests, and hospitals.[7]

Except in California, the upper Midwest, and a few other regions, most doctors who accepted these contracts had no idea how to practice within a budget. They'd been operating in a nearly unrestricted fee-for-service environment and usually still had as many fee-for-service patients as HMO patients. So they tended to practice the way they'd been practicing all along. And if they were in a small group that was taking financial responsibility for all professional services, they were guaranteed to fail. Not only did they not have enough doctors to share the economic risk but they lacked the infrastructure to manage it.[8]

As a result, few groups outside California made money on risk contracts, and many lost their shirts. Moreover, there was widespread public opposition to the "gatekeeper" approach. By the time that the HMOs decided that delegating financial responsibility to physician groups and IPAs was more trouble than it was worth, many physicians had already come to the same conclusion.

The California Experience   West Coast physicians had been practicing in a managed-care environment since the 1980s, and those in Kaiser Permanente, for much longer. So the idea of prepaid care was not strange to them, and it seemed quite natural to take on insurance company functions like physician credentialing and utilization review. Some groups that had professional risk or full-risk capitation contracts (which also covered hospital care) did quite well for a time.

"Everybody thought they could control the cost," recalls Ronald Bangasser, a family physician who practices in a 145-doctor multispecialty group in Redlands, California. "We began looking at how long people stayed in the hospital, and moved them out of the hospital if they didn't need to be there. Then we started talking about alternative levels of care, and how you could put somebody who was on IV antibiotics in a nursing home or have them on IV antibiotics at home. That kind of stuff dramatically shifted the cost of care from the hospital to the outpatient side. Huge chunks of money were being saved in the mid- to late eighties. I remember we were earning a significant amount of money because of the reduction in hospital utilization. Later on, pharmacy risk came in, and that was just the opposite. We were never able to control that."

Capitation Rates Plunge   By the time physician groups started taking financial responsibility for prescription drugs in the late 1990s, the economics of the delegated-risk model were careening out of control, mainly because in 1997, California HMOs began cutting capitation rates. Over the next three years, HMO payments to physician groups dropped between 20 and 30 percent.[9] As a result of this decline and of the turmoil created by investor-driven physician practice management companies, scores of IPAs and groups went out of business. Many other physicians were also severely affected by the reduction in health care spending.

Since then, capitation rates have mostly recovered—although they haven't gone up as fast as insurance premiums. The groups that survived are doing much better economically. For example, the Bristol Park Medical Group, an eighty-three-doctor primary care organization in Irvine, California, is now earning $1 on HMO contracts for every 60 cents it makes from fee-for-service PPO plans.[10]

Bristol Park takes professional risk and shares financial responsibility for inpatient care with a local hospital system. It's large enough to afford a clinical information system and case managers, and it has a utilization management committee that keeps a close eye on how resources are used. The group encourages its family physicians, internists, and pediatricians to do as much as they can for each patient, and it contracts only with specialists who practice cost-effectively.

After all the ups and downs of managed care, the internist Andrew Siskind, Bristol Park's former president, still believes in it. "We think it's the only system where the incentive is to keep the patient healthy," he says. "There is no other system that has that incentive. So we like that. To us, it's the most ethical way of practicing medicine."

Physician-Managed Care

In the view of some experts, however, the disaster that hit California groups in the 1990s proved that physicians couldn't manage care by themselves. "We tried this, and it failed miserably," Uwe Reinhardt of Princeton University says. "When capitation rates fell to levels where physician groups couldn't cover fixed costs, they went bankrupt."

Reinhardt is right, yet the physicians were not to blame for the plunge in capitation rates. When prepaid groups in California and elsewhere decreased hospital utilization, keeping the difference between their budgets and the actual costs, the HMOs figured they could get away with paying doctors less. That allowed them to hold down their premiums and increase their own profits at the groups' expense. So even where doctors did learn how to manage care, their success became their undoing. Group budgeting was not inherently a flawed concept; health plans and self-insured employers just wanted to keep the savings themselves.

Group capitation could be part of the solution, however, if groups could set their own budgets and if patients could choose among them, using published cost and quality rankings. If doctors knew that by de-livering better care at a lower cost, they could attract more patients and earn more money, the health care system would have a fundamentally different dynamic.

In his 1993 book *Strong Medicine*, George Halvorson, now CEO of Kaiser Permanente, proposes a system of competing "prepaid account-able care teams." According to Halvorson, prepayment is infinitely supe-rior to fee for service, which provides an incentive for doctors to do more rather than to provide better care. However, he adds two caveats: The system would have to be designed to encourage quality measurement and continuous improvement, and individual physicians would have to be protected from excessive financial risk.[11]

Controlling the Risk   One of the black holes of risk is hospital care, which can be hugely expensive. In California, the typical approach is for prepaid groups to share inpatient risk with HMOs or hospitals. But global capitation has fallen out of favor with hospitals everywhere. Even if they were willing to participate, this form of risk sharing would limit where patients could be admitted and would prompt a new round of practice purchases by hospitals, making markets less competitive.

For these reasons, the groups in our reform model should be respon-sible only for professional services, including primary care, specialty care, outpatient tests, and outpatient drugs. If tests or procedures were done in a hospital's outpatient department, the ambulatory services would be part of hospital charges. But the primary care groups would take risk for all physician services, except for those furnished by hospital-employed radiologists, anesthesiologists, pathologists, emergency-medicine special-ists, and hospitalists.

Pharmacy risk was challenging in the past because drug capitation rates were set too low, doctors found it hard to deal with multiple for-mularies (lists of approved medications), and groups had no access to drug claims data, which made it difficult to track costs. But in this model, each group would maintain its own formulary and would have access to all pharmacy claims data. In addition, as I show later, regional buying cooperatives would enable the groups to obtain good prices on most prescription drugs.

Even if a physician group were financially responsible only for pro-fessional services, it could have higher-than-expected costs because of a few very expensive cases. To deal with the possibility of catastrophic costs, each group should be required to buy stop-loss insurance, which kicks in after the cost of a case passes a certain point. If the groups were fairly large, the cost of this insurance would not be prohibitive.

To even out the risk of one group—particularly one with superior quality scores—attracting sicker patients than another, capitation payments to groups should be "risk-adjusted." This means that the amount budgeted for care by each group should be ratcheted up or down, depending on the expected costs of caring for the patients who signed up with that group.

Contracting with Specialists   All primary-care groups would have to be guaranteed equal access to available specialists. Besides being a medical and a competitive necessity, this requirement would also allow a wider range of patient choice. Thus, no group or hospital could contract exclusively with any specialist. Groups must be free to contract with the best, most cost-effective specialists, and specialists must be able to walk away from deals that would pay them too little.

To create or preserve this negotiating space, the federal government must exercise its antitrust power. A limit should be placed on the size of specialty groups in relation to the market, and unrelated surgeons and subspecialists should be prohibited from colluding to force up reimbursement from primary-care groups.

Capitated groups in California have discovered how difficult it can be to bargain with outside specialists or with specialist members of IPAs. Steve Howard, a family doctor in San Carlos, California, recalls that when the HMOs cut his IPA's capitation rate, "the surgeons said, 'We need a 30 percent raise, otherwise you won't have surgeons next week.' " The IPA had no choice but to pay the surgeons what they wanted, he says, and then all the other specialists lined up for theirs. "That happened with every IPA. And after a while, the IPAs found themselves unable to maintain payments. They all fell behind."

A Refined "Gatekeeper" Approach   To manage their resources well, primary-care physicians must do as much as they can for patients before referring them to specialists. While this approach carries the "gatekeeper" stigma, it's absolutely necessary to contain costs and provide high-quality care. Patients oppose any limitation on their ability to see specialists; yet they might not object as much if they were allowed to go directly to specialists in return for higher out-of-pocket payments.

Surveys indicate that as more of the cost of care has been shifted to consumers, they've become more receptive to the gatekeeper concept. A 2004 poll conducted by the National Opinion Research Center revealed that 52 percent of consumers would go through a gatekeeper to see specialists if that would keep their health expenses down.[12] And in a 2003 survey of insured adults, the Center for Studying Health System Change found that 59 percent agreed with the statement: "I'd be willing to accept a limited choice of physicians and hospitals if I could save money on my out-of-pocket costs for health care."[13]

The reform model I'm proposing, moreover, would be much less restrictive than traditional HMOs with narrow networks. In addition to being able to self-refer to specialists for an additional cost, patients could select any primary-care physician they liked. Their choice would not be limited to the physicians in a particular group; they'd be able to switch groups at regular intervals. So, while they'd have less freedom of movement than patients in PPOs do now, they'd have a greater overall choice of physicians.

Patients would also be able to see obstetrician/gynecologists without a referral, and they could obtain referrals to certain specialists for extended periods; for example, a patient with a heart condition would be able to see his or her cardiologist whenever necessary. Similar arrangements could be made with ancillary providers such as nutritionists and physical therapists, and patients would be able to seek care in urgent care centers or retail clinics without a referral. But all of these providers would have to keep the patient's primary-care physician informed about what they were doing for the patient and the patient's health status.

Under this system, each person would have a "medical home"—a physician who coordinates that person's care and guides him or her through the health care system. Few specialists can do that well.[14] Yet today, many people rely on specialists and rarely, if ever, see a family physician or a general internist. So for this approach to succeed, we'd have to mount a massive public education campaign about the importance of primary care and the proper role of specialists.

Preventing Conflicts of Interest   Capitation can influence doctors to withhold care from patients, just as fee-for-service can predispose them to do unnecessary tests and procedures.[15] These conflicts of interest can be reduced if doctors work in larger groups and their compensation blends different incentives. For example, doctors in pre-paid groups may be paid a combination of salary (which doesn't reward overuse) and productivity-based compensation (which motivates them to work hard).[16] To further discourage doctors from underusing, over-using, or misusing services, key indicators of quality and access would be continuously measured, as Halvorson has urged. So patterns of poor care would not remain invisible for long.

Some experts point to the inherent conflict between a physician's duty to each patient and the expectation of managed care that he'll carefully husband the resources available to all the patients in his group or health plan. The problem, according to E. Haavi Morreim, a medical ethicist at the University of Tennessee, is that "the physician cannot both favor his patients' interests and also distribute resources impartially."[17]

When physicians must do "bedside rationing" of scarce resources or deny clearly beneficial care to patients, this conflict can be quite troubling. Henry Aaron and William Schwartz explore the dilemma in a penetrating book that analyzes rationing in the United Kingdom and its implications for the future of U.S. health care. In the United Kingdom, they note, physicians tend to justify their rationing decisions by lowering their standards. "Faced with tight budget constraints, doctors gradually redefine standards of care so that they can escape the constant recognition that financial limits compel them to do less than their best."[18]

As Aaron and Schwartz observe, this type of rationing would be very difficult for U.S. physicians to do. But fortunately, we haven't yet reached the point where we have to limit care to that extent. If physician groups could make their own budgets, rather than have them determined by a profit-making HMO, they could set them at a level that allowed them to provide all care that was covered by a standard benefit package.

Ultimately, published quality and cost indicators like the ones de-scribed in the next chapter would enable patients to hold the physician groups accountable for their financial decisions. While many patients wouldn't look at quality scores, the groups would be aware of them and would want to rank as high as possible.

The Positive Side of Control   Some physicians have discov-ered that being in charge of a health care budget can be liberating. For example, Kenneth Gjeltema, a family physician who belongs to a prepaid IPA in the San Francisco Bay area, told me a story several years ago: "I have a patient who's dying in the hospital," he said at the time. "I could transfer him to the skilled nursing facility at the hospital, send him to an outside nursing home, or send him home with hospice care. I know what each of those costs, but I get to make the choice, depending on what the family wants. The family is more comfortable with him being at the hospital's skilled nursing facility, and though the outside facility is $50 a day cheaper, it's not worth the difference. I get to make the decision, and that's really nice. It helps the patient and helps the family."[19]

While Gjeltema has had to make choices that are much harder than this one, he has the satisfaction of knowing that an HMO cannot over-rule him. "I'm the one who has to face the patient and say, 'I want you to do this.' In some cases, it's not nice to be the rationer of care; but I'd rather have it be me than the HMO medical director."

15 A Real-World Model for Reform

On January 1, 2005, a grand social experiment ended in Minneapolis. On that day Medica, one of the city's three dominant health plans, incorporated Patient Choice—which it had purchased in 2004—into its line of insurance products.[1]

Inaugurated in 1996 by the Buyers' Health Care Action Group (BHCAG), a coalition of big, self-insured companies, the Patient Choice program was the most extensive attempt by U.S. employers to contract directly with health care providers.[2] Although Patient Choice used third-party administrators to enroll employees and pay claims, BHCAG's members were, in effect, contracting with about two dozen physician groups and independent practice associations (IPAs)—known as "care systems"—for all patient care.

The groups, which included most primary-care physicians in the Twin Cities, set their own budgets and managed care by themselves. They contracted with specialists and hospitals and competed for patients on the basis of published measures of cost and quality. These report cards had a real impact, because Patient Choice members paid more of the premium if they picked higher-priced care systems.[3]

Patient Choice has not disappeared. Ann Robinow, who ran the operation before its sale and is now vice president and general manager of Medica's Patient Choice division, says Medica will be able to grow the program with its superior marketing ability. And Aaron Reynolds, executive vice president of the health plan, promises that Medica will leave the unique aspects of Patient Choice alone. But to doctors who've grown tired of dealing with health plans that cut their reimbursement and limit their clinical autonomy, Patient Choice was a breath of fresh air that's been shut off.

"Patient Choice tried to get everyone's incentives aligned appropriately," says Rolf Skogerboe, MD, a longtime member of the eighty-doctor Columbia Park Medical Group in Minneapolis. "And you have to applaud that, because the incentives of a health plan are not typically aligned with either the patient's or the doctor's incentives. They're at cross-purposes to both, so they make everybody mad. This was an honest attempt by employers whose interest was to do the best job they could for their employees."

Physician Loyalty Remains   At its height in 1998, Patient Choice had about 150,000 enrollees;[4] when Medica purchased it, that number had shrunk to around 80,000, mainly because some of the larger employers had been lured away by rival health plans that promised to cut their premiums.[5] Efforts to transport the idea to other cities and regions across the country failed. And despite all of BHCAG's efforts, health costs are now growing just as fast in Minnesota as they are elsewhere. So why is this experiment relevant to health care reform today?

One reason is that physicians like it. Although Patient Choice never contributed more than 5 percent of the business of most groups that participated in it, all of them stuck with it even after it was acquired by Medica.[6] That in itself speaks volumes about the interest and the hope it spawned among physicians.

"The concept and the model are good," says Mark Fisher, CEO of the Minnesota Healthcare Network, an IPA with about four hundred primary-care physicians. "Most, if not all, providers saw this as a good thing to be part of and stayed with it."

Physicians appreciate Patient Choice, he adds, because it lets them show what they can do to improve care and restrain costs without interfering with their clinical autonomy. "Patient Choice is head and shoulders above other plans we work with," Fisher says. "Because right from the beginning, its leaders recognized that they had to work with the doctors and the clinics and the care systems to let their quality shine through."

Employers See Savings   Employers also realized cost savings from the program. In 1998, two years after the provider groups started competing with one another for patients, the average cost to companies for employees who enrolled in Patient Choice was 20 percent below the average commercial rate of Minnesota HMOs.[7] Cost increases for the BHCAG employers from 1997 to 1999 were 5–6 percent a year. By comparison, state employees, who had a choice of health plans that didn't include Patient Choice, saw their premiums rise 6–13 percent a year in the same time period.[8]

From 1999 to 2003, Robinow says, Patient Choice's annual cost hikes averaged about 6 percent a year, two points below the market average. In 2003, the cost increase was almost 7 percent, she says. By comparison, total HMO premium revenue in Minnesota jumped 8 percent in 2003, according to Allan Baumgarten, a Minneapolis-based consultant who tracks HMO data in several states. The real figure, he adds, was probably closer to 10 percent, since Medica, the state's largest HMO, gave some of its profits back to customers in that year.

Robinow attributes much of the difference in cost growth to the migration of patients to more efficient providers over the years. Some of the absolute cost difference, she adds, stemmed from the program's very low administrative cost—only 5 percent of total spending.

Regulatory Barrier to Growth   Why didn't Patient Choice keep growing on its own? Aside from the ruthless competition of the market's three giant plans,[9] the program was limited to companies that were big enough to take the insurance risk for their employees. Without a state insurance license—which would have required the maintenance of large financial reserves—Patient Choice couldn't offer a fully insured product to small and medium-sized employers.

Also, Robinow explains, the initial use of a standard benefit package deterred many employers that wanted to offer different benefits or that had to provide certain benefits under union contracts. In 2000, Patient Choice relented and started offering multiple benefit packages.

The number-one reason Patient Choice failed to spread beyond Minnesota is that there are no other markets where most physicians belong to group practices. Also, physicians in most parts of the country don't know how to manage care. In contrast, Minnesota doctors are thoroughly familiar with managed care and have internalized the goal of practicing cost efficiently.

Jonathan Weiner, of Johns Hopkins University, cites the "conservative nature of practice" in Minnesota. "If you look at the John Wennberg studies [of practice variations] and Medicare data, it's always Minnesota at one end of the spectrum. And the reason for that is group practice and the HMOs, which have always been a big piece of how they practice in Minnesota."

Weiner co-authored a paper on the BHCAG experiment that shows that, from 1997 to 1999, Patient Choice "appeared to perform reasonably well in containing costs, without measurable adverse effects on quality."[10] Arguing in a 2004 interview that the program was still "first rate," he cited its pioneering use of diagnosis-based risk adjustment to pay physician groups and its role in founding the Institute for Clinical Systems Improvement, which helped develop statewide clinical guidelines (see Chapter 7). Patient Choice's use of report cards on provider groups, he added, has spread to the local health plans as well as the state employees' system. As a result, consumers have more information about doctors and hospitals in the Twin Cities than they do anywhere else.

Employers Try to Break Through   Patient Choice emerged from earlier efforts by BHCAG to do "value-based purchasing." A coalition of fourteen of Minneapolis's largest employers, including General Mills, Honeywell, Pillsbury, and 3M, BHCAG tried to get the area's group practices and integrated delivery systems to bid for the employers' business by providing evidence that they delivered appropriate care. In 1992, BHCAG contracted with a consortium that included Health Partners (which is a physician group as well as an HMO), the Mayo Clinic, and the Park Nicollet Clinic. Health Partners administered a "point of service" plan for BHCAG, using a network of seventy group practices that included about nine hundred doctors. The providers were reimbursed on a fee-for-service basis, and BHCAG employers took the insurance risk.[11]

In response to Health Partners' coup, other local insurers consolidated into two big plans, Blue Cross and Blue Shield of Minnesota and Medica. This move presented BHCAG with a problem: Its employer members wanted to encourage competition among provider groups, based on their quality and efficiency, but now they were dealing with three dominant health plans that had widely overlapping networks and that averaged all of the groups' data together. Unable to distinguish among these plans or their networks, BHCAG firms decided to try something bold and different: While keeping the option of enrolling in traditional health plans, they'd let their employees choose from a menu of "care systems" instead. BHCAG defined a care system as a group of primary-care physicians affiliated with specialists and hospitals.[12]

Health Partners initially provided administrative support to this fledgling effort, which would become Patient Choice. But later, the HMO withdrew after deciding Patient Choice was a rival.

The Emergence of Tiering   Each care system was required to submit a bid that was essentially a budget to provide all care for enrollees in the ensuing year. Nineteen care systems tendered offers in March 1996, and seventeen of the bids (two from organizations outside of Minneapolis/St. Paul) were accepted. Ranging from $80 to $105 per member per month, these "targets" were 9.5 percent below the costs BHCAG employers had projected for 1997.[13]

Of the fifteen Twin Cities care systems that originally participated in Patient Choice, five were organized by physician groups, five by hospitals, and five by health plans.[14] (Today, of the sixteen care systems in Minneapolis/St. Paul, six are physician-owned, nine are operated by hospitals and physicians, and one is owned by a health plan.)[15] But however it was structured, the core of each care system consisted of the primary-care physicians who were exclusive to it. When a patient signed up with Patient Choice, he chose a doctor in one of the groups, and the cost of the care he received was attributed to that group, regardless of which specialists or hospitals were used.[16]

Using its members' claims data, BHCAG slotted the care systems into low- , medium- , and high-cost categories or "tiers." Of the twenty-four employers involved, seventeen paid the total cost for employees who chose groups in the low-cost tier. Workers who picked one of the high-cost groups had an average of $37 a month deducted from their paychecks.[17]

Virtual Capitation   Only a licensed insurance entity could legally prepay the groups. So, to make the care systems financially accountable, BHCAG adopted a payment method known as "virtual capitation." Each group was required to submit an annual budget for patient care. If the group's costs fell below that target in a particular quarter, BHCAG would raise the doctors' fee-for-service reimbursement; if the group exceeded the target, the amount paid for each service was cut proportionately.[18]

If a group attracted more sick patients than it had expected, it would overspend its budget for reasons beyond its control. So BHCAG added another pioneering feature known as "risk adjustment." Using a system devised by experts at Johns Hopkins University, the coalition's administrators adjusted payments to each group based on the differences among the diagnoses and acuity of illness of its patients.[19] This approach is significantly different from that of most HMOs, which vary capitation payments only on the basis of age and sex.

Besides increasing the fairness of reimbursement, risk adjustment also made it possible for employers to compare the performance of groups. "If you don't take into account the variations in how sick different organizations' populations are, you're not measuring anything meaningful," Ann Robinow says. "You're just measuring who dodged risk the best."

Backing Away from Risk   After decades of living with HMOs, many Twin Cities physicians did not have a problem with virtual capitation. In the early going, BHCAG made it more palatable to doctors by protecting them from financial losses until they had a certain number of patients in the program.

In the late 1990s, however, as the HMOs cut physician reimbursement, capitation began to acquire a distinctly unpleasant aroma. Concurrently, HMOs were under attack from the public. So Minnesota, like most of the rest of the country, backed away from prepaid care. Between 2000 and 2003, the percentage of provider revenues that came from capitation contracts plummeted from 35.7 percent to 8.4 percent.[20]

Patient Choice responded by removing the element of financial risk from its reimbursement method in 2000.[21] Although care systems still submit annual budgets—expressed as the pricing of services—their reimbursement is no longer tied to whether they meet those targets. Instead, they set their own fees and project the other costs of care, and each care system's "bid" is combined with the prior year's claims to determine whether the group belongs in the low- , medium- , or high-cost tier. If a group lowers its utilization and raises its prices commensurately, it will remain in the same tier, and vice versa, Robinow says.

Rating Groups on Quality   Patient Choice bases its published quality ratings on indicators of clinical quality, patient satisfaction, access, and service. Initially, the program used patient surveys to measure group performance. In 2004, it began asking the physicians to voluntarily submit clinical data in areas such as diabetes, coronary artery disease, and preventive care. That year, about a third of the groups submitted quality information.[22] Currently, the big Minneapolis plans, including Patient Choice parent Medica, send auditors into medical offices to harvest data from patient records.[23]

Three-quarters of Patient Choice enrollees who responded to a 1998 survey said they used information about care systems provided by their companies. Respondents said they relied mainly on ratings of a care system's overall quality and service. Detailed aspects of the ratings were less helpful to them. High quality-scores attracted some respondents, regardless of whether they had to pay more to join a particular care system. But most employees were sensitive to premium differences.[24]

In 1998, the four lowest-cost clinics scored the biggest enrollment gains, ranging from 15 to 57 percent. Five mid-cost groups saw their enrollment increase between 2 and 20 percent, and one mid-cost care system with high quality ratings attracted 30 percent more members. The Allina Medical Group, which was in the high-cost tier, lost almost 20 percent of the employees of BHCAG companies who had to pay more out of pocket to belong to Allina. But the group had a net gain of Patient Choice enrollees because some employers still paid the same portion of premium, regardless of which group the worker picked.[25] (By 2004, all employers that offered Patient Choice required employees to pay more for higher-cost care systems.)[26]

Recent studies, Robinow notes, show that enrollees don't pay much attention to patient satisfaction ratings unless they've already decided to change care systems. But the data consistently indicate that employees do change groups based on cost, she says. This is not surprising, points out Patrick Taillefer, an administrator of the Quello Clinic, considering that the difference between choosing a care system in the top and bottom cost tiers can be $30 to $60 a month for a single person.[27]

Today, Robinow says, about 70 percent of Patient Choice enrollees belong to care systems in the lowest-priced tier, which has grown as more groups have reduced their costs. Additional providers would have improved their performance, she says, if Patient Choice had constituted a larger portion of their business.

David Wessner, CEO of the Park Nicollet Clinic, agrees. "If Patient Choice could have achieved a higher market share, the effect on the marketplace would have been real and significant," he says. "Because it didn't, the effect was not nearly what it could have been."

Patient Choice did, however, prove one thing, he observes: It showed that care systems could compete with one another on the basis of value. "Making that possible without being a health plan was the thing that Patient Choice brought to the marketplace."

Who Needs Competing Plans?

Patient Choice's success in lowering costs by having consumers choose among provider groups rather than health plans raises an important question: Why do we need competing health plans?

Unless we switch to a government-run system, private insurance entities of some kind will be needed to enroll patients, process claims, and contract with health care providers. Insurance companies must actuarially project the costs of care and combine them with administrative costs to determine how much the insured must pay in premiums. They also have to maintain financial reserves to absorb the ebbs and flows of health care outlays. It's certainly possible for a single insurance company to perform these functions in a given market. But, if we want competition among physician groups to replace health-plan competition, such an entity would have to be structured differently than today's health insurers are, and it would have to develop a whole new set of goals.

The Insurance Game   The primary aim of any insurance company—whether it calls itself for-profit or not-for-profit—is to make money. As George Halvorson puts it in *Strong Medicine*: "The hard reality is that the business goal of insurance companies is to collect more premium revenue than they have to pay out in claims and administrative costs. We do not pay insurers to improve health care, efficiency, or quality, and we do not reward them for spreading risk across large populations."[28]

Halvorson knew whereof he spoke: He was then head of Health Partners (he's now CEO of Kaiser Permanente). Among the strategies that insurers use to avoid risk, he noted, are cherry-picking the healthiest employer groups, charging higher premiums for older people and women, using pre-existing condition exclusions, and "experience-rating" consumers based on health status, past history of illness, family history, or occupation. These underwriting methods are used to deny insurance to small employers with sick employees or charge them such high prices that they can't afford insurance. Insurers have also been known to drop small firms when one employee becomes seriously ill.

The other problem with the insurance market is that it's inherently inefficient. Large companies pay much less for insurance than small ones do, because they have a better spread of risk and because it costs less per enrollee to market to them and administer their plans. Administrative expenses for small companies average about 20 percent of premium and can range up to 40 percent, according to Halvorson.

As single-payer advocates point out, this inefficiency is a large part of the reason our health care system is so expensive. Managed-care companies pay about 85 percent of their premium revenues, on average, for medical care. The other 15 percent goes to administration, sales and marketing costs, and profits.[29] By contrast, recall that Patient Care spent only 5 percent of its customers' money on functions unrelated to patient care.

Administrative Cost Savings   What are the implications of this for our health care reform model? Total U.S. health spending in 2004 was $1.88 trillion;[30] private health insurance covered $658 billion of that. If the health plans' administrative and marketing costs and profits had been only 5 percent, instead of 15 percent, we'd have saved 10 percent, or about $66 billion. That would have gone a long way toward covering the uninsured.

And this is only part of the savings that could be achieved if we didn't have multiple insurers. The average physician practice contracts with between ten and twenty health plans and handles many more benefit packages tailored to particular employers.[31] As a result of all the paperwork generated by this and by managed care, the number of staffers needed to support each doctor has risen exponentially in the past several years.[32] A recent study of California practices showed that billing and insurance-related costs soaked up 13.9 percent of revenues in multispecialty groups and 14.5 percent in primary-care groups. In California acute-care hospitals, these administrative costs ranged from 6.6 to 10.8 percent.[33]

Jacque Sokolov, MD, a veteran health care and benefits consultant who used to run the health plan of Southern California Edison, believes that direct contracting in the Minneapolis mold could save up to 10 percent of total costs on the insurance side and 5–7 percent on the provider side. If the administrative savings added up to 15–17 percent, they'd cut $95 billion-$107 billion from our national health care bill at its 2004 level.[34]

In a world without competition, the savings on the provider side would increase the incomes of physicians and hospitals, rather than lower costs for consumers and employers. But in the competitive markets envisioned in this reform model, physician groups would have a strong incentive to give up some of those savings in the form of lower prices to increase market share.

High Profits, Less Spent on Care   By contrast, a large chunk of this decade's huge increases in insurance premiums have gone into the pockets of insurance companies and their top executives. In 2005, the top seven U.S. health insurers earned a combined $10 billion, which was nearly triple their profits five years earlier.[35] The nation's Blue Cross and Blue Shield plans, similarly, saw combined profits rise 15 percent to $8.5 billion, an increase of 204 percent since 2001.[36] Net income for all managed-care companies was predicted to jump 15 percent in 2006, despite flat membership in HMOs and PPOs.[37]

Chief executives have profited the most. In 2004, Jack Rowe of Aetna received $4 million in salary and $18.2 million from stock options. Howard Phanstiel of PacifiCare received $13.8 million. And William McGuire of the UnitedHealth Group received $10.2 million in salary and $114.5 million from exercising stock options.[38] (In total, McGuire had stock options worth $1.6 billion if exercised in 2006.) But he resigned under fire after it was disclosed that some of his and other executives' options had been backdated to increase their value.[39]

Meanwhile, the biggest, most profitable insurers spent less of their revenues on health care in 2005 than in 2004.[40] The "medical-loss" ratio between patient-care expenses and premium income was 76.9 percent for Aetna, 82.3 percent for CIGNA, 83.2 percent for Humana, 78.6 percent for United, and 80.6 percent for WellPoint.

One reason these companies have been able to get away with this is that they have ever less competition. In 2004, Blue Cross and Blue Shield plans and three nationwide carriers—UnitedHealth Group, Aetna and CIGNA—controlled more than 60 percent of the health insurance market in 34 states and more than 70 percent in 23 states.[41] That calculation includes the late 2004 merger of WellPoint and Anthem, two Blue Cross/Blue Shield companies that together cover 27.7 million people.[42] It also factors in United's acquisition of Mid Atlantic Medical Services and Oxford Health Plans in 2004 but not its 2005 buyout of PacifiCare, which brought United's total enrollment to 25.7 million.[43] Even in 2004, however, one or two firms controlled at least half of the HMO/PPO market in nearly every metropolitan area.[44]

This market dominance has enabled the insurers to make big rate hikes stick in many regions. So, even as they've passed on the rapidly rising prices of consolidated hospital systems, the percentage of the premium dollar spent on health care has actually dropped.[45]

Are There Real Differences?   Even where there is price competition among plans, their physician and hospital networks have become nearly indistinguishable. Pressed by employers to broaden those networks in response to the managed-care backlash, the plans have embraced almost every willing provider.[46] At the same time, the distinction between how HMOs and PPOs manage care has blurred.

If plans share common networks and have the same basic approach, what makes one better than another? Peter Kongstevdt, MD, a partner in Accenture's health care consulting division, says it's "a matter of execution. The plans differ as to how well they do this stuff. Some process claims better and faster, some have better disease-management programs than others. And some have a bigger network, just because their fee schedule is different. When you get into how they do what they do on a day-to-day basis, there are differences."

Differences also appear in the quality scores of health plans that are measured by the National Committee for Quality Assurance (NCQA). These "HEDIS" ratings, which are used by very large employers, compare plans on patient satisfaction and various elements of preventive and chronic care.[47] But if the majority of doctors in every plan's network are the same, quality differences amount to little more than whether a particular plan reminds patients to get the care they need, provides self-care education, and posts some very limited information on the comparative value of providers.[48] Most of the other differences in quality scores can be attributed to variations in benefit designs that make it harder or easier for patients to obtain care.[49]

NCQA data show that, in many categories, the quality scores of the reporting, NCQA-accredited health plans improve every year. Disease-management programs have contributed to that improvement; but if managed-care organizations were really doing a good job, there wouldn't be studies showing that Americans don't get recommended care nearly half of the time.

One Step Forward, Two Steps Back   To be fair, there's a lot of physician resistance to change. Doctors resent efforts by payers to tell them how to practice, especially when those same companies have been whittling away at their incomes for years. It's not surprising, therefore, that they suspect the plans are more interested in saving money than in raising quality. But if they want things to change, they're going to have to take responsibility for managing care themselves.

If all primary-care physicians were in groups equipped with electronic health records, and if they had incentives to deliver the best care at the lowest cost, they could do everything the health plans want them to do and more. So if we could create financially accountable groups and a mechanism for funneling resources to them, we wouldn't need competing insurers that duplicate each other's functions and suck huge wads of cash out of the system. The insurance system that we know, with all of its wasteful administrative costs and obscene profits, could be eliminated without adversely affecting health care delivery. The next chapter shows how this could be done.

16 The End of Insurance as We Know It

How do we transform health insurance? It cannot be done gradually, because the insurance industry would find ways to counter any measure that merely changed how it did business. The only way to ensure radical transformation—short of a government takeover—is to take rapid steps that fundamentally redefine the insurance companies.

The first step in this process is to follow the Patient Choice example and have consumers choose among financially accountable physician groups rather than health plans. The primary-care groups would be ranked in tiers, based on their total cost of care, and patients' share of the premium would depend on which group they picked. While consumers probably wouldn't pay more attention to quality scores than most of them do today, those rankings would get the attention of physicians, prompting them to improve quality more than pay for performance ever could.

The second step is to allow only one health insurer to operate in each city or region. Such an insurer would operate like a state-regulated power utility. While this "utility insurer" could be a private for-profit or a not-for-profit company, it would act mainly as a conduit between payers and providers and as a financial reservoir. It could not negotiate or set prices, and its only role in managing care would be to measure the performance of physician groups, specialists, hospitals, and other providers. The federal government would decide which companies could bid for insurance contracts with regional health boards that would include physician, hospital, employer, and consumer representatives. The government would also specify a maximum profit margin for insurers and the maximum amount that their top executives could earn.

This approach would have several advantages. First, it would reduce administrative costs enough to provide most of the money needed to reach universal coverage (see Chapter 18). Second, everyone in each region (except for Medicare beneficiaries) would become part of one big insurance pool. By returning to the community rating system that was used before insurance became a big business, the utility insurers would spread coverage costs equally across the healthy and the sick, regardless of how large their employer was or whether they had a job. And third, without interference from the insurance companies, but with accountability to the public, physician groups would be able to strike an acceptable balance between serving the needs of the population and those of the individual patient.

Provider Payments   While each physician group would set a monthly budget for all professional services, it wouldn't dole out the money itself. The utility insurer would prepay the group for primary-care services and would also pay the claims of specialists, labs, and other providers. Money that was left over at the end of a quarter or a year would go back to the group; shortfalls would be debited against the group's budget for the following period. (This overspending, however, could not rise above the level at which it would trigger stop-loss insurance in individual cases.)

Using claims and encounter data, the utility insurer would adjust the size of each group's budget for the severity of the cases its doctors treated. So if a particular group had more than the average number of very sick patients, its budget would be increased without affecting its place in the cost rankings.

If insurers couldn't bargain with hospitals on price, it might seem as though there'd be nothing to stop hospitals from charging whatever they wanted. But the primary-care physicians and their contracted specialists would help patients decide which hospital to use, just as doctors do today. If the groups' tiering on public report cards were based on total costs, their doctors would have a strong incentive to admit patients to more efficient hospitals.

This approach, however, would be insufficient to control growth in hospital charges, especially if there were few hospitals in an area. So the government would have to extend Medicare's prospective payment systems for inpatient and outpatient care to the utility insurers. Public and private payers could work out some mixture of per diems and case rates that would limit cost growth while accommodating hospitals' need for flexibility. (For details, see Chapter 19.) Similarly, Medicare's prospective pricing system for nursing homes, inpatient rehab facilities, and home health care could be extended to the private sector.

Some allied health providers, such as podiatrists, nutritionists, chiropractors, vision providers, and physical therapists, might be included in the physician groups' budgets to enhance the coordination of care. But if dental care were a standard benefit—as it should be—dentists would have to form their own groups and be responsible for their own budgets, because patients would want to go directly to their dentists in an emergency.

Finally, there's the question of how to negotiate with pharmaceutical companies. A single primary-care group couldn't do it; even a utility insurer would be too small to have much impact on prices. But a buying cooperative that represented, say, a dozen insurers could get a drug firm's attention. If a co-op were purchasing drugs for several million people, it would have as much leverage as the Veterans Administration system, which obtains much bigger discounts than pharmaceutical benefit managers do on many common drugs. And unlike pharmaceutical benefit managers, buying co-ops wouldn't tack on a hefty charge for their efforts.

Say Good-bye to Self-Insurance   The advent of utility insurers would make employer-sponsored health plans unnecessary and counterproductive. Today, large companies self-insure partly to escape state insurance mandates, which would disappear if there were a national standard benefit package. Employers also self-insure to control their cash flow, earn interest on money set aside to pay claims, and avoid liability under state laws. But none of these advantages compares with the amount companies would save under this system; and if everyone under sixty-five is going to be in the same community-rated insurance pool, employees of large companies—who tend to be among the healthier members of the community—should not be exempt.

The federal government would no longer insure the health costs of Medicare patients; instead, it would pay the utility insurers a fixed, risk-adjusted amount for each Medicare patient. As explained later in this chapter, Medicaid would be folded into the private plans, although the states and the federal government would continue to share its cost. The poor, nonelderly population would be part of the overall community risk pool, but Medicare beneficiaries would remain in a separate insurance pool.

Why not include seniors in the same pool as those under sixty-five? The main reason is that health care for the elderly costs two to three times more than care for younger people.[1] So if Medicare beneficiaries were dumped into the same insurance pool as everyone else, people under sixty-five would rebel at the huge increase in their premiums. Even if the rates were modified by age, the subsidy required of working-age people would still be enormous.

Eventually, it would be preferable to have everyone in the same risk pool and for people under sixty-five to subsidize their elders directly. But Medicare's transition to a different financing mechanism would be complex and difficult. So this reform model would be easier to implement if we retained dual financing systems.

Medicare HMO Approach   Although they'd be in a different insurance pool, Medicare patients would have the same benefits and the same choice among provider groups that privately insured patients did. The government would continue to administer Medicare and would contract with the utility insurers, just as it does today with Medicare HMOs.

There are two differences, however, between this approach and the government's dealings with senior HMOs. First, while the government's annual contribution to Medicare would be fixed, Congress would no longer determine that amount; it would be based on the budgets submitted by utility insurers, which would depend partly on physician group budgets. Just as in the non-Medicare market, competition would moderate spending on professional services, because seniors would pay lower premiums to receive care from less expensive groups.

The second key difference is that, while a utility insurer would be taking the insurance risk, it would delegate the financial responsibility for professional services to physician groups. While this approach is common in California, and both Medicare and Medicaid HMOs have done it, it would be a switch for the government to depend so heavily on physicians to manage care.

Give Medicaid Patients Equal Access   People who are now on Medicaid should have the same benefits and belong to the same community-rated health plans as everyone else. This step should be taken, first of all, for the sake of social equity. While Medicaid benefits in many states are relatively good, physicians are paid so little for these patients that many will no longer care for them. In some areas, primary-care physicians can't find specialists who will take referrals of their Medicaid patients.[2] That is a national disgrace. Only when physicians are paid the same for Medicaid and commercial patients will the poor have equal access to the health care system.

The Clinton health-reform task force considered mainstreaming Medicaid. Although this idea didn't make it into the final proposal, Drew Altman, president of the Kaiser Family Foundation, commented at the time that it was the right thing to do. "There are really serious problems in putting Medicaid into the new system, but that's what we ought to do," he said. "A separate program for poor people will always be a poor program, underfunded and neglected."[3]

Equal access would enable Medicaid recipients to get proper preventive and chronic care. And that, in turn, would save states a significant amount of money, because fewer of these patients would end up in the emergency room or the hospital. In addition, with universal coverage, states that now pay hospitals a subsidy for charity care would save large sums. So they could afford to pay more to make sure that Medicaid patients received better care.

It wouldn't be much of a stretch to move Medicaid recipients into managed care. Fifty-nine percent of the nation's 43 million Medicaid enrollees belonged to HMOs in 2003.[4] And, in an effort to expand insurance coverage, some states have also placed low-wage workers and their families in Medicaid HMOs.[5]

It might be argued that combining Medicaid and private enrollees in the same insurance pool would raise the cost of coverage for everyone. But right now, providers who lose money on Medicaid charge more to private payers and individuals to make up for it.[6] That cost shift would be eliminated if providers were paid the same for Medicaid and privately insured patients.

One problem with this scenario is that long-term care now absorbs 35 percent of Medicaid spending.[7] To prevent this component of Medicaid from driving up the cost of private health coverage if both were combined in a single pool, long-term care would have to be segregated from Medicaid, and the government would have to find another way to pay for the care of institutionalized seniors.

The issues of long-term care go beyond the scope of this book. Suffice it to say that long-term care is a problem facing all advanced countries as their populations age. Some nations have decided to raise worker health insurance contributions to prepare for the coming crunch. Whether the United States will ever take this step is impossible to predict. Perhaps we'd subsidize long-term care within the Medicare program instead. But we'd probably be better off focusing on universal health care—which these other nations already have—before we worry about long-term care.

Size of Service Areas   How large an area would a utility insurer cover? That would depend on the population density and on the number of patients that the competing physician groups would need to be financially viable. Taking both of these factors into account, a carrier might insure between 150,000 and 500,000 lives in smaller cities and suburban/exurban areas. In large metropolitan centers, it might cover 500,000 to one million people, and there would be multiple, contiguous insurance regions in big cities. Rural regions might include as few as 100,000 people, enough for two or three IPAs.

Because most health care is local, the home address of an individual, not his or her work address, would determine which insurance region he or she belonged to. This requirement would create some "boundary issues." For example, the borders of an insurance region might separate some patients from their doctors; an exception would have to be made for them. Also, some people might want to see specialists in a different part of the city, and those doctors might admit them to a hospital outside their regular insurance area. In these cases, utility insurers would have to make reciprocal arrangements so that their physician groups wouldn't get stuck with bills for providing care to patients from outside the area.

In large metropolitan areas, some people who lived in one insurance region would commute to other areas for work. So in theory, they and their employers would be paying premiums (or "healthcare contributions") to a different utility insurer than the one that would pay their medical bills. But as I show in Chapter 18, the money would be collected in the form of payroll taxes and distributed to the correct insurers.

Providers would also have boundary issues. For example, a physician group might have clinics in multiple insurance territories. If so, it would contract with the carrier in the area where its headquarters were located. If it had enough physicians in another territory to compete with the other groups in that region, its branch there could contract with the other utility insurer, as well.

To prevent too many groups from clustering in a particular area, such as an affluent suburb, the regional health board could limit the number of groups in a territory. Other groups would have to set up shop and recruit physicians elsewhere in the insurance region. Nevertheless, even if they were caring for inner-city residents or sicker people, risk adjustment would ensure that their compensation would be equal to those of groups in other areas.

Roots of Reform   Aside from Patient Choice, there are few precedents for this reform approach. The delegated-risk model of California managed care has a long history, and, despite its well-publicized problems, many group practices and independent practice associations are still doing well with it. The publication of group performance data has also proved its utility in California. But the idea of having physician groups determine their own budgets would be alien in the homeland of HMOs.

The United Kingdom's National Health Service tried a form of managed competition in the early 1990s. Trying to inject some entrepreneurial spirit into the country's struggling single-payer system, the National Health Service gave capitated primary-care practices known as "fund-holders" extra money to pay for elective surgery, diagnostic tests, and prescription drugs. This measure was supposed to make the system more efficient by increasing competition among physician groups, and, to some extent, it did.[8]

The Blair administration has replaced fund-holding with "primary-care trusts," larger groups of physicians that now control about 75 percent of health care purchasing. The results of that experiment are not yet clear.[9] But it is clear that the situation of our doctors is not remotely similar to that of doctors in a government-run system with a national health budget.

In this country, as mentioned in Chapter 1, the theory of managed competition gave rise to the Clinton reform plan. The reform model in this book shares some characteristics with that proposal, including the use of community rating and standard benefits. But under the Clinton approach, consumers would have chosen among health plans, not physician groups.

Some experts think the concept of utility insurers is feasible. Walter Zelman, a health care adviser to President Clinton, recalls that in 1990 he was on a commission that explored ideas for achieving universal coverage in California. The choices eventually narrowed to managed competition or a statewide single-payer system. In the single-payer model, Zelman says, the government would have contracted directly with doctors and hospitals. However, he adds, the commission could have merged that model with the managed-competition approach, which relied on regional insurance-purchasing cooperatives. "A [regional] single payer of health plans could also contract directly with doctors and hospitals," he observes. "That would have been a competitive mechanism."

So the utility insurer model is a credible alternative to a government-run health care system. Combined with the kind of financially accountable care systems that have already proved their mettle in Minneapolis, it offers a powerful model that could put the management of health care where it belongs: in the hands of medical professionals and patients.

Government's Role

While the federal government would not run this system, it would have a large role in shaping and overseeing it. Perhaps its most important function, which we return to in the final chapters, would be to create a national technology assessment board that would determine what should be included in the standard benefit package and would update it as new technologies are developed. Once established, however, this national board would be independent of the government, just as the Federal Reserve is.

To move from our current system to the new model, the first thing that Washington would have to do is take over insurance regulation from the states, using its power to regulate interstate commerce. Without taking that step, Washington would be powerless to set up utility insurers or to prohibit health plans from continuing to operate as they do now.

Moreover, state regulation of insurance would become outmoded under the new system. A national benefit package would preempt state laws that require coverage of specific benefits. Other state laws covering the licensure and regulation of insurance entities would also become obsolete. For example, each state has different capital requirements for insurers, and some have guaranteed-issue and community-rating laws of various kinds. State managed-care consumer protection laws, similarly, vary a great deal. Because many companies operate in multiple states, all of these regulations would have to be standardized, and only the federal government could do that.

Setting Up Utility Insurers   The government would have to designate insurance regions that included a certain number of people. As suggested previously, the range might be 150,000 to one million people. Those living in outlying areas would be included in the nearest city's insurance region.

Next, the federal government would establish criteria for companies that wanted to become utility insurers. To make sure that a few giant insurers didn't dominate the business, the government would have to limit the number of insurance regions that each could serve. Some companies would inevitably lose revenue or go out of business, and some would sue the government. Not-for-profit insurers would be on weaker legal ground, because they don't have stockholders who could be harmed, and because they're supposed to serve the public interest. But for-profit carriers might sue on behalf of their stockholders, claiming the government was unjustly seizing private property.

To avoid these suits, the conversion should be done in a way that could potentially compensate shareholders. One option is to let them trade their stock for shares in the utility insurers that their companies form. That stock could be valued on the basis of how many individuals the new insurers covered and their projected profits, which could be considerable.

There would, of course, be winners and losers. Both for that reason and because the government would limit the utility insurers' profit margin, their stock prices would initially decline. But shareholders wouldn't necessarily see a long-term drop in value. The regional health boards would decide whether to renew insurer contracts at regular intervals. That would mean that some of the losers in the first round could turn into winners. Also, the insurers could branch into disease management and actuarial work. So the companies could grow revenues and profits, gradually boosting stock prices.

Regional Boards Would Be in Charge   Each insurance region would be governed by a quasi-governmental health board that would equally represent employers, providers, and consumers. The federal government would establish a uniform process for the people in each community to select their representatives. Presumably, the employer and provider sectors would choose board members by mutual agreement, while the people in each region would vote for consumer delegates.

The most important duty of each board would be to pick and oversee a utility insurer. That company would have to make its books available to the board upon request. At regular intervals—say, once every two or three years—the board would decide whether to renew the contract or to hire another insurer. While the carrier would have to obey all federal mandates, it could also be required to meet certain goals specified by the board. For example, if the previous insurer had been slow to pay providers, the board could specify that payment be made within a certain period.

The board would also supervise the insurers' collection and dissemination of provider performance data. And, like the proposed regional health information organizations, it would play a key role in the development of an electronic infrastructure tying together all of the providers in its region. The infrastructure would have to conform to federal standards so that providers in one region could communicate online with those in other areas.

Finally, the board would decide whether the community needed hospital building projects, as well as physician- or investor-owned specialty hospitals and ambulatory-care facilities. But in metropolitan areas where these facilities might serve patients in more than one insurance region, the regional boards should consult with each other on projects. State certificate-of-need laws would be superseded, but states would be involved in health planning and in resolving differences among regional boards (see Chapter 21).

Getting Physicians to Join Groups   One of the biggest challenges to building this reform model is persuading individualistic, entrepreneurial doctors that their interest lies in joining group practices. Here the government must be firm: It must tell primary-care physicians that after, say, three years, only those in prepaid groups of a certain size would be allowed to contract with Medicare. If that weren't enough, the government could prohibit utility insurers from contracting with primary-care physicians who remained independent. So even if doctors cared only for privately insured patients, they would have to join a group—unless they could build a practice composed purely of cash-paying patients.

The federal government would also have to help rural physicians form clinically and financially integrated networks. Wherever possible, these independent practice associations would join with those in nearby cities so that they'd include enough primary-care physicians to be competitive.

To entice physicians to join groups, the government could provide grants for purchasing electronic health record (EHR) systems to all primary-care groups that met its criteria. Even if all existing EHRs were replaced and there were no volume discounts, the cost to the government would be only $8.1 billion at current prices[10]—and, by increasing efficiency, this move would save public programs far more than that. Moreover, rather than waiting for physicians to purchase EHRs, a program of providing government grants could be implemented immediately. And physician groups could afford the kind of robust technical support that few small, privately owned practices now have access to.

One EHR would not, of course, fit all practices, as the U.K. government has learned the hard way. So groups should be able to choose among a number of products that satisfy government criteria for functionality and interoperability. If they wanted to buy an EHR that cost more than the average, they should be able to do that, too, by making up the cost difference themselves.

Specialists might complain that the federal government wasn't buying EHRs for them, but they can afford these systems more easily than primary-care physicians can. In any case, they wouldn't have a choice. If the primary-care groups had EHRs, they'd require the specialists they worked with to have them, too.

When every practice was equipped with computerized records, we'd have the building blocks for regional health information networks. Then, and only then, could we begin to harvest the huge efficiency gains from health information technology that experts have predicted.

Avoiding Overconsolidation   In Chapter 13, I discuss the minimum size of physician groups, based on the experience of prepaid practices. A maximum also should be placed on the number of primary-care physicians in each group, depending on the size of the market; otherwise, physicians would form cartels and stifle competition. Similarly, as noted earlier, specialists must be prohibited from forming supergroups that the primary-care groups would be forced to contract with.

Besides limiting the size of groups, the government should also prevent the kind of investor speculation that fueled the rise and fall of physician practice management companies in the 1990s. If such speculation were repeated, the Wall Street-driven mania to merge practices and extract profits from them would only hurt physicians and inhibit the formation of truly integrated groups that were dedicated to providing high-quality care.

The solution is three-fold: First, the government should guarantee loans to provide doctors with the capital to form larger organizations without seeking it from investors. Second, Congress should pass a national "corporate practice of medicine" law that would prohibit nonphysician ownership of medical groups, either directly or through "foundations." And third, the government should prohibit the sale of any primary-care practice that contracts with utility insurers, although mergers with other contracting groups would be allowed. This feature would have implications for physician equity that I explore in the next chapter.

17 Getting Down to Nuts and Bolts

"Doctors do not come together well," says Gary Matthews, a veteran health care consultant in Atlanta who has done a lot of physician-practice mergers. "They all want to practice medicine in their own individual way. And even if they're in a group, they don't want to be told how to practice."

That having been said, there's no doubt that if primary-care physicians knew they'd have to join a group or be out of business in three years, they'd start to merge with their colleagues. The question is, could groups of the requisite size be put together in that time?

Matthews and other consultants say yes. But those groups would have to be assembled in a two-stage process: First, tiny practices would merge into groups of eight to ten doctors, and then these practices would join together to form larger aggregations. Normally, the medium-sized groups would cohere and recoup their merger costs within a couple of years after coming together, the consultants say. So, in three years, it would be possible to create groups that could take financial responsibility for professional services and compete within a utility-insurer market.

Specialty Mix Is an Issue   What kinds of doctors should belong to these groups? The answer is not as simple as it might appear. To begin with, we have to define "primary-care physician." By common agreement, family physicians, general practitioners, general internists, and pediatricians would all qualify. Many people also regard obstetrician/gynecologists as primary-care physicians for women. But even if an ob/gyn practices only gynecology, his or her training and knowledge are limited to a relatively narrow range of medical problems. In addition, ob/gyns are in great demand in most regions. So they should be available to everyone, and they wouldn't be if they belonged to competing primary-care groups.

Each physician practice must be able to treat both adults and children to compete with other groups. Thus a practice that included only pediatricians or only internists wouldn't work. A group of family physicians would meet the criterion, but internists are arguably better at treating patients with more complex medical conditions; that's why internists tend to have larger Medicare practices than family physicians do. Also, if a group consisted only of family physicians, the number of family physicians available to other groups would be reduced.

Establishing a specialty-mix formula would be difficult because of the wide regional variations in particular specialties. There's a big disparity between the Northeast, where general internists make up 54 percent of active primary-care physicians (including ob/gyns), and the West, where they make up only 41 percent. Similarly, while family physicians and general practitioners account for 31 percent of active primary-care physicians across the country, only 17 percent of generalists are family physicians or general practitioners in the Northeast.[1]

Because of these disparities, the specialty-mix formula for primary-care groups would have to be adjusted state-by-state, and it would have to be flexible enough to accommodate local conditions. Wherever possible, family physicians should be included (general practitioners are a dwindling minority); but it's also desirable to have both pediatricians and internists in the mix.

Finding Merger Partners   Now that we've established what kinds of physicians should be in our groups, let's see what doctors in small practices must do to join together.

First, they'd have to decide with whom they wanted to practice. That could be a daunting prospect, notes Kenneth Kubitschek, an internist who belongs to a nine-doctor group in Asheville, North Carolina. "Doctors are concerned about the competency of the people they're joining with," he points out. "If everyone has to join a group, you'll be forced to practice with people you don't want to practice with."

Especially in small towns and cities, physicians are well aware of their colleagues' reputations. While Kubitschek guesses he could form a first-class group with about twenty doctors whom he knows in the Asheville area, "a number of people would be left out if we made our own choice," he says.

This would be a problem everywhere, but it's imperative that doctors choose their own partners from the available pool. If their choices were limited because some of the physicians they respected had joined groups that were full, they'd simply have to merge with other physicians and work with them to achieve a uniformly high standard of practice. In fact, even the best physicians in town would have to join with other physicians who weren't in the elite circle, because these groups would be too large to include only the best.

If the size of groups in a particular market were limited by regulation, a group would never attract so many physicians that it became dominant. And rarely would a group lose so many doctors that it was no longer viable. But in case that did happen, an orderly procedure would have to be established so that the remaining doctors could join other practices.

Equity Considerations   When practices merge, they usually bring different amounts of equity or net worth. The three main components of practice equity are "hard assets" (i.e., equipment and fixtures), accounts receivable, and an element called "goodwill," which is related to intangibles such as location and reputation. Today, because there are few buyers for primary-care practices, they have much less goodwill value than they used to; in some areas, they have none.[2]

With regard to practice mergers, this reduced goodwill value is a good thing. It means that the practices mainly have to equalize the value of their hard assets—rarely worth more than $25,000 per primary-care physician—and accounts receivable. So no money changes hands in a typical primary-care merger. Instead, the doctors in the practice who own less valuable equipment and are owed less will simply have a slight reduction in pay for the first year or so after the merger.[3]

The reduction of goodwill in practice valuations not only facilitates mergers but also fits well with our reform model. It means that most primary-care physicians would have little practice equity to lose when they joined a group. When they retired or left the group, the other partners could buy them out for relatively little. Eventually, buy-ins and buyouts would disappear, because if the group couldn't be sold (see Chapter 16), it would have no market value.

Merger Costs and Return on Investment   Even if the participating physicians don't exchange much money, practice mergers are expensive. Between the fees of consultants, accountants, and lawyers, a merger of small practices might cost $8,000–$12,000 per doctor, Gary Matthews estimates—and that doesn't include the cost of a new computer system for billing and scheduling, which can add another $10,000 per doctor.

Today, primary-care physicians who form groups often do so to get better terms from health plans or to invest in ancillary facilities. Extra income from labs or bone densitometry units, combined with higher insurance reimbursement, can help these groups generate a return on their investment.[4] But for a prepaid group, ancillaries would be cost centers, and the size of a practice would not affect its relationship with a utility insurer.

Groups would, therefore, have to recover their merger costs by increasing efficiency. The use of electronic health records would certainly contribute to increased efficiency by cutting transcription costs and eliminating record handling and duplicate tests. Also, there would be far less administrative work than practices have today. No longer would staff members be on the telephone with insurers, trying to get referral or test authorizations, verifying coverage, or finding out why a claim hasn't been paid. While "encounter data" would still have to be submitted electronically to the utility insurer, they would all be in a single format and could be generated by the electronic health records. Specialists and other professionals would send their claims directly to the utility insurer, which would debit the primary-care group's budget.

Should Doctors Work in One Place?   Physicians would tend to remain in their own offices, both because they're used to practicing that way and because patients in most parts of the country prefer smaller offices. Some groups have found that they can save money by centralizing their operations in a single location. But, whether they do that or not, most mergers don't produce economies of scale.

"Usually, there's not going to be an overhead reduction," says Geoffrey Anders, a practice management consultant in Plymouth Meeting, Pennsylvania. "Every doctor needs pretty much the same number of square feet of office space, the same number of support staff. You might save a little bit in the billing operation, but there's no cost that gets spread better across the group. Even legal and accounting prices go up when you get a bigger, more complicated group. So on a per-doctor basis, there really are little or no savings."

Mergers do make some staff members redundant because their job functions are eliminated or because they lack required skills. In some mergers, Anders notes, the staff of one practice will turn over completely in eighteen months, because the culture of the other practice has taken over. Especially considering that many doctors are married to their office managers, these human factors can pose serious challenges to group formation.

Also, if physicians continue to work in their own offices, it can be difficult for them to feel as though they're part of the same group, rather than competitors. But prepaid practices have discovered that, by making the doctors dependent on each other, shared financial risk can generate a lot of the "glue" that's needed to form independent doctors into a group.[5]

Group Management While physicians should always remain in control of both the clinical and business aspects of their group, functions such as contracting, budgeting, personnel, and supply purchasing can be outsourced to entities known as management service organizations (MSOs). Especially during the transition from medium-sized to large groups, and during those groups' early years, MSOs could be indispensable.

Some caveats, however, are in order. Because investors expanded MSOs into physician practice management companies with the regrettable results cited earlier, MSOs must be as carefully regulated as utility insurers are. They should not be allowed to own or control physician groups; they must be prohibited from contracting with more than one group per insurance region; and, to prevent them from becoming too powerful, the government should also limit the number of regions they can do business in.

Without strong physician leadership, however, there would still be a danger that groups could degenerate into loose collections of doctors run by MSOs. So the groups should adopt model bylaws that describe the responsibilities of each party. Ultimately, physicians have to step up to the obligations of self-governance. Only by doing so can they create a real group culture that will encourage quality improvement and good care coordination.

Change Is Messy

Roughly 10 percent of physicians in the country already practice in groups of twenty or more physicians.[6] Some of these groups are single-specialty units; others include many specialties. If the model proposed in this book is implemented, these groups should be preserved wherever possible. The reason is simple: their physicians understand how to work in groups, and many know a great deal about managing care. Their experience and knowledge would be an inestimable resource for other doctors.

Existing primary-care groups could form the nuclei of the new groups that would compete with one another for patients. But multispecialty groups pose a ticklish problem, because they may be primary-care-driven or specialty-dominated, medium-sized or large. Those in which primary-care physicians were a majority would fit into the utility insurer model without much trouble. But if a group comprised mainly specialists, it couldn't take financial responsibility for all professional services, because its doctors wouldn't be in a position to coordinate care. Therefore, the utility insurers wouldn't contract with such a group, and it would have no choice but to allow its generalists to join primary-care groups.

Some multispecialty groups, such as those of Kaiser Permanente, Health Partners, and the Mayo Clinic, are so big that they'd overwhelm the primary-care groups in our model. But it would be difficult to split them up because of their group cultures and their massive investments in infrastructure. The same would be true for integrated delivery systems such as Allina in Minneapolis, the Carle Clinic in Bloomington-Normal, Illinois, and Sharp Healthcare in San Diego. Large, heavily capitated independent practice associations, such as California's Hill Physicians, Brown & Toland, and Greater Newport Physicians, have less infrastructure but have extensive information systems.

Most of these multispecialty groups and IPAs cover wide metropolitan areas. Thus, their primary-care physicians could form subsidiary practices that would contract with different utility insurers while continuing to share the larger group's infrastructure. The specialists in the multispecialty groups would be able to contract with any primary-care group in the regions where they practiced. Any outside income they earned would go into their group's bonus pool.

Dissolving HMO ownership of some of these groups or their exclusive contracts with the physicians, however, would be difficult because in group-model HMOs, the financing and the provision of care are closely linked. The solution might be to transform group-model HMOs into utility insurers in the few regions where they're currently strong. In that scenario, they could delegate financial risk to primary-care groups formed from their own employed physicians, as well as other groups; and, if they proved their worth to regional health boards, they could remain in that role indefinitely.

Hospitals Must Spin Off Groups   Including the big, integrated systems mentioned earlier, hospitals still employ tens of thousands of mostly primary-care physicians. Because practices must be able to admit to any hospitals they choose to, the institutions would have to spin off their groups under our reform model.

For most health care systems, such a divestiture should not be much of a sacrifice. According to the Medical Group Management Association, hospitals lost a median $58,000 on each employed physician in 2005.[7] That was an improvement over the $89,500 median loss they suffered in 2000, when many hospitals were giving primary-care practices back to their physicians. The 2005 figure would also be smaller if the employed doctors' use of hospital-owned ancillary services such as labs and imaging facilities were included in the calculation. Nevertheless, many hospitals should be glad to get rid of their remaining practices.

Why, then, do so many hospitals hang onto them? Usually, it's to guarantee admissions to the hospital and referrals to the specialists who practice there. This competition can be especially fierce in less populated areas, where rival hospitals may employ a large portion of the primary-care physicians. Also, recent changes in the federal self-referral regulations have made it difficult for hospitals to help local practices recruit physicians, even in areas where they're in short supply. So in many instances, the hospitals are hiring them directly, and their competitors are being forced to do the same.[8]

Despite all of this activity, the market value of primary-care practices remains low across most of the country.[9] This means that federal "inurement" and anti-kickback rules would not stop hospitals from returning previously purchased practices to physicians for little more than accounts receivable. (The Internal Revenue Service's inurement regulation prohibits not-for-profit hospitals from providing anything of value to referring doctors if they want to keep their tax exemptions. The anti-kickback law covers all hospitals that do business with Medicare or Medicaid.)

Health care consultant Michael LaPenna explains that, if a hospital consistently loses money on a practice, it doesn't have the fair market value that it had when it was purchased. Hence, there may be no inurement if the physicians take back ownership. Todd Greenwalt, a Houston-based attorney, agrees. "From a fair value perspective, the hospital is making a better deal by letting physicians go their own way. And from the IRS viewpoint, there's no inurement issue."

Based on this experience, it's fair to assume that there would be no need to compensate hospitals for the loss of their primary-care practices.

First Steps in Managed Care

Once all of the financially accountable groups were in place, they'd immediately face the challenge of how to manage their resources wisely. The physicians in each group would first have to agree on protocols for referring patients to specialists. As we've seen, this is an area where scientific evidence is still slim, but groups with managed-care experience have devised some rules of thumb.

Among those rules is that primary-care physicians should do as much as they can for patients before referring them to specialists. The problem in applying this principle is that primary-care physicians in different parts of the country view their "scope of practice" variously. While the training physicians receive is not markedly different in California than in, say, Georgia or New York, their expectations—and those of their patients—vary with regional practice patterns.

For example, 25 to 30 percent of family physicians across the country still deliver babies, but nearly 50 percent of those in Minnesota do, while fewer than 20 percent in Florida do.[10] Similarly, there are more family doctors in the West and Midwest than in the East,[11] and their scope of practice is wider outside of the East Coast. It's not uncommon for West Coast family physicians to do colposcopies or Holter monitoring or to freeze off warts. But in the East, they tend to refer patients to specialists for procedures and tests like these. They're also more likely to refer patients with chronic conditions such as asthma, diabetes, and arthritis.

"If you look at what's referred back East, it's a lot different," says Andrew Siskind of the Bristol Park Medical Group in Irvine, California. "We have internists who do fine needle aspirations of the thyroid. You'll never see that back East. We have a broad spectrum of skills, and we try to keep patient care within the group."

Dividing the Wheat from the Chaff   From the perspective of a primary-care group in our model, the number of specialists required to take good care of patients would depend largely on its system for coordinating care.

As George Halvorson explains in *Strong Medicine*: "If . . . we change the incentives for all providers . . . by choosing to prepay our care providers as teams of caregivers, then those caregiver teams themselves will make their own decisions about the numbers of specialists and subspecialists they need. They will only want to pay for as many specialists as each health team really needs to achieve its targeted outcomes. If the teams are truly held accountable for the actual cost and outcomes of their care, then they will recruit the number of specialists needed to achieve those outcomes—but no more. Accountable teams of providers will not support redundant subspecialists or their ability to generate unnecessary services."[12]

Let's say that our competing primary-care groups took Halvorson's advice and contracted only with the best, more cost-effective specialists. What would happen to the redundant consultants? Would they migrate to areas that had few physicians in their specialty?

Experience shows that most physicians are reluctant to leave comfortable urban or suburban situations to practice in rural or inner-city areas, even if they're offered premium compensation for doing so.[13] Some don't want to practice in towns where they're frequently or always on call; others don't want to live in places where there are fewer cultural opportunities or jobs for their spouses. Many smaller hospitals also lack the advanced technology that specialists use.

Jonathan Weiner of Johns Hopkins University, who believes there's an adequate supply of physicians in the United States, says that unneeded specialists might relocate if the utility insurer system were "hermetically sealed." But Edward Salsberg, director of the Center for Workforce Studies of the American Association of Medical Colleges, argues that we're heading toward a serious physician shortage. So while he agrees that physicians would move to underserved areas if they couldn't find work in a metropolitan region, he doubts that that would happen. "If there's going to be a big shortage, then there will likely be opportunities in both places," he says.

One thing, however, is clear: If primary-care physicians were in charge of the professional-services budget, and if they could earn more by controlling costs, their incomes would probably rise, relative to those of specialists. Under that scenario, it's likely that more physicians would go into primary care, just as they did during the heyday of HMOs.

Controlling Drug Costs   Besides limiting specialty costs, the primary-care groups could also have a big impact on drug expenditures. They wouldn't try to negotiate drug prices—that, as discussed earlier, would be the province of buying cooperatives formed by the utility insurers. But the groups could influence the use of prescription drugs.

They would, for example, draw up lists of preferred medications known as formularies. Each group would create its own formulary, because that would be the best way to get member physicians to use it. If groups were financially responsible for drugs, they'd undoubtedly encourage the use of generics and less expensive therapies. Physicians could prescribe other drugs, but they'd have to justify their decisions in their electronic records. And if a doctor prescribed unapproved drugs too often, the group's utilization management committee would probably question him or her about it.

Drug companies, of course, would try to influence the formulary-setting process and individual prescribing decisions. Their representatives would talk to each group's pharmacy and therapeutics committee, and they'd continue sending detailers to individual physicians' offices. But if a group's physicians were smart, they'd agree not to see drug reps, for two reasons: The more brand-name medicines a doctor prescribed, the more it would cost the group. And, as we've seen, detailers are not an objective source for information on new drugs.

Process Reengineering

To provide better, safer, more cost-efficient care, primary-care physicians have to change how they work. A big part of this change involves using electronic health records to follow evidence-based guidelines and avoid medical errors. But as pointed out in Chapter 5, electronic health records alone will not solve the problems of health care. Computerizing inefficient, disorganized work processes will only produce greater inefficiency. And assembling physicians into groups won't change anything unless those practices redesign their work processes to minimize waste and to maximize the intelligent use of their resources.

Groups can draw on many proven techniques to reengineer their work processes. Donald Berwick's Institute for Healthcare Improvement has promoted some of these in its "Idealized Design of Clinical Office Practice" program, which has involved dozens of group practice sites.[14] The American Academy of Family Practice and the American College of Physicians have proposed other reforms to help bring ambulatory practice into the twenty-first century.[15] The following sections describe some of the approaches that physician groups have implemented successfully.

Same-Day Scheduling   Many medical offices book appointments to see doctors for nonurgent problems weeks or even months ahead. Waits are longest for specialists, even in areas that are well supplied with them: In Boston, for example, it takes an average of thirty-seven days to see a cardiologist, fifty days to see a dermatologist, and forty-five days to see an ob/gyn. But primary-care physicians are often booked up, too. It can take a couple of weeks to see a primary-care physician for a chronic problem, and two months or more to schedule a physical.[16]

One solution, developed by Mark Murray, MD, when he worked at Kaiser Permanente in the early 1990s, is called "same-day" or "open-access" scheduling. Under this system, every patient is offered an appointment the day he or she calls in, regardless of how sick he or she is. Obviously, not everyone can come in the same day, so some appointments are booked ahead. But more patients are seen when they want to be seen.

Because the demand for a physician's time is more or less constant, Murray and other doctors who use open-access scheduling have found that their work hours are no longer, on average, than they were when they booked all nonurgent visits in advance. But their patients are much happier and receive care that's better, in many instances, because it's more timely.[17]

"Max-Packing"   One way for doctors to moderate the volume of same-day visits is to implement what Murray calls "max-packing." This means that when a patient comes in for a flu shot or with a sore back, the physician checks on other aspects of the patient's condition: Has she been taking her cholesterol medication? How is her blood pressure? If she's a diabetic, has she had her eyes checked recently?

Today, neither physicians in mostly fee-for-service nor practices that are mostly prepaid use this system consistently—a major reason for the poor quality of care. The fee-for-service doctors are too busy trying to see more patients, and they get paid more when a patient visits more often. The capitated physicians are also trying to see as many patients as possible so they can handle large panels. Both are focused more on acute medical problems than on chronic disease care.[18]

Partly as a result of pay for performance, some of the larger groups have built registries of chronic-disease patients. These registries tell doctors what patients with particular conditions need and whether they've received those services. Our reform model would ensure that every group used electronic registries and that doctors tried to provide all necessary care during every visit. They'd also be equipped and motivated to provide continuous care between visits.

Nonvisit Care   Some physician innovators, such as Joseph Scherger and Peter Basch, say that only 30 to 40 percent of patients who call their offices for an appointment really need to come in. But, as mentioned earlier, fee-for-service physicians are reluctant to communicate with patients online or on the telephone, because they're paid only for office visits or they're paid less for e-mail consultations. Prepayment makes it much easier to provide nonvisit care.

Scherger is a leading proponent of using secure online messaging services to transform primary care. In his experience, patients don't overuse e-mail, and he's been able to help them by answering their questions about self-care, how to take drugs, and so on. In the future, he says, physicians will be able to deal with many minor problems online, reserving office appointments for patients who really need to be seen.

While Scherger's vision is not widely shared among practicing physicians, there's a growing recognition among experts that nonvisit care is not only essential to care coordination but also cost effective. As Berwick notes, "The more you can move demand away from office visits, the more time you'll have to deal with patients who really need personal interaction."

Disease Management   Although this topic is covered in Chapter 3, it's worth making a few points here about how primary-care groups would handle disease management under our reform model. First, doctors would have an incentive to engage in disease management, because their income would depend indirectly on keeping patients' chronic conditions under control. Second, the groups could use the chronic-care model that involves caregivers across a variety of settings and specialties. To improve the coordination of care, they could create multidisciplinary teams that included particular kinds of specialists, as well as nurses, pharmacists, nutritionists, and other health care professionals.

David Lawrence, in his book *From Chaos to Care*, describes similar care teams.[19] The teams he envisions are drawn from the many disciplines found in big multispecialty groups like those of Kaiser Permanente. Nevertheless, there's no reason primary-care groups could not orchestrate similar collaborations with contracted specialists and allied health care providers. They could also reward particular team members who do an outstanding job of care coordination.

Most health plans outsource disease management to specialized vendors, rather than build their own programs; so it's unlikely that physician groups of even fifty to a hundred doctors could afford to do it all by themselves. But Lawrence Casalino of the University of Chicago has a vision of the future in which reorganized physician practices follow the chronic-care model with the assistance of disease-management companies.[20] By adding these vendors' capabilities in outreach and patient education to strategies based on the doctor-patient relationship, physician groups could have the best of both worlds.

Team-Based Care   The Institute for Healthcare Improvement's reengineering program emphasizes the use of a different kind of care team within the primary-care practice itself. This approach is especially important in larger groups, which tend to produce atomization and a "not my job" attitude.

Care teams would consist of two or three physicians and four or five staff members who are cross-trained to back each other up.[21] The physicians can help each other meet the fluctuating demands of open-access scheduling, and the staffers can be assigned to jobs that are best matched to their skills. Care teams would also rely heavily on nurse practitioners and physician assistants, who are already common in both primary-care and specialty practices. These highly trained "midlevel" professionals can do many of the things that physicians do, including prescribing and seeing patients for minor problems and routine exams. If they were properly utilized, they could take much of the strain off of doctors, freeing them up to handle more complex cases.[22]

As the number of midlevel practitioners has soared in recent years, some observers have speculated that they might be the foundation of a new approach to practice. For example, physician workforce expert Edward Salsberg believes that one primary-care physician working with three or four nurse practitioners or physician assistants could provide high-quality, efficient care. But medical society leaders reject such a possibility.

"Midlevels are critical to working in a team approach and providing the best care for people with multiple chronic diseases," says internist Lynne Kirk, president of the American College of Physicians. "But it's important that it be a team approach and that physicians be ultimately responsible for the care."

Group Visits   Recognizing that physicians don't always have time to meet all the needs of patients in individual visits, some large group practices have introduced "group visits," or a variant known as "drop-in group medical appointments." The goal of this approach is two-fold: to increase physician productivity and to improve care for patients who have chronic diseases. Group visits also provide a more supportive model for patients with psychosocial needs than a typical office visit does; in some cases, a behavioral health professional co-leads the sessions with the patients' physician.[23]

Doctors are always present at these weekly visits, which typically run from sixty to ninety minutes. A doctor may invite all those patients he or she thinks would benefit from this approach or may segment the group visits by type of condition, such as diabetes, asthma, or hypertension. The "drop-in" variant also encourages patients to attend prescheduled group visits without an appointment.

Group visits do not replace individual appointments; patients always have the option to see their doctors privately. But group visits do seem to reduce the number of telephone calls and visits by "frequent flyers" who crave a doctor's attention. They also help patients share experiences and reassure each other. This group feedback has helped doctors deal with some difficult patients, and, along with advice on prevention, nutrition, exercise, and healthy lifestyles, it has helped patients manage their own health better.

Teaching Managed Care

Most physicians have never learned how to manage care. In fact, they don't know even know how to work together in groups. So if they were thrust into prepaid, competing primary-care groups, they'd need some expert guidance. Here are some ideas about how to bring physicians up to speed quickly to practice in an environment unlike any they've ever been in.

Managed-care college. The Bristol Park Medical Group and a number of other prepaid groups offer a kind of "managed-care college" for young doctors who've recently joined the practice.[24] Other physicians around the country could serve rotating apprenticeships in these groups and attend these training courses. Then they could return to their groups and teach their colleagues.

HMO medical directors. The number of health plans would be dramatically reduced in the transition to utility insurers. As a result, hundreds of HMO medical directors would have to make a career change. Perhaps some of them might establish traveling seminars to help impart their knowledge of managed care to primary-care physicians. Most of these HMO executives were practicing physicians at one time; some still practice part-time. So they should be able to connect with their peers, despite their erstwhile association with the insurers that doctors loathe.

Recertification programs. After physicians complete their training, they must pass rigorous board certification exams in their specialty, and they must be recertified at specified intervals. Unless they're certified, doctors in most areas cannot join hospital staffs or contract with health plans.[25]

In 2004, reacting to the public outcry over patient safety and poor health care quality, all twenty-four of the specialty certification boards—including those in primary-care specialties—agreed to require physicians to show competence in six areas as part of the recertification process.[26] Before residents can sit for initial board certification, they must also prove their competence in the same six fields: patient care, medical knowledge, practice-based learning and improvement, interpersonal and communication skills, professionalism, and "systems-based practice."[27]

To prove competence in systems-based practice, doctors must show they know how to use local health care resources effectively. A primary-care physician, for example, must be able to work well with specialists or with health plans to get what patients need. But the definition could be expanded to demonstrating the ability to manage care effectively.

This redefinition would have an immense impact. It would change how primary-care residents are trained, and it would trigger the creation of continuing medical education programs to teach doctors already in practice how to manage care.

A Competitive Market   Converting physicians to the idea of managed care and accustoming them to work in groups would take much longer than assembling those groups. Many hurdles must be passed, and a great deal of physician leadership would be required. But if the government provided the proper regulatory framework, physicians could create a competitive market.

Coupled with the administrative savings of the utility-insurer model, a competitive market in health care could create the basis for comprehensive, universal coverage without a government takeover of the system. And, as explained in the next chapter, comprehensive insurance is the only kind that can provide equitable access to health care.

18 Universal Health Care

     Some well-meaning people have suggested that universal coverage would be a major step forward, even if the insurance covered only catastrophic care or only primary care. Why comprehensive insurance is needed—and why anything less would keep driving costs up for all of us—becomes clear when one considers who the uninsured are.

     Eight in ten uninsured people are wage earners or members of working families, and two-thirds are low-income individuals or members of families with incomes of less than twice the federal poverty level ($38,614 for a family of four in 2004). Thirty percent have incomes between 100 percent and 200 percent of the poverty line, which usually makes them ineligible for Medicaid.[1] The typical uninsured person is someone who works at a fast-food restaurant, drives a cab, answers phones, lays bricks, harvests apples, or does any of the millions of low-paid service jobs that keep our economy running.

     If we covered the uninsured with high-deductible plans, many of them would not get primary care. We know from the RAND insurance experiment[2] and other studies that people use fewer medical services when they have to pay more for them; this tendency is more pronounced among the poor and near-poor who constitute the majority of the uninsured. High out-of-pocket costs limit access to care for millions of Americans, both insured and uninsured, and place heavy financial burdens on 11 percent of families.[3] So bare-bones universal coverage would not solve the problem. Conversely, covering only primary care for the uninsured would perpetuate our system of hit-or-miss charity care for those who are really sick and need help.

     Still, it would be a boon if everyone had access to the preventive and chronic care that the well-insured receive. Many of the uninsured don't even have a regular physician. And when people can't afford to see a doctor at all, they tend to wait until they're very sick before seeking medical care at an emergency department. That's the most expensive venue for treatment, and emergency care often leads to hospitalization. Similarly, if chronically ill people without insurance are unable to buy the medications they need, they may end up requiring emergency treatment and hospital care.[4]

In 2005, the cost of providing health care to uninsured people, beyond what they paid out of pocket, was about $43 billion. (That doesn't include the cost of uncompensated services provided to under-insured people who couldn't pay their share of the bill.) Government programs and philanthropy covered about a third of the cost of this uncompensated care. The rest was passed on to employers and consumers. A Families USA report estimates that, in 2005, this cost shift added $922 to the average premium for families with private insurance, and $341 to the average insurance cost for individuals.[5]

What these figures mean is that we're all paying for the uninsured. Whether or not you believe that everyone is entitled to health care, you're already subsidizing care for the uninsured through your taxes and your share of insurance premiums. As the number of uninsured and the amount of uncompensated care grow, so will the costs for the rest of us. So universal, comprehensive coverage is not only a moral imperative but an economic necessity.

Playing the Benefits Game   Except for certain large categories, such as prescription drugs and dental, vision, mental-health, and home care, most commercial health plans vary little in the services they cover. To some extent, all plans (other than "mini-plans") pay for doctor visits, preventive care, lab, radiology, and cardiology tests, and hospitalization; they all cover cancer care and heart operations. They all pay for noninvestigational organ transplants, and most cover chiropractic care. Most plans exclude coverage of cosmetic surgery, alternative therapies such as acupuncture, and treatments that are deemed "experimental."[6]

In contrast, insurance benefits, which spell out who pays how much for what, vary tremendously. Different benefit packages offer a broad range of deductibles, copayments, and coinsurance, as well as very different limits on annual out-of-pocket costs and lifetime benefits. An insured person's financial cost for in-network and out-of-network care can also vary widely.

The insurance business thrives on these myriad variations in benefits. The differences in benefit structures allow the plans to distinguish themselves from their competitors and permit employers to be selective about what they provide to their workers. By offering so many benefit designs, the insurers give all but the sickest and poorest individuals and the riskiest employer groups the opportunity to buy insurance at a more or less affordable price. But the limitations of that insurance mean large differences in access to care.

Standard Benefits: Pros and Cons   A standard benefit package, in contrast, would offer everyone the same set of services with similar out-of-pocket costs. (However, the poor would pay little or nothing for care.) A standard plan would give all insured people equal access to health care if it were combined with community rating and personal spending were capped at an affordable level.

The services covered under a standard benefit package should be comparable to good private insurance benefits offered by large companies. While some might object that that would be too expensive, the Institute of Medicine argues in a report on insurance that comprehensive benefits are essential: "Benefit packages that include preventive and screening services, outpatient prescription drugs, and specialty mental health treatment in addition to outpatient medical and hospital care are more likely to facilitate the receipt of appropriate care and better health than insurance that does not include these features."[7]

Although the Institute of Medicine doesn't specifically endorse standard benefits, it states, "Health insurance should enhance health and well-being by promoting access to high-quality care that is effective, efficient, safe, timely, patient centered and equitable."[8] It's hard to see how this goal can be reached without providing a standard package that has broad coverage and affordable out-of-pocket costs.

Clinton Plan's Benefits Package   The last time this country seriously considered adopting national standard benefits was during the debate over the Clinton reform plan. The Clinton team's package included comprehensive benefits that the American Medical Association generally approved of. The proposal also would have allowed people to buy supplemental insurance.[9]

Walter Zelman, the former Clinton adviser, recalls that members of the health-reform task force did not fiercely debate what should be in the benefit package. "It wasn't the most difficult issue, but it was somewhat difficult. There were some who felt that the guaranteed benefit package should be very broad. Others were more concerned about the cost and how we were going to fund this over time. But nobody was advocating something radically bigger or smaller than the standard HMO benefit package."

Paul Ginsburg, president of the Center for Studying Health System Change, argues that the time for standard benefits has passed along with the original premise of managed competition, which was based on competing health plans with different provider networks. "The main reason to standardize the benefits was to make it easier for people to choose among plans," he says. Now that insurers are moving toward "consumer-directed" care, which focuses on having people choose among providers, "there's no need to standardize the benefit package anymore," he maintains.

Ginsburg's comments are right on target in the current environment. But a utility insurer system would require standardized benefits. If consumers are going to select physician groups on the basis of cost and quality, they should have access to the same services at the same out-of-pocket cost, just as in the original Patient Choice. Individual insurance contributions should vary with the efficiency of the group rather than with the level of benefits.

Supplemental Benefits   Joseph Scherger of the University of California, San Diego, has long favored a standard benefit package that would be available to all. "A universal benefit package is essential to universal health care," he says.

Scherger also observes, however, that Americans like the ability to upgrade themselves. Just as some people decide it's worth the extra cost to fly first-class, he says, there will always be people who want more health care. So he supports the idea of letting people buy things that aren't included in the standard package. "Everything else would be an upgrade or add-on, which wouldn't be essential for good basic health care."

This upgrade could take several forms: People could buy cosmetic procedures or whole-body CT scans out of pocket, as they do now. Or they could purchase supplemental insurance that might cover experimental procedures, acupuncture, and other alternative therapies. One could also envision multiple standard packages that would entitle those who paid more to some extra services.

Whatever the details, the contents of a standard benefit package would have to be determined by some kind of national health board, preferably with consumer input (see Chapter 22). And to make sure that standardization did not deter innovation, those benefits would have to be regularly updated.

Financing Universal Coverage

The Institute of Medicine's report on health insurance posited four ways to achieve universal coverage: a major public program extension with a new tax credit; an employer and individual mandate with a government premium subsidy; an individual mandate and a tax credit; and a single payer system.[10] As explained in Chapter 2, the United States is not ready for single-payer. The expansion of public programs in some states has failed to produce universal coverage, and the tax credits discussed so far have been far too small to have much impact. An individual mandate combined with larger tax credits would be a nonstarter if it required employees to pay taxes on the value of employer-provided insurance.

That leaves the combined employer and individual mandate with government subsidies. On one hand, this solution has the advantage of familiarity, and it builds on a system that still covers the majority of nonelderly Americans. On the other hand, our employer-based system of private insurance is swiftly unraveling, and many businesses remain firmly opposed to a mandate, especially if they employ low-wage workers.

"For industries with low-wage workers, mandating insurance means a huge payroll tax," Princeton University economist Uwe Reinhardt explains. "Think of a semi-skilled worker who makes $35,000 a year. An insurance policy for a family now costs $10,000. If that grows by 10 percent a year, 10 years from now, it'll be $20,000 or $25,000. But the wage base will be, at most, $50,000 for workers who now earn $35,000. So you're requiring business to take half of the wage base and turn it over to the health system."

Even on a higher wage base, companies are increasingly finding that the provision of health benefits is making them less competitive. That was one reason GM and Ford cut back recently on health coverage.

Employers' concern about their competitive position, however, has not stopped some states from trying to force them to pay for health care. Hawaii has had an employer mandate for full-time workers in effect since 1983.[11] Twenty years later, California passed an employer mandate law that was repealed in a referendum in 2004.[12] Other states have since introduced similar legislation, and in 2006, Massachusetts passed a universal coverage statute that, among other things, requires companies to offer insurance or pay a fine.[13] Before we look at that, let's see how the employer mandate has affected Hawaii and why businesses opposed the California law.

A Qualified Success   At one point in the early 1990s, only 4 percent of Hawaii's population was uninsured, less than in any other state.[14] By 2002, that rate had shot up to 10 percent, which placed Hawaii behind seven other states with lower rates of uninsured people.[15] Yet that's still far below the national average, and the mandate didn't kill the state's small businesses, as some had predicted.

Hawaii's Prepaid Health Care Act requires employers to cover most full-time and some part-time workers. It excludes people who work fewer than twenty hours a week, workers covered by union contracts, seasonal agricultural workers, and a few other categories. And it doesn't require dependent coverage.

Employers and employees are expected to share the cost of insurance equally, but the workers' share is limited to 1.5 percent of their wages. Employees are not allowed to decline coverage. The law also specifies a standard benefit package.[16]

The State Health Insurance Program (SHIP), which started in 1989, extended government subsidies, on a sliding scale, to people who remained uninsured but earned too much to qualify for Medicaid. By 1993, SHIP was providing coverage to twenty-two thousand enrollees, or about two-thirds of this "gap group." That was far more than the additional number of people who received coverage because of the employer mandate.[17] The biggest impact of the mandate, says Gerard Russo, an assistant professor of health policy at the University of Hawaii, is that it required a standard benefit package.

Nobody Left Hawaii   Small employers, though not thrilled about the mandate, did not exit Hawaii en masse after its passage. Recently, like their brethren on the mainland, they've been complaining about the steep growth in insurance costs. But John Lewin, MD, former health commissioner of Hawaii, says that few of them would want to go back to the old days before the employer mandate.

A 2003 survey by the Hawaii Uninsured Project, a program of the Hawaii Institute for Public Affairs, lends some credence to this claim.[18] According to this survey, most employers believe that health insurance attracts and retains employees, and three-quarters of companies paid the total cost of insurance premiums for full-time employees. However, Lewin admits, employer support for the law is declining, partly because the employer share of the insurance cost keeps rising, while the employees' portion is still fixed at 1.5 percent of earnings.

Although 77 percent of employers offer dependent coverage to workers,[19] it has grown so expensive that many workers can no longer afford their share, Lewin observes. That's one reason for the rising rate of uninsured in Hawaii. Also, when SHIP was combined with Medicaid in 1993, it became too expensive for many people, because SHIP had previously offered more limited coverage than Medicaid did.[20] In addition, rapid growth in the number of part-time workers reduced the percentage of insured workers.[21] Some observers say employers have hired fewer full-time people to avoid the mandate.[22]

Despite these problems, Lewin notes, Hawaii remains the only state where nearly every busboy, store clerk, and taxi driver has good health insurance. The employer mandate has raised the cost of goods and services, he admits. "But when everybody has to provide insurance, it levels the playing field. If Wendy's provides it, so do McDonald's and Burger King."

Struggle in California   California's "play-or-pay" act would have required mid-sized and large employers to provide health insurance or pay into a state insurance fund. Employees' share of premiums would have been limited to 20 percent. The workers' contribution couldn't exceed 5 percent of their wages if their income was below 200 percent of the federal poverty level.[23]

If the law hadn't been rescinded, it would have gone into effect January 1, 2006, for employers with 200 or more workers, and would have kicked in for companies with 50–199 employees in 2007. Firms with 20–49 workers would have had to pay the fee or buy insurance only if government subsidies were available, and those employing fewer than 20 workers would have been exempt. Observers expected the law to expand coverage to about a quarter of the state's uninsured residents.[24]

The California Chamber of Commerce led the successful fight to repeal the law. The organization claimed that the legislation would have cost employers $7 billion a year, would have killed jobs, and would have driven many companies out of the state.[25] "Instead of covering more employees, this will result in a greater loss of coverage," Sara Lee, a spokesperson for the Chamber of Commerce, said before the referendum.

Raising Employers' Contribution   Ninety-nine percent of California firms with 200 or more workers and 94 percent of companies with 50–199 workers already offered insurance to their employees in 2002.[26] But Lee noted that "what the bill mandates is different from what employers offer" and also required coverage of some part-time workers. Moreover, she said, "employers have to pay 80 percent of the premium, and that's a very high threshold."

While 80 percent of employers with more than fifty workers already paid at least 80 percent of their employees' premiums, the other 20 percent would have had to increase their contribution.[27] A UCLA study of the potential impact of the employer mandate found, however, that companies covered by the new law would have had a median after-tax increase in business costs of $1,343 for each newly insured worker. That translated into a 0.2 percent increase in median operating expenditures.[28]

The California experience shows that the business opposition to a mandate remains very strong. But it's not monolithic: According to the UCLA study, 64 percent of the state's businesspeople favored a "play or pay" type of mandate. Even more surprising, 59 percent of respondents who didn't offer health insurance supported the coverage requirement. (A national survey, similarly, found that 54 percent of employers that didn't provide insurance favored an employer mandate.)[29]

California almost reached universal coverage by a different route in 2006. The Democrat-dominated legislature passed a bill that would have required the state to cover everyone through a single-payer system.[30] But the party-line vote on the measure showed the strength of the business opposition, and Republican governor Arnold Schwarzenegger vetoed the legislation.[31]

Early in 2007, Schwarzenegger proposed another route to universal insurance. Borrowing some elements from the Massachusetts plan, the governor would require individuals to buy policies and would require businesses with ten or more workers to either offer coverage or pay 4 percent of their wages into a state insurance fund. Medicaid coverage would be expanded, and providers would have to pay a tax to help fund higher payments to those who treat Medicaid patients. The plan to cover the state's 6.5 million uninsured people would cost $12 billion, according to the governor's office. Around half of that amount would come from the federal government and a redirection of state funds that now go to charity care.[32]

Hard on the heels of California's initiative, Democratic governor Edward Rendell of Pennsylvania proposed another variation on the Massachusetts plan. Rendell would set up a community-rated insurance pool to lower costs for small businesses that don't offer coverage and that pay wages below the state average of $39,000. He'd allow uninsured adults to join the same program, with state subsidies for those who make under 300 percent of the federal poverty level. Everyone who earns more than that (but not their employers) would be required to buy insurance, and companies of fifty or more employees would have to pay a "fair share assessment" if they didn't cover their workers.[33]

Massachusetts Makes Its Move   This flurry of state-level reform efforts began in 2006, when Governor Mitt Romney of Massachusetts, a Republican, signed a measure that made his state the first in the country to require individuals to buy health insurance. Passed with bipartisan majorities in the state legislature, this much-discussed law penalizes people who supposedly can afford insurance but don't acquire it by July 2007. In 2007, they'll lose their state personal tax exemption; in 2008, they'll forfeit tax refunds equivalent to half of the premium for the lowest-cost "acceptable" insurance policy in their area.

In contrast, businesses with eleven or more employees have to pay only $295 per worker per year if they don't offer health insurance; smaller firms pay nothing.[34] Governor Romney later watered down even that modest penalty by letting employers off the hook if they paid at least a third of the insurance premium.[35] So the onus is clearly on individuals, not companies, to purchase insurance—a point I will return to later.

The Massachusetts reform law is expected to extend coverage to up to 95 percent of its 550,000 uninsured residents. The state is using a combination of tax incentives, insurance subsidies, and an expansion of current government programs to get there. Federal funds and redirected state appropriations will cover most of the estimated $1.2 billion cost of the program.[36]

The Massachusetts law directs the state Medicaid program to enroll about fifty thousand people who qualify for coverage but aren't receiving it; the state signed up thirty-four thousand of those by the end of 2006.[37] The state is also providing insurance subsidies, on a sliding scale, to people who earn less than 300 percent of the federal poverty level; for the first three years, they'll have four Medicaid HMOs to choose from.[38]

Another key provision of the initiative allows small businesses, as well as working people who don't have employer-sponsored plans, to buy coverage through a state insurance pool. The state has given insurance companies incentives to offer low-cost plans to people in this pool.[39] Since these plans have to meet state-mandated benefit requirements, some experts expect them to have high deductibles or restricted provider networks or both.[40]

At the time of this writing, the four state-approved HMOs were just starting to sign up people earning between 100 and 300 percent of the poverty level. The premiums for individuals range from $18 to $170 a month, depending on their income and the plan they choose. How much the plans for higher-income people will cost isn't yet clear. State officials said that most people could afford to pay $200 a month for insurance and that health plans could offer high-deductible policies with "comprehensive benefits" for that much.[41] But in Massachusetts, nonsubsidized individual policies cost at least $600 a month, and family insurance, $1,000 a month or more.[42]

This discrepancy underlines the fact that the law fails to define what an "affordable" health plan is or how large a subsidy the state will provide to poorer residents. The higher the subsidy, the more it will cost Massachusetts, and the fewer people it will be able to cover without having to find new funding sources. But if the subsidy is too low, or if the plans are too skeletal, people either won't be able to afford insurance or won't want to pay for it.[43]

Individual versus Employer Mandate   Massachusetts is making a good-faith effort to provide some coverage for most of the uninsured. But it sets a very troublesome precedent by placing the burden for buying insurance mostly on individuals. Coupled with state subsidies for low-income workers, it leaves open a very wide escape hatch for employers who want to drop coverage—and, as the cost of health care rises, many undoubtedly will. A fine of $295 won't stop any employer from ditching an insurance policy that costs $6,000 a year. Even if a high-deductible policy through the state pool costs half of that, paying the fine is still the obvious course. Moreover, as John Holahan and Linda Blumberg of the Urban Institute point out, the requirement that all employers offer "Section 125" flexible spending accounts that enable employees to buy insurance with pretax dollars "reduces the incentive for small employers to offer coverage to their workers independently."[44]

If an individual mandate spread nationwide, it would mean poorer coverage at greater expense for most people. And, while businesses might save if the cost of charity care were no longer shifted to them in the form of higher insurance rates, in the long run they'd pay more in taxes for government subsidies to help people buy insurance. There's no free lunch. Every other advanced country requires employers to contribute to the cost of health care; and, one way or another, the United States will have to do the same.

Combination Mandate "Plus"   Despite business resistance, a combined employer and individual mandate, with government subsidies for small firms and lower-income people, still seems to be our best hope for attaining universal, comprehensive coverage. Even though this was part of the discarded Clinton plan, the utility insurer model offers many advantages that that proposal lacked, including more local control, a better alignment of financial incentives, and a built-in nest egg from administrative savings. If businesses could be convinced that universal coverage was in their best interest, and currently insured workers could be assured that they wouldn't lose part of their coverage, this financing approach could gain majority support.

Here's how it would work in our reform model: Every company and every employee earning more than a minimum amount would have to make a health care contribution in the form of a payroll tax, and every self-employed individual would pay quarterly health taxes, similar to estimated income taxes. People with enough income to make a contribution—including Medicare beneficiaries who now pay Part B premiums—would pay more to enroll with a high-cost physician group than with a lower-cost group.

The government would subsidize insurance payments on a sliding scale, based on a person's income. Nobody would have to contribute more than a certain percentage of his or her earnings for health insurance, and no company would have to contribute more than a set percentage of its payroll. However, firms that could afford it would have to pay up to 80 percent of the toll.

There are some good reasons to have the Internal Revenue Service collect the health care contributions. First, as Julius Richmond and Rashi Fein have pointed out, the IRS "has the competence to perform this function. Furthermore, since it has information on the income of individuals and household units, it is in a position to administer a system that varies the premium in relation to income."[45] And for low-income families and transient workers, this mechanism is much less complex than figuring out how to collect insurance premiums from them.[46]

While this approach bears some resemblance to single-payer financing systems, it would not give the government control over health care. All of the funds collected for health care would be distributed among the utility insurers, and the size of employer and employee contributions would be based partly on the budgets that the insurers submitted to Washington, rather than vice versa. While the government could limit overall health spending by reducing its subsidies, all sectors of society would strongly resist such a move. Political protests haven't stopped Medicare and Medicaid cuts, of course, but it would be harder to curtail subsidies if every voter were affected.

Loss of Tax Deductions   The move from employer-provided insurance to a system of payroll taxes would be largely invisible to employees. The portion of the premium that's now deducted from their paycheck would merely go to the IRS rather than to an insurance company. The only change that most employees would see would be in the amount of their contributions—and for many, that wouldn't be significant.

Employers, however, would be losing a major tax deduction; so would the self-employed who buy their own policies. So, unless we want them all to pay substantially more for insurance—a political nonstarter—their contributions would have to be adjusted to compensate for the loss of that deduction.

Take a company that now pays 80 percent of $6,000 a year for an employee's health insurance, or $4,800. The tax deduction for that amount might be worth $1,600. Let's assume that, under the new system, the firm's insurance contribution remained the same. In that case, the employer would pay the IRS $3,200, which would equal the former premium minus the former tax benefit. So the employer wouldn't be paying any more for health insurance than it was before, and the government would be taking in $1,600 more in general taxes that it would have to put into the utility insurers' pool.

Where Would the Money Come From? With the health care system as it exists today, government subsidies of the magnitude discussed here would entail a big tax increase that would be politically unacceptable. But, if health care financing and delivery were restructured along the lines proposed in this book, we could achieve universal coverage without raising general taxes, except in the short term.

The uninsured now receive health care worth about $100 billion a year.[47] If everyone had coverage equivalent to that of good private plans, their additional use of health care would cost about $69 billion a year (in 2001 dollars), according to one study.[48] However, the economist Uwe Reinhardt notes that this estimate is low for three reasons: Some of the uninsured population's current out-of-pocket spending would shift to the government budget; providers would be paid for care that's currently uncompensated; and some already insured people might give up their private coverage to join subsidized public programs.[49] While this last wouldn't occur under our reform approach, there would be additional costs from paying providers more to take good care of Medicaid patients. So it might cost $100 billion extra to reach universal coverage, as Reinhardt indicates.[50]

Previously, we figured out that the utility insurer system could save that much in administrative costs alone. But these savings wouldn't be available to expand coverage if providers and employers pocketed them. So the difference between the administrative costs of the utility insurers and those of the former health plans wouldn't be returned to employers and individuals in the form of lower contributions. Instead, that money would decrease the government's cost of subsidizing insurance for the working poor.

There would be no direct way to capture the administrative savings of physicians and hospitals. But, as noted earlier, the budgets submitted by competing physician groups would reflect some of those savings. This hypothesis is supported by the experience of Patient Choice, which, to repeat, had premiums that were 20 percent lower than those of local HMOs. Only part of that difference could have come from lower costs for health plan administration.

Even in the best-case scenario for administrative savings, there would be no extra money to improve Medicare benefits (by adding more generous drug coverage, for example). And, as the Institute of Medicine points out, a standard benefit package would inevitably raise insurance costs for people whose current plan provides less than those standard benefits.[51] To provide the subsidies that would be needed to cover these extra costs, the government would have to raise taxes in the short term, perhaps by repealing some of President Bush's tax cuts for the rich. In time, however, those subsidies would steadily drop as the competing, prepaid physician groups squeezed out waste.

Group Practice Benefits   As discussed in Chapter 13, prepaid group practices can provide better, more cost-effective care than small, fee-for-service practices can. Organized care delivery, coupled with financial accountability, should lead to better use of resources, the ability to care for patients continuously, better coordination of care, and greater use of evidence-based clinical guidelines.

If variations in care could be reduced to an appropriate level, and if most of the waste and redundancy in the system could be eliminated, health costs might drop by 30 to 40 percent, according to Donald Berwick of the Institute for Healthcare Improvement and Arnold Milstein, MD, medical director of the Pacific Business Group on Health.

In explaining his estimate, Berwick emphasizes the extra costs generated by supply-induced care. "The work of John Wennberg and Elliott Fisher at Dartmouth shows that the more intensive services are available in a community, the more they're used without effect on the quality of care," he says. "So supply drives demand. It's a monster cost driver without value added."

The other reason he believes that an efficient health care system could save this much is his experience with single-payer systems. "When you go to the U.K. or Canada or Sweden or Norway or the Netherlands, you're seeing systems that have half our cost but function just as well or better than ours."

Industrial Reengineering   Milstein derives his estimate of potential savings both from the Dartmouth studies and from the experience of other industries that have cut costs by 30 percent through continuous quality improvement. By reducing waste and improving quality, he figures, the health care industry could halve its costs; even after subtracting the costs of reengineering and information systems, he says, health care would cost 35 percent less than it does today.

The health care consultant and cardiologist Jacque Sokolov doubts that variations in care will ever be reduced enough to decrease U.S. health spending by that much. "At most, we'll get half of the way there in reducing the variability," he says. "And the reason why is that it's not totally related to quality. There's just a variability of practice in the way people treat patients."

Let's assume that the truth lies somewhere between Sokolov's and Milstein's estimates. This would mean that a quarter of current U.S. health spending—about $500 billion a year—could be safely eliminated. If we could save even a large portion of that colossal sum, we'd have more than enough money to provide good, comprehensive care to everyone.

The competition among physician groups that we'd count on to produce much of these savings, however, does not pertain in the hospital sphere today—and wouldn't under our model, either. Some markets have only one hospital; and in other places, hospital competition leads to increased costs. Hospitals are also so much stronger than any other kind of health care provider that they can bend the market to suit themselves. So with hospitals, as the next chapter explains, government intervention must take a different form.

19 Toward Uniform Hospital Pricing

In our reform model, utility insurers are not allowed to negotiate hospital prices. So hospitals would have every incentive to charge as much as they could get away with politically. Publishing their charges and quality ratings, as many politicians and employers now advocate, would have relatively little impact on prices. Most consumers pay scant attention to such information today (see Chapter 6), and they'll never be able to understand the arcane details of hospital pricing. Moreover, the majority of people go where their doctors send them, and they don't want to travel very far from where they live.

The prepaid physician groups in this system would have an incentive to eliminate unnecessary hospital admissions, tests, and procedures that drove up professional costs. If inpatient expenses were counted in the total cost of care that determined a patient's cost for choosing a particular group, the groups would have a reason to use cheaper hospitals. However, doctors would still have to consider geography and individual needs and preferences in deciding where to admit patients. For example, if a patient wanted to use a particular cardiac surgeon who practiced at a certain hospital, that's where he or she would go, regardless of the hospital's prices. And if physician groups limited inpatient utilization, some hospitals might raise their prices to compensate for the decreased volume.

Consequently, there seems to be no alternative to some form of administered hospital pricing—which means that payers predetermine what they'll pay for a service, group of services, or duration of service. While administered pricing has its own set of problems, it has the great virtue of insulating payers from the market power of any hospital system, no matter how large.

The End of Cost-Shifting   Historically, hospitals have tended to shift costs from public payers, which don't negotiate with them, to private payers, which often do. According to the American Hospital Association, in 2003 hospitals had an aggregate cost-to-payment ratio of 95 percent on Medicare business and 92 percent on Medicaid. That means that they lost 5 percent on Medicare and 8 percent on Medicaid. Partly to compensate for this shortfall, they induced private insurers to pay them 22 percent above cost.[1] (Hospitals also pass on uncompensated care costs equal to about 4 to 5 percent of their revenues to private payers; but that should go away with universal, comprehensive coverage.)[2]

In the utility insurer system, there would no longer be any cost shifting. While each insurer would maintain separate pools for Medicare patients and people under sixty-five, it would pay every hospital the same risk-adjusted amount for each service, case, or duration of stay. So there would be nowhere for the hospital to shift costs, except to its outpatient department, a subject taken up in a later discussion. The key challenge would be to figure out how to merge the current public and private payment systems. To understand how that could be done, it helps to know a little about the history and the approach of each system.

History Lessons

The federal government and the states have taken different approaches to administered pricing. A few states have adopted "all-payer" laws specifying what hospitals could charge insurers. From 1983 to 1996, for example, New York set rates that were supposedly high enough to cover the hospitals' costs and provide them with a slim profit margin. But the law backfired, because it punished well-run hospitals by lowering their rates, while rewarding inefficient hospitals with higher rates.[3]

New Jersey passed an "all-payer" law setting hospital rates for all health plans in the 1970s. According to Terrence French, executive vice president of Newark's Cathedral Healthcare, the legislature did this to "stabilize hospital over-capacity." In other words, no hospital was allowed to go out of business, so hospitals had no reason to become more efficient. After the state ended rate-setting in 1992, some hospitals began to encounter serious difficulties. By 1999, even the state hospital association was saying that twenty-five facilities needed to be closed.

The Centers for Medicare and Medicaid Services (CMS) has used a different method to fix hospital prices. Since 1983, Medicare has paid fixed prices for "diagnostic-related groups" (DRGs) of services. This "prospective payment system" (PPS) covers all inpatient services, and a different payment regimen now governs reimbursement of hospital outpatient departments.[4]

"DRG Creep"   The prospective payment system did not restrain hospital spending for long. After an initial drop-off in the early 1980s, hospital-cost growth accelerated again until 1994, when managed care began squeezing costs out of the system. Then in 1999, the upward march resumed.[5] Although hospital admissions and average length of stay declined substantially in the 1980s and 1990s, total hospital spending has continued to expand.[6]

"While the introduction of the Medicare prospective payment system (PPS) in 1983 provided a respite from double-digit hospital inflation, most of the savings were due to declines in admission volume," John Ashby and Craig Lisk wrote in *Health Affairs* in 1992. "By the third year of PPS, the yearly increase in operating cost per case returned to about 9 percent, where it has remained."[7]

One reason for this increase was the phenomenon of "DRG creep," which results from hospitals' "upcoding" diagnoses so that they can charge Medicare for a better-reimbursed DRG. From 1985 to 1989, according to a Medicare advisory group, DRG creep accounted for more than a third of the change in Medicare's case-mix to more serious types of diagnoses.[8] A 1997 government report found DRG creep to be endemic throughout the hospital industry.[9] And since large sums of money are at stake, there's every reason to believe that hospitals—aided by a small army of consultants—are still upcoding to milk Medicare for extra payments.

There's also some evidence that DRGs are a disincentive to hospital quality improvement efforts. If a patient has a complication in the hospital, for example, his case goes into a higher-reimbursed DRG. Conversely, notes Brent James, MD, of Intermountain Healthcare in Salt Lake City, providing better care has cost his hospital money by reducing its average level of DRGs.[10] But this problem could be mitigated if DRGs were risk-adjusted and their number significantly increased, as explained in a later section.

Out-of-Whack Payments   Besides having only limited success in cost containment, DRG payments have drifted out of proportion to the costs of providing services over the years. This fact came to light in the course of the policy debate over specialty hospitals, which have been accused of draining the most lucrative business away from traditional hospitals. In a 2005 report on specialty hospitals, the Medicare Payment Advisory Commission (MedPAC) found that one reason specialty hospitals threaten full-line institutions is that they specialize in procedural DRGs that are more profitable than many services provided by traditional hospitals.[11]

MedPAC recommended that CMS eliminate the differences between the relative profitability of different DRGs. It also said that CMS should adjust payments based on the severity of each case within a DRG. MedPAC viewed this risk-adjustment as essential to preventing specialty hospitals from skimming less complex cases, leaving the sicker patients to full-line hospitals. These two changes, MedPAC suggested, would increase the fairness of the competition between specialty and full-service hospitals.

Other experts agree that the DRG system has gotten out of whack, and not just in the battle between specialty and traditional hospitals. "Virtually all hospitals use surgical DRGs—and cardiac ones in particular—as winners and nonsurgical DRGs as losers," Robert Berenson of the Urban Institute says. "Finally, MedPAC has documented that and shown that it causes market distortions."

Paul Ginsburg of the Center for Studying Health System Change shares this view. In a recent article, Ginsburg and coauthor Joy M. Grossman stated, "Differences in the profitability of individual services appear to be contributing to important changes in care delivery, as both physicians and hospitals expand their capacity to compete to deliver the most profitable services."[12]

To its credit, CMS embraced MedPAC's suggestions. In April 2006, the agency proposed basing the relative values of DRGs on hospital costs, rather than basing them on charges, as it does now.[13] To the extent that CMS could obtain reasonably current cost data, this method would be more accurate, and it would result in a payment system that was less procedure-oriented.

By 2008, CMS said, it also wanted to replace the current system of 526 DRGs with one that included 861 "severity-adjusted" DRGs.[14] According to Joseph Newhouse, an economics professor at Harvard, increasing the number of categories to recognize differences in health status would be an improvement on the current system. "It would mitigate this tendency of specialty hospitals to draw low-cost patients within each DRG."

However, there would be winners and losers, he adds. "Hospitals that tend to get fairly straightforward cases within any DRG would lose, and hospitals that get relatively complicated cases would win."

Under CMS's plan, payments for some complex procedures would have decreased by 20 to 30 percent. Unsurprisingly, fierce lobbying by groups representing doctors, hospitals, consumers, and medical device manufacturers forced CMS to water down these efforts substantially. In August 2006, the agency issued a final rule that cut procedural payments only slightly and added just a handful of new DRGs, while setting a three-year phase-in of cost-based payments.[15]

But CMS didn't give up the fight to reduce the profitability of some DRGs. In April 2007, the agency announced a plan to create 745 new severity-adjusted DRGs to replace the current ones. CMS predicted that, in fiscal 2008, hospitals would still receive an average increase of 3.3 percent, close to the expected rate of inflation. However, the American Hospital Association said that the real increase would be less, and specialty and rural hospitals remained opposed to the change.[16]

Private Payment Methods

Whereas Medicare hospital reimbursement is mainly DRG-based, private payers may use capitation, percentage of cost, per diems or case rates (which are similar to DRGs). However, observers agree, there has been a big drop-off in global capitation. And few plans reimburse on a percentage of cost anymore, because it exposes them to higher payments whenever hospitals raise their charges.

Michael LaPenna says hospitals tend to prefer per diems because their accounting systems are set up to track costs daily. However, case rates are becoming more common for some kinds of cases. Edward McKillip, finance director for the Main Line Health System in Bryn Mawr, Pennsylvania, has noticed this trend in the Philadelphia area, and Deborah Chanen, senior director for managed care and network development for Adventist Health Managed Care in Glendale, California, has observed the same thing in her region. "We still have a number of per diem rates for general medical cases," she says. "In the surgical areas, there are a lot more case rates."

While case rates have long been common for obstetrical/gynecological and cardiovascular procedures, Chanen is now seeing more of them in other areas such as bariatric and neuro-interventional cases. In California, fewer case rates are in place for joint replacements. "More often," she says, "hospitals would have an implant exclusion—they'd get paid a per diem plus the cost of implants."

On the East Coast, however, joint-replacement case rates are common, and hospitals welcome them. "With a hip procedure, we're pretty sure the patient is going to stay between three and five days," McKillip notes. "We know how much the hardware costs, we know how much physical therapy they're going to need, and so on. So we have a pretty good idea of what goes into taking care of that patient.

"We wouldn't ask for a case rate for a category that has a wide variation in the types of cases within it. For example, I wouldn't recommend putting a case rate around tracheotomies, because a patient can stay anywhere from fourteen days to one hundred days in an acute setting. So it's really a lot more risk. And it's hard to come up with a case rate where there's so much variability."

"Front-Loaded" Cases   The best candidates for case rates, the hospital executives say, are those that incur a lot of cost in the first day. "A hip patient could stay for four days, and if I have a per diem rate of $1,500 or $1,800, I'm not even going to be able to cover the cost of the implant, unless they really jack the per diems up," McKillip says.

Chanen agrees that hospitals prefer case rates on admissions that have a lot of "front-loaded" expenses. "Some case rates can be for a one-day stay—angioplasty or cardiac catheterization, for example. It's better to have a case rate, because you're going to build in a lot of operating room time or high-tech equipment that you pay for. You bill the rate based on your cost; with a per diem, you try to get to that, but it's hard."

A large percentage of such cases are surgical, including joint replacements and heart procedures. But Donald Liss, a regional medical director for Aetna, says that his company is also paying case rates on an increasing number of general medical admissions, such as those for pneumonia and heart failure.

Liss doesn't believe hospitals are taking a big risk on these cases, because they're used to dealing with DRGs. And if a patient stays in the hospital a certain number of days, he notes, Aetna will pay a per-diem beyond that point.

Another way that hospitals try to protect themselves is to have health plans reinsure them against catastrophic costs. But plans aren't always willing to provide this reinsurance; even if they are, some West Coast plans are demanding that hospitals swallow more of the cost before this "stop-loss" coverage kicks in.[17]

Similarities with Medicare In trying to merge Medicare and commercial payment systems, we would have to strike some kind of balance between per diems and DRGs/case rates. While the DRG is Medicare's predominant mode, it does pay per diems in lieu of full DRG payments to hospitals that transfer patients to skilled nursing facilities too swiftly. For 223 DRGs,[18] the hospital gets either half of the total DRG payment or twice the usual per diem rate on the first day. It receives per diems for each subsequent day of the hospital stay until the total bill reaches the DRG amount. (If the patient goes home in less than the average amount of time for the DRG, however, the hospital receives the full case rate.)[19]

This is the only situation in which Medicare pays per diems. But, as we've seen, private plans are increasingly paying hospitals on the basis of case rates. So it seems possible to harmonize the two approaches.

Paul Ginsburg notes that private payers already use Medicare's relative-value system as the basis for setting physician fee schedules. Since this is fee for service, it's not comparable to Medicare's inpatient prospective payment system. But the DRG system does use relative weights, Ginsburg says, that could be applied to case rates used by private payers. After Medicare revamps its DRGs so that they track more closely to costs, he adds, they might look more attractive to commercial insurers.

"In the mid-eighties, when the Medicare prospective payment system began and managed care was in its early days, a lot of people were surprised that plans didn't use DRGs," he recalls. "The real reason was that they had a lot of anticipation of what they could accomplish with their own managed-care methods. They felt those could be more effective than a case-rate system, which is more dependent on the hospital to do the economizing. Now that managed care has less of an ability to do utilization management than it used to, and Medicare is more committed to making its payments accurate, it might be more natural for insurers to use DRGs."

Unified Payment System Amid the rubble of strictly managed care, Ginsburg sees advantages in a unified administered pricing system for public and private insurers. While he admits that the history of hospital rate-setting by states is not encouraging, he observes that, under universal coverage, the states would no longer have to funnel money to inefficient hospitals to subsidize charity care. If all hospitals received the same adjusted payments for the same procedures, the inefficient ones would be more likely to cut their costs or go out of business.

At the same time, he acknowledges that allowances must be made to achieve desirable public policies. CMS would continue to subsidize teaching hospitals, for example. "Also, there are standby costs that must be recognized. Running a trauma center loses money; so in an administered pricing system, you'd have an allowance to pay for that."

Ginsburg views a compromise between the public and private approaches as inevitable. "It would probably be a better system if you worked out a uniform mixture of payments, so that some services would be paid on a case rate, and others on a per diem basis. That makes a lot of sense."

Outpatient Care Growth Whatever inpatient payment system is devised, it won't exist in a vacuum. An increasing amount of acute care is being provided in hospital outpatient clinics and other ambulatory facilities. The more closely inpatient reimbursement is controlled, the more incentive hospitals have to move whatever care they can to the outpatient side. And the new technologies enable more and more procedures to be performed in an ambulatory setting.

Outpatient spending accounted for 13 percent of hospital revenues in 1980, 23 percent in 1990, and 35 percent in 2003.[20] And those figures don't fully indicate the increasing importance of outpatient departments to hospitals. According to the health-policy expert Jeff Goldsmith, ambulatory clinics now contribute 60–70 percent of hospital profits.

Kenneth Thorpe of Emory University doubts that the figure is that high. "If you have a big trauma unit and a walk-in AIDS clinic, and are treating a lot of uninsured patients—those factors aren't a great recipe for making money [on the outpatient side]," he says. "But if you're in a different market and you have better control of who walks into the emergency room, outpatient services can certainly be profitable."

After paying more and more for outpatient services every year, CMS introduced an outpatient prospective payment system in 2000.[21] While this system has similarities to the DRG setup, it uses a relative-value-based fee schedule like the one that CMS uses to pay physicians. For surgical procedures, the agency pays case rates that bundle fees for operating and recovery room services, most pharmaceuticals, anesthesia, and surgical and medical supplies. CMS pays separately for imaging and lab tests.[22]

ASC System in Flux   With ambulatory surgery centers, CMS also uses a fee schedule to pay for a bundle of facility services, such as nursing, recovery care, anesthetics, and supplies. But up to now, these fees have not been based on the relative use of resources. CMS is now proposing to pay ambulatory surgery centers the same type of prospective case rates that it pays hospital outpatient departments (see Chapter 9).[23]

Combined with the ongoing reform of the DRG system, these steps should help level the playing field between hospitals and specialty hospitals, as well as between outpatient departments and ambulatory surgery centers.

This brief outline indicates that utility insurers could pay case rates for all outpatient procedures, whether done in an ambulatory surgery center or an outpatient department. How they would reimburse hospital outpatient departments, dialysis centers, and other clinics for nonsurgical care is a trickier question; but there's no doubt that public and private payers could create a uniform payment system.

The bigger issue is how to control overall hospital costs, which, like drug outlays, are the product of price and volume. As has been suggested, part of the solution is to have primary-care groups ride herd on specialists. But to truly keep tabs on what specialists and surgeons do in the hospital, and to oversee the care coordination that is so essential to controlling costs, another type of physician will be required. That physician, already present in a large and growing number of hospitals, carries the inelegant moniker of "hospitalist." But, as we'll see in the next chapter, he or she can have a great impact on the quality and efficiency of care.

20 Let "Hospitalists" Take Charge

On a balmy spring morning, internist Charles Meidt is making his rounds at Bryn Mawr Hospital in Bryn Mawr, Pennsylvania. One of his patients, Roger Johnson, a very pale, eighty-three-year-old man who came here from a nursing home the day before, has blood clots in his legs. He also has a history of gastrointestinal bleeding. Normally, his internist at the nursing home would have given him a blood thinner (also known as an anticoagulant) to dissolve the clots, but she was concerned about a recurrence of the gastrointestinal bleeding.

When Johnson was admitted yesterday, Meidt consulted a gastroenterologist, and they considered the options together: try an anticoagulant and carefully monitor the patient for signs of recurrent internal bleeding, or put in an IVC filter to prevent the clots from entering the pulmonary arteries. Johnson doesn't want invasive care, which rules out the IVC filter. So he's now on injectable heparin, a blood thinner, and Meidt is starting to phase in Coumadin, an oral anticoagulant. Meidt takes a look at Johnson's legs and comments that the swelling has gone down.

Having seen in the patient's chart that the gastroenterologist has checked the patient's test results, Meidt calls Johnson's daughter. He tells her that the blood thinners are working without causing internal bleeding. Her father will be here two or three more days while the Coumadin in his blood rises to a therapeutic level. When he's discharged, Meidt will call his nursing home doctor.

A New Breed of Physician One of the new breed of "hospitalists," Meidt coordinates the hospital care of patients referred to him by office-based primary-care physicians and specialists. The soft-spoken, forty-seven-year-old internist also takes "unassigned" patients who don't have any regular physician.

Meidt is chief of the hospitalist service of Main Line Health, which includes three acute-care hospitals—Bryn Mawr, Paoli, and Lankenau—and a rehabilitation facility. Besides caring for patients, he supervises thirty-two hospitalist physicians at Bryn Mawr and Paoli Hospitals. (Lankenau Hospital has internal-medicine residents who serve as hospitalists.) Each full-time hospitalist works seven twelve-hour shifts in a row and then gets a week off. As a group, the inpatient physicians are on the medical floors twenty-four hours a day, seven days a week.

According to Meidt, who helped Bryn Mawr Hospital found its hospitalist service in 1996, nearly every hospital in his area now has one. As a result, he says, patients now expect to have a hospitalist manage their care when they're admitted. So do doctors. Three-quarters of the primary-care physicians on Bryn Mawr's staff refer to him and his colleagues.

A "Bargain" for Bryn Mawr   Because they do "evaluation-and-management" work, most hospitalists don't bring in enough fee-for-service income from insurers and Medicare to justify their salaries. Yet Main Line Health prizes Meidt and his fellow hospitalists enough to make up the difference.

"They're very cost-effective because of the differences we see in length of stay, and the fact that there's availability and responsiveness of physicians on a regular basis," explains Claire Baldwin, Bryn Mawr Hospital's vice president of nursing administration. "There's someone there who's coordinating care. And they can give feedback on the patient to the nursing staff and the regular hospital staff. They can get orders done. They're just great."

Before the hospitalist program started, Baldwin notes, "We were having problems with excessive length of stay, basically because physicians weren't able to get in here from the office. Physicians were covering for each other, and if someone started covering on Friday, they wouldn't discharge a patient over the weekend."

While Bryn Mawr's overall length of stay has dropped since then, the community physicians are still keeping patients in the hospital longer than the hospitalists are. The average length of stay for Meidt and his colleagues is 3.9 days, compared with 5.3 days for office-based physicians.

Meidt emphasizes that he and his colleagues receive salaries and have no incentive to discharge patients any sooner than they should. One of the other hospitalists, Matthew Cahill, concedes that the hospital does put a "big emphasis" on expeditious discharges. But he adds, "I don't know if I'd call it pressure, because it's my objective, too. I don't think people are particularly well-served to be kept in the hospital. They'd rather be going home, and they're often better off if they can transfer to a rehab facility or something that's more appropriate to what they really need to get back home."

Why Hospitalists?   In 1996, Robert Wachter, MD, and Lee Goldman, MD, faculty members at the University of California San Francisco, shook up the medical world with an article in the *New England Journal of Medicine* about the then new field of hospitalists.[1] They noted that some large medical groups—especially in California—were either using full-time hospitalists or having primary-care physicians take turns doing nothing but hospital care for a week or a month at a time. As Wachter and Goldman observed, this trend was largely a response to HMOs' demands for greater efficiency in inpatient and outpatient care. As long as it affected only big groups in areas where a lot of people belonged to HMOs, it was no big deal to most physicians. But the authors predicted that it was just the beginning of a new division of responsibilities between generalists who followed patients in the hospital and those who cared for them in the office.

"As a result [of managed care]," they wrote, "we anticipate the rapid growth of a new breed of physicians we call 'hospitalists'—specialists in inpatient medicine—who will be responsible for managing the care of hospitalized patients in the same way that primary care physicians are responsible for managing the care of outpatients."

Physicians Support Hospitalists   Wachter and Goldman's prediction has come true, but for reasons somewhat different from what they anticipated. HMOs' demand for efficiency played a role, but most plans were unable to mandate the use of hospitalists because of fierce physician opposition.[2]

Nevertheless, a lot of doctors started using hospitalists voluntarily. Office-based physicians began to realize that they were spending a lot of time traveling to the hospital to round on a few patients when they could be back in the office making money. As managed-care plans cut physician reimbursement ever more steeply, increasing the pressure on them to see more patients, this view gradually dominated. A 2002 *Medical Economics* poll of primary-care physicians revealed that 61 percent of respondents were referring patients to hospitalists, and only 9 percent were doing so because it was mandatory. Moreover, 85 percent of the physicians rated the hospitalists' care of their patients as excellent or good.[3]

Many doctors also used hospitalists because it spared them from having to take emergency calls. "Malpractice cost pressures in some markets [have] made hospitalist programs attractive to hospitals and medical groups, by contributing to physicians' avoidance of inpatient care and emergency department (ED) call because of the perceived increased liability risk associated with these settings," researchers from the Center for Studying Health System Change note.[4]

Meanwhile, hospitals were starting to perceive the advantages of hospitalists, too. By reducing the length of hospital stays and pharmacy, supply, and test costs, hospitalists cut total hospital costs by 10 to 15 percent.[5] These cuts helped hospitals make more money under Medicare's prospective payment system and also under the case rates that more health plans were imposing on them.

Trend Expected to Continue   For all these reasons, the number of hospitalists jumped from a few hundred in 1996 to about eight thousand in 2003 and to as many as twenty thousand today. The Society of Hospital Medicine (SHM), which counts 40 percent of them as members, predicts there could be thirty thousand hospitalists by the end of this decade.[6]

The number of hospitals that use inpatient physicians has also grown rapidly. Among hospitals with two hundred or more beds, SHM reported in 2004, 55 percent had hospitalist programs; 45 percent of those with one hundred or more beds did.[7] But that still left a lot of institutions that didn't have hospitalists—one reason for the expectation that growth in the field would continue.

According to a 1997 survey, most hospitalists were internists; of these, 51 percent were generalists and 38 percent were internal-medicine subspecialists, including pulmonologists and critical care physicians.[8] By 1999, however, only 15 percent of all hospitalists were subspecialists; 74 percent were general internists, and most of the rest were pediatricians or family doctors.[9]

Who Employs Hospitalists?   Hospitals employed 34 percent of hospitalists in 2003, according to the SHM survey. About 25 percent of inpatient physicians worked for hospitalist-only groups, including multistate companies and local physician groups. Academic hospital medicine programs employed 18 percent of hospitalists, and 16 percent belonged to multispecialty groups. That was down from 23 percent just two years earlier and from 31 percent in 1999.[10]

The sharp decline in physician groups' use of hospitalists may be partly related to the concurrent drop in capitation. When groups stop sharing financial responsibility for hospital care, they have less of an economic incentive to employ hospitalists.

But James Pizzo, a partner in Accenture's Health and Life Sciences practice, notes that some groups that are mainly paid fee-for-service no longer employ hospitalists, either. "Originally, it was thought that the extra income generated back in the office [by other physicians] would be more than enough to offset the cost of the hospitalists," he points out. "But the volume at the hospital for their own patients wasn't large enough."

In contrast, all but the smallest hospitals have enough patients to justify the use of hospitalists. While hospitals directly employ only a third of inpatient physicians, Robert Wachter estimates that institutions subsidize the salaries of 70–80 percent of hospitalists. For example, his own hospitalist group is part of the medical school at the University of California at San Francisco, but it's financially dependent on the hospital where he and his colleagues work.

Similarly, Cogent Healthcare, a multistate hospitalist company that employs two hundred hospitalists, relies on hospitals paying it more than it can collect by billing for its doctors' services. "A hospitalist program can't support itself with fee-for-service collections," Ronald Greeno, Cogent's medical director, says.

Local groups of internists also set themselves up as hospitalists, often without the hospital's permission, Greeno notes. Since they depend entirely on billings, they may be following twenty to thirty patients at a time[11]—far above the national average of twelve to fifteen.[12] Greeno doesn't think they do as good a job of caring for each patient as they could if they had fewer patients.

Greeno is not a disinterested observer. But Wachter also hears that some hospitalists are caring for too many patients. "Anecdotally, I tend to hear this a little more from hospitalists who are working either for private companies or for themselves," he says. And as Mark Sprangers relates in his anecdote about Florida hospitals in Chapter 8, the use of freelance hospitalists who don't follow the patients closely can result in very poor care coordination.

"Voltage Drop" in Communications   The possibility that hospitalists might interrupt the continuity of care has been a concern from the beginning. Wachter admits that the discontinuity of care between the inpatient and outpatient spheres is a drawback of the hospitalist model. There's always a "voltage drop" in communications, he says, "caused by movement of information from the office to the hospital ward and back again." But because they're conscious of this problem, he argues, hospitalists tend to pay extra attention to communication with referring physicians.[13]

Nevertheless, in a recent interview, Wachter said he was concerned that some hospitalists don't always keep primary-care physicians informed. "There are plenty of programs that don't do it as well as they should. When you're too busy and running around too fast, I'm afraid this may be one of the things that people say is partly elective."

In the *Medical Economics* survey of primary-care physicians, nearly half of the respondents agreed with the statement, "I'm occasionally or frequently surprised that a patient had been admitted or discharged, or has had a serious incident while under the care of a hospitalist." But 55 percent agreed with, "Hospitalists keep me in the loop when my patients are hospitalized."[14]

Doctors May Be Hard to Reach   Charles Meidt says that he and the other Bryn Mawr hospitalists always try to inform a patient's regular physician about the patient's admission, discharge, and important changes in health status or diagnosis. They may also consult the primary-care physician if they're conferring with a patient's family about whether to pursue an aggressive course of treatment.

The devil is in the details. For example, Meidt notes, he and his colleagues dictate discharge summaries within twenty-four hours after a patient is discharged. These reports are usually transcribed in a few hours and faxed to the referring doctors. Yet some doctors who complained about poor availability of discharge summaries had told the transcription service not to fax anything to them.

When Meidt tries to phone referring doctors, he reaches someone who knows the patient only about half the time. Usually the patient's physician is busy with other patients, out of the office, or on vacation.

Covering physicians often have no direct knowledge of the patient or access to his or her records, he says.

Satisfaction, Quality, and Safety   Patients who are cared for by hospitalists are just as satisfied as those who see their own physicians in the hospital. According to Wachter and Goldman, "patients may be willing to trade off the familiarity of their regular physician for the availability of the hospitalist."[15]

While a number of studies have shown that hospitalists reduce costs without lowering the quality of care, it's less certain that they provide better care than traditional attending doctors do. The Main Line hospitalists' readmission rate, Meidt says, is one-third that of the rest of the medical staff; but peer-reviewed studies have been equivocal on this point.[16] A randomized controlled trial involving joint replacement cases did demonstrate that those who were co-managed by hospitalists had significantly fewer complications.[17]

A pair of studies published in 2002 found that patients cared for by hospitalists had lower mortality rates both during their hospitalization and for thirty days afterward; these benefits became more significant as the hospitalists gained experience. But an accompanying editorial notes that only a handful of hospitalists were studied, raising the question "whether the results were due to these particular physicians or to the fact that they functioned as hospitalists."[18]

It would seem obvious that having hospitalist doctors available twenty-four hours a day, seven days a week should improve patient safety. Yet this is not an open-and-shut case, either. The number of medical errors in hospitals has hardly budged since the Institute of Medicine issued its famous report in 1999, and recent analyses of hospitals' safety records have dwelt on issues such as systems design, information technology, and error reporting, rather than hospitalists.[19] In an article on the subject, Wachter admits that hospitalists have created yet another safety challenge by generating a new discontinuity of care. But he also cites the advantage of having expert inpatient physicians available all the time and notes that "hospitalists have emerged as important advocates for safety and systems thinking."[20]

Impact on Specialists

The Park Nicollet Clinic in Minneapolis was one of the first large groups in the country to adopt a hospitalist system. When the 380-doctor multispecialty group started down this path in 1994, most of the hospitalists were internists or family physicians who took off time from their outpatient practices to care for hospitalized patients.[21] While Park Nicollet still uses this system of rotating outpatient doctors, the majority of generalist physicians who care for inpatients are now full-time hospitalists.[22]

Richard Freese, MD, of Park Nicollet reports in an article published in 1999 that the group shifted to the hospitalist model partly because office-based physicians were often absent from the hospital when they were needed. He also cites "preventive, frequently unnecessary consultations with specialists." These consultants were often called, he says, "because primary care physicians wanted care to proceed while they themselves were unavailable during the hospital day."[23]

Two years after implementation of the new system, Freese writes, 89 percent of the group's internists and family physicians believed that it was "better or much better" than the old system. And consultations with medical specialists and surgeons had decreased by 17 percent. "It was our perception," he says, "that the change to the hospitalist model led to fewer but more appropriate consultations." For example, in the earlier system a cardiologist would have been routinely called in to examine a patient with chest pains, because his primary-care physician might not be available. "The need for this type of consultation dissolved," he adds, "when a hospitalist is constantly available."

Because specialists were always on the floor, hospitalists were able to have impromptu conferences with them more often, Freese points out. And as the hospitalists gained experience with inpatient care, they had to consult the specialists less and less often. Partly as a result of these changes, Park Nicollet's average length of stay declined by nearly a day, and its overall costs for the twelve most expensive diagnoses dropped by 25 percent.

Nationwide Trend   Park Nicollet's early experience has been replicated nationwide. According to Wachter, the use of hospitalists reduces the amount of consultation with specialists by 10 to 30 percent.[24] While this estimate is based on anecdotes from other hospitalists, a 2001 study in *CHEST* supports his point.[25]

Examining the treatment of Medicaid patients in a community hospital, the study found that hospitalists consulted with specialists in 17 percent of cases, while private-practice attendings consulted with them 38 percent of the time. There were even larger differences between the percentages of hospitalist and nonhospitalist patients for whom two or three specialists were called in.

While the study wasn't designed to measure comparative quality, the authors did not detect markers of poor care such as greater "inpatient mortality, clinically indicated ancillary therapies, or delays in minor procedures" for hospitalist patients. Also, despite shorter lengths of stay, "we did not detect increased hospital readmissions, home-care referrals, transfers to extended care facilities, or use of rehabilitation facilities." In the researchers' view, this meant that the increased efficiency of hospitalists did not lead to increased costs outside the hospital.

Specialists' View   Most specialists at Park Nicollet liked the hospitalist service, according to Freese. A survey showed that 76 percent thought the change was "positive to tremendous," and only 12 percent believed it was detrimental. However, the group's specialists were salaried, so "their incomes did not diminish with the decrease in consultation-related volume."[26]

Wachter notes that busy specialists tend to appreciate hospitalists because they don't consult them on the minor things that primary-care physicians often call them in for. These consultations aren't very lucrative, because there are no procedures involved. "Also, most specialists don't like to do consults that they don't think require their expertise," he adds.

He admits, however, that the situation is different in areas that are oversupplied with specialists who need to find more work. "In those areas, hospitalists are less popular," he says. While predicting that nearly every hospital will eventually have hospitalist programs, he states that in some places, "it's the specialists worrying about those consults that force the program not to form."

Richard Afable, MD, executive vice president and chief medical officer of Catholic Healthcare East, a major hospital chain, agrees that specialists can be an obstacle. Noting that hospitalists have led quality improvement efforts in some of his facilities, he says, "The only guys that are unhappy with hospitalists are the cardiologists or pulmonologists who used to get unnecessary consults."[27]

Some Specialists Like Hospitalists   In the Philadelphia area, out-of-control malpractice insurance costs and low reimbursement rates have produced a shortage of consultants and surgeons, Charles Meidt observes. So the specialists are generally supportive of the hospitalists, he says.

He and Matthew Cahill have noticed some differences, however, between the consultants' attitudes at Bryn Mawr and Paoli Hospitals. At Paoli, which has somewhat younger patients and more family physicians on its staff, fewer primary-care physicians wanted to round on their patients before the hospitalist program was introduced. As a result, Meidt says, patients who came to the emergency room were more often handed off to specialists than were Bryn Mawr patients.

Even now, five years after the hospitalists arrived, the Paoli specialists don't work as closely with them as the ones at Bryn Mawr do. "At Paoli," Cahill says, "when somebody comes in and you get one consultant, they consult two more people. Here, if you consult a specialist, they wouldn't do that; they may suggest you might want to consult somebody else."

Because of the physician shortage and the desire of specialists to do more procedures in their offices or ambulatory surgery centers, they increasingly rely on the hospitalists to do things they used to do. For example, Meidt points out, the gastrointestinal specialists used to admit all patients with gastrointestinal bleeding; but now, they let the hospitalists take those cases. The same thing has happened in cardiology. "We're taking chest pain patients who used to go to cardiology." The hospitalists still call in specialists for consultations when necessary, he adds.

Most hospitalist patients are admitted from the emergency room. In past years, says Meidt, many of these patients would have gone to ENT specialists or surgeons, but "they're so stretched now that they need help admitting." His service is taking nearly all ENT patients and even some neurosurgical patients. Neurosurgeons will look at patients with intracranial hemorrhages, but if they're not going to operate, they'll let hospitalists co-manage the patient. Similarly, a hospitalist will order a CT scan on a patient with unspecified belly pain; unless it turns up something that requires surgery, he'll handle the case.

Hospitalists' Role in Reform   For all the reasons enumerated, it makes eminent sense for hospitals to hire or contract with hospitalists. But as we've seen, there's much less of a business case for physician groups to employ full-time hospitalists. So in our reform model, hospitalists should work for their institutions and should take patients from all physician groups equally.

While the use of hospitalists would remain voluntary, the primary-care groups should strongly encourage physicians to refer patients to them wherever possible. Assuming that the hospitalists prioritized communication with office-based physicians, that would be an important step forward in the battle for better coordination of care and fewer medical errors. And it could help the groups stay within their budgets by curbing unnecessary specialty consults.

In 2002, when there were about five thousand hospitalists, Wachter and Goldman estimated that they were collectively reducing inpatient costs by about $2.4 billion a year.[28] Hospital spending has risen 33 percent since then,[29] and there are now about twenty thousand hospitalists. Applying Wachter and Goldman's estimate to the current workforce and level of hospital spending, hospitalists might have saved roughly $13 billion in 2006.[30] And that's a conservative estimate: If hospitalists could save a quarter of inpatient costs, as they did for Park Nicollet's most expensive diagnoses, the figure would be $32.5 billion;[31] and if we had thirty thousand hospitalists, the savings could be as high as $49 billion at the 2006 level of spending.[32]

While that's a lot of money, it's still only a small fraction of total hospital spending. To reduce the bulk of the waste, in both inpatient and ambulatory care, we'd also have to limit excess capacity in the health care system and increase the amount of evidence supporting evidence-based medicine. The key to progress in these two areas, as described in the next two chapters, is working through communities. Chapter 21 looks at how local communities can help control the proliferation of unneeded health care facilities and programs. And Chapter 22 explains how the physician community can develop a better system to find out what works best in practice.

21 Health Planning and the CON

If variations in medical utilization are correlated with the number of hospital beds in a market, and if variations in surgical procedures are correlated with the availability of diagnostic equipment, an excess of either will inevitably lead to inefficient use of health care resources. That's why leading experts such as John Wennberg, Donald Berwick, and George Halvorson have called for more rational planning of hospital capacity.[1]

The federal and state governments have been trying to restrain the expansion of hospital and outpatient capacity for three decades. Their main tool in this never-ending struggle is certificate-of-need (CON) laws, which require state approval for new health care facilities, equipment, and programs. Three-quarters of the states still have these regulations. Yet, as noted earlier, we're seeing an explosion of new hospitals, ambulatory surgical centers, imaging centers, and other facilities. To what extent do CON programs restrain the market's tendency to grow health care capacity, and what effect does that have on spending?

Critics of CON regulations say they don't contain costs but do help hospitals stifle new competition. "The only reason CON exists is because of the hospital lobby," health-policy expert Jeff Goldsmith says. "Businesses long ago abandoned these laws as providing any real check on health costs. But hospitals found them to be convenient in protecting their franchises. So hospitals have captured the regulatory system, and when they do come forward with proposals for new construction projects, they usually get them approved."

Gloria Bazzoli of Virginia's Commonwealth University is less skeptical of CON laws. While she can't prove that they cut costs, she notes that they have limited facility construction. "The markets that have no certificates of need are the ones that have the most building going on," she says. "That includes specialty facilities, specialty hospitals, and ASCs [ambulatory surgery centers]. And hospitals are expanding their existing services. CON has always been a barrier to new facility development."

CON regulations do pose an obstacle to ambulatory surgical centers in some states. "The CON boards are really oriented to the hospital health system model of delivery," Craig Jeffries, president of the American Association of Ambulatory Surgery Centers, says. "Therefore, they have a bias against other entities such as surgery centers that might impact hospital health systems."

Similarly, few specialty hospitals are located in states that have CON programs.[2] Even now that the federal moratorium on these facilities has been lifted, "the path of least resistance is to expand in states where there is not a certificate of need," says Robert Homchick, a Seattle-based health care attorney.

CON laws, however, do not necessarily prevent traditional hospitals from expanding or purchasing expensive equipment. In the 1970s, when Texas adopted its CON law (which has since been repealed), CT scanners and MRIs were just emerging, Gary Eiland, a Houston health care attorney, recalls. "There were some hard-fought CON battles, and there were some losers that didn't get an MRI or a CT on the first round. But once those new technologies became the standard of care, usually those hospitals that applied again a year or two later were more successful. That's happened to a lot of equipment and other technology. When it becomes the standard of care, it's hard for regulators to say, 'You can't have it.'"

The Federal Trade Commission opposes all CON laws. In a 2004 report, the agency stated, "On balance, CON programs are not successful in containing health care costs, and . . . they pose serious anticompetitive risks that usually outweigh their purported economic benefits."[3] The American Health Planning Association, which represents directors of CON programs, shot back that the Federal Trade Commission had provided little evidence to support this statement or "to demonstrate that market forces have had . . . the positive effects in the health-care system that the authors claim or assume."[4]

This heated exchange highlights a long-running theme in the battle between proponents and detractors of "health planning." A form of government intervention that seeks to match the supply of health care with the needs of each community, health planning was once trumpeted as a means to control spending. Now it has mostly shrunk to CON laws, which are themselves under attack everywhere. But whatever one might say about CON, the fact that it ignites such fierce debates shows that it still has some relevance.

Vulnerable CONs on the Defensive   Under legislation passed in 1974, the federal government was empowered to reduce Medicaid funding for any state that lacked a CON law covering a wide range of health services.[5] So by the late 1970s, every state had such a statute.[6] The government also required states to do health planning and established regional health services agencies to advise the states and review proposals for new projects.[7] But a few years later, the Reagan administration withdrew the mandate for CON and cut back on federal support for health services agencies.

Today, only a few states still do health planning, and fourteen states have rescinded their CON laws.[8] Meanwhile, some states that kept their CONs have restricted their scope. In Florida, for example, all major medical equipment was taken out of review in 2001.[9] And New York, which still has an extensive CON program, has enforced it much less strictly over the past decade, observers say.[10]

Budget cutbacks in many states have left CON programs vulnerable because they're controversial, says Thomas Piper, head of the Missouri CON program and a past president of the American Health Planning Association. Besides the resistance of health care entrepreneurs to CON, he says, "we've had a major shift toward conservative government, which wants less regulation. So philosophically, there's been a strong effort to reduce regulation."

Nevertheless, CON laws still cover more than thirty types of health services, ranging from acute-care hospitals, long-term care facilities, and ambulatory surgery centers to cardiac catheterization labs, CT, MRI, and PET scanners, and lithotripters. Some states regulate only nursing homes, while others also apply CON to medical office buildings, home health care, and renal dialysis. Many specific hospital services are covered, including obstetric services, open-heart surgery, organ transplants, burn care, and psychiatric services.[11]

Gaming the System   Health-care entities have found ways to game every type of government regulation, and CON is no exception. "You have more and more talented entrepreneurs who are finding ways around regulations," Piper notes. "In Alabama, for instance, they were able to pass special legislation for a digital hospital. They were doing what a regular hospital does, only with computers and electronic medical records."

Some hospital owners get state regulators to let them close money-losing inner-city facilities; then they're permitted to build suburban hospitals with the same number of beds without submitting to CON review.[12] Existing hospitals in those suburbs tend to fight this invasion of their turf, but they often lose.

Another common dodge is to lobby the state to change the dollar threshold for reviewing the purchase of an MRI or a PET scanner. "In a lot of cases, the certificate-of-need program has raised the threshold of approval high enough that they don't cover those major equipment purchases," Jeff Goldsmith says. In Rhode Island, for example, medical gear is reviewable only if it's worth $1 million or more. "We believe there are a lot of MRIs that cost just under $1 million," says Michael Dexter, chief of the state's Office of Health Systems Development.

Do CON Laws Do Any Good?   When hospitals oppose the introduction of a new facility or program, they don't always win. But at least the state is forced to consider whether new health care services are needed. For example, a CON application for an open-heart program at a Rhode Island hospital was granted even though two Providence hospitals that had similar programs opposed it. Landmark Hospital, about fifteen miles north of Providence, received approval for the program in 2000, at a time when it was hemorrhaging cash.[13] (It has since executed a modest turnaround.)

Why were three cardiac surgery programs needed in the region? Landmark was located in an area with "higher rates of cardiovascular disease and lower usage rates of cardiac services," Dexter replies. It was also going to be staffed by physicians from a Harvard-affiliated group. And before they were allowed to start doing surgery, Landmark had to open a diagnostic catheterization lab and show that it was performing at least a hundred cardiac "caths" each month.

Attorney Robert Homchick doesn't think that the Landmark case proves that CON laws are ineffective. "You could say, 'Why would you do that for a failing hospital?' But unless you've got a lucrative service line like cardiology, you're not going to be able to cross-subsidize the range of other services that are so important to keep a failing hospital open."

High Volume, Better Outcomes   CON supporters note that outcomes tend to be better in hospitals where a particular procedure is performed more often. By limiting the number of facilities allowed to do that operation, they argue, a CON program can raise the volume of surgery at each hospital and, therefore, the percentage of patients who have good outcomes.[14]

Little research has been done to compare outcomes in CON and non-CON states, but what there is suggests that CON advocates are on the right track. A 2002 study of more than nine hundred thousand Medicare patients who underwent coronary artery bypass graft surgery in over a thousand hospitals found that more of these patients died in states without CON laws.[15] Another example is New York State, which has a CON and requires that at least five hundred coronary artery bypass grafts a year be performed in any hospital permitted to do the procedure.[16] New York, which also publishes report cards on cardiac surgeons, has the lowest mortality rate from this procedure of any state.[17]

CON Track Record   Despite this positive feature of CON laws, they haven't been shown to reduce overall cost growth very much. A paper published in 1976 found that "they slowed construction of hospital beds, but that other capital expenditures increased and the net effect was negligible."[18] The Harvard economist Joseph Newhouse says that the studies done on CON programs in the 1980s also showed that "they weren't that effective."

In a 1998 study, Christopher Conover and Frank Sloan of Duke University found that "mature" CON programs produce a 5 percent long-term reduction in acute-care spending per capita, "but with no significant reduction in total per-capita spending." In fact, both Medicare's prospective-payment system and HMO cost-cutting appear to have had more impact than CON on the number of hospital beds per one thousand people and the average cost of a hospital admission.[19]

Kenneth Thorpe of Emory University offers a slightly more positive perspective. "In states that have CON laws, spending is a little bit lower, and the growth in beds per population is probably lower, too," he says. "But the CON laws vary so much that it's hard to generalize."

Pennsylvania's Conundrum   One test case is Pennsylvania, which repealed its CON law in 1996. "Now there are heart programs in every nook and cranny," says Claire Baldwin, vice president of nursing administration for Bryn Mawr Hospital. Her hospital and its two sister institutions, Paoli and Lankenau, have their own cardiac programs, she adds. However, fewer coronary artery bypass grafts are being done in those hospitals than in the past, she says, because interventional cardiologists are doing more angioplasties instead.

The decline in open-heart surgery has also been accompanied by a rise in cardiac catheterizations. Although more hospitals now have catheterization programs, however, many have failed to generate adequate volume to ensure high quality.[20]

Meanwhile, Pennsylvania's ambulatory surgery centers are having a field day. Between 2001 and 2003, the number of patient visits to ambulatory surgery centers increased 83 percent, and forty-eight new surgery centers opened from July 2003 to May 2004.[21]

Nevertheless, Mark Pauly, a health economist at the Wharton School in Philadelphia, maintains that if the CON regulations had remained, hospitals would have just expanded their programs more to meet the demand.

"If the demand is there, in terms of insurance coverage, constraining certain elements of capital through CON just forces the money to go somewhere else, but it doesn't go away," Pauly explains. "In general, the idea of trying to restrain health care costs by limiting a particular input, such as capital, has got to be up there among the world's dumbest ideas. The metaphor is that you've got this pot that's boiling, and you're going to try to keep it from boiling over by sitting on the lid. That's very uncomfortable and not very effective."

Health Planning Redux   John Steen, a former health services agency executive in Georgia and New York, doesn't dispute the fact that CON laws have been ineffective in limiting health costs. But he argues that the original idea of health planning went far beyond cost-cutting. "Certificate of need is less about cost containment than it is about access and quality, and above all, about giving a voice to the community—shedding the light of day on matters that otherwise wouldn't be touched," he says. "One of the principal reasons for health planning agencies was to give a role to ordinary community spokespeople in helping the state and local health departments plan a health system that would be more appropriate for their needs and would better represent the public interest, instead of only private interests."

Can anything be salvaged from the wreckage of health planning programs that might work better than CON alone? For an answer to that question, let's turn to Rochester, New York, which has one of the oldest health services agencies in the country, and one of the few that's still functioning in its original role.

A Spirit of Cooperation

In 1992, when Bill Clinton was running for President, he praised Rochester as a community that had found the secret to keeping health costs low while providing good access to care. The national media gave Rochester rave reviews.[22]

The city's indicators looked excellent back then. In 1991, Rochester's total cost per employee for health care was $2,378. That was about two-thirds of the national average and only 55 percent of New York State's average. Meanwhile, only 6 percent of Rochester's population was uninsured—less than half of the national mean of 14 percent.[23]

What the pundits largely overlooked was the fact that Rochester's success stemmed from a decades-long tradition of health planning and community cooperation. Some of that cooperation was made possible by the local dominance of Rochester (now Excellus) Blue Cross and Blue Shield, which controlled (and still has) 70 percent of the area's private health insurance market. Also, nearly all contracts offered by local insurers were then community-rated. That gave local firms an incentive to work together to control health costs.[24]

Unfortunately, the Rochester "miracle" didn't last. Local employers demanded—and got—insurance premiums based on the health status of their employees, and the resultant premium increases in other sectors of the market led to a sharp rise in the number of uninsured. [25] Local hospitals, which had once thrived under global-capitation contracts with Medicare, Medicaid, and the Blues, chose to accept prospective payments from those payers on a per-diagnosis basis.[26] After the state deregulated hospital payments in 1996, they were free to negotiate their rates with insurance companies.[27]

In this freewheeling environment, the hospitals started an all-out "arms race." Whereas before, there had been only a couple of open-heart programs, one burn unit and one neonatal intensive-care unit in town,[28] suddenly every hospital wanted to offer new lines and have the latest imaging equipment. Also, there was no limit on the amount of new services and facilities that could be offered outside of hospitals in the early 1990s.[29]

Fast forward to today. While Rochester struggles with the same health care inflation that afflicts the rest of the country, its health spending is still about 10 percent below the national average.[30] Part of the reason is that the closing of two hospitals left the others in the city operating at full capacity.[31] It also has something to do with the efforts of a local independent practice association to get physicians to practice more cost-efficiently.[32] But a large part of the credit must go to the Finger Lakes Health Services Agency—a survivor of the 1970s reform movement—and a unique local organization called the Community Technology Assessment Advisory Board (CTAAB). Representing employers, insurance companies, hospitals, physicians, and consumers, CTAAB has played an important role in matching health care resources to community needs.

Insurers Won't Pay if the Board Disapproves   Since its formation in 1993, CTAAB has evaluated the appropriateness of new health care technology and facilities in the Rochester area. While CTAAB only advises applicants on whether the community needs their proposed facility or service, area insurers generally follow the board's recommendations.[33] Health-care entrepreneurs know that if they build something not approved by CTAAB, there's a high likelihood that the health plans won't pay for care delivered there.[34]

CTAAB has achieved results. In 2003, according to Leonard Redon, chairman of CTAAB and a vice president of PayChex, the MRI test rate for the Finger Lakes region (where Rochester is located) was 19 percent lower than the national rate and 28 percent under the state rate.[35] Local observers think that's related to CTAAB's rejection of many proposed MRI purchases, particularly by radiology groups. CTAAB has also recommended against the building or acquisition of new imaging centers, sleep centers, catheterization labs, lithotripters, and ambulatory surgery centers. And it has weighed in on new technologies such as PET scanning, ThinPrep cervical cancer tests, and novel treatments for prostate cancer and bone fractures.[36]

Ambulatory surgery centers proliferated in New York after the state loosened its CON regulations in 1996.[37] But CTAAB has taken a stand against some of them, and there seem to be somewhat fewer centers in

Rochester than elsewhere, says Edgar Black, MD, regional vice president and chief medical officer for Excellus Blue Cross and Blue Shield's Rochester region.

Right-Sizing Health Care   Employers and insurers, naturally, like CTAAB. In a 2004 op-ed piece in the local newspaper, for example, Sandra Parker, president and chief operating officer of the Rochester Business Alliance, urged increased support of CTAAB as one means of reining in cost increases.[38]

Hospitals have also been supportive, but that may be partly because CTAAB has largely stayed off of their bread-and-butter turf. While the board has reviewed their proposed equipment purchases, it has usually approved them.[39] And Black notes that CTAAB doesn't look at hospital service lines like birthing centers or orthopedic units, which are under the state CON's purview. But in 2003, the organization did oppose a request for a catheterization lab at Geneva Hospital in nearby Geneva, New York, and the state upheld CTAAB's decision.

Since then, CTAAB has probed further into hospital territory. For example, in 2005 it was considering Strong Memorial Hospital's application for renovations to an adult intensive care unit and an intermediate care unit, as well as for a third electrophysiology lab. Park Ridge Hospital also asked for CTAAB's blessing to add a second catheterization lab.[40]

Bonnie DeVinney, executive director of the Finger Lakes Health Services Agency, sees less duplication of hospital service lines in Rochester than elsewhere. But it could easily have turned out otherwise, she says. Recalling the arms-race mentality that pervaded the area several years ago, she notes that the competition was starting to spread to outlying communities. "We had rural hospitals that wanted to have cardiac caths and heart services. We've seen a stepping away from that. People have realized that this medical arms race is not serving anyone. It's not clear where we're headed with that. But we're starting to see some of the health care leaders adopting a collaborative approach."

Hospitals Accept Oversight   Raymond Mayewski, MD, vice president and chief medical officer for Strong Health, one of the city's three major hospital systems, calls CTAAB's approach "reasonable. It's designed to give information to support payment by payers. And to the extent that it provides a forum to discuss new technology, we support it."

Rochester doesn't have a lot of excess outpatient capacity, says Mayewski, and CTAAB is one of the reasons for that. "It's an extra pair of eyes on top of the state CON process. A lot of people are looking at what you're doing in terms of big pieces of equipment and so forth."

On the inpatient side, he notes, Rochester has only about three hospital beds per thousand people. That's about a third of what Buffalo has and far less than many other cities have, he says. But this has nothing to do with CTAAB, he acknowledges. It's a result of Rochester's tradition of health planning and of the elimination of two hospitals, St. Mary's and Genesee.

"We've always been somewhat low on capacity compared to other cities, but when those hospitals went out, we were really low," Mayewski says. "Our hospital is 100 percent full all the time, as is Rochester General. And our ERs are really filled, because when Genesee Hospital closed, thirty-three thousand visits had to be spread over the other emergency rooms." As a result, he adds, Strong has had to expand its emergency department. Yet Mayewski and DeVinney agree that the city's hospital capacity would be adequate if there were intermediate-care facilities to accommodate people who don't need to remain hospitalized but can't get into nursing homes.

Physicians Are Mixed on CTAAB   While hospitals see CTAAB as a good thing, on balance, physicians aren't so sure. "It's a love-hate relationship," says Louis Papa, an internist and president of the Monroe County Medical Society. For example, when CTAAB said that Rochester needed only one PET scanner, he recalls, "Doctors said, 'Three months from now, that's not going to be the case.'" And indeed, there are now several PET scanners in Rochester.

Papa believes CTAAB's approach has improved. "In the past, there have been some concerns about the real limiting of care and access to new technology. I think that's changed in the way they look at the technology. CTAAB's technology assessment committee looks at the literature on it and how other communities are experiencing the technology, and sees whether there's some value for the cost."

On the whole, he adds, doctors have respect for CTAAB and believe that it's working for the good of the community. "You'll hear grumbling all the time, because there are those who don't like someone else deciding what care will be available in the community. But it's helped

Rochester avoid having CT scanners, PET scanners, and sleep centers on every other corner."

All Health Care Is Local   Rochester's health leaders view community action as central to the health planning process. They don't believe that a state CON program, no matter how well designed and implemented, can do it as well. "A community-based approach is better than any state approach that I know of," Mayewski says. "It's more focused on this community and its needs as a higher priority than the region and the state. The state looks at what's good for the state first."

Rochester is different from most other cities. It has a health-planning outlook that took shape over many years. It has a single dominant insurer, so health-plan competition is not a big stumbling block. And it has a health-planning agency with extensive experience in doing the research required to match supply to demand.

Yet what Rochester has done is certainly doable within our reform model. If health-services agencies were restored, and they gathered the data needed to make good decisions on health care resource needs, the regional health boards that supervise the utility insurers could act on that information. And, since they'd comprise the same kinds of stakeholders that are in CTAAB, the regional boards could make decisions with the confidence that they truly represented the community. Of course, the states would still have a say in bigger projects that extended beyond particular cities or insurance regions. But wherever possible, the local boards would control health planning in their own communities.

Edgar Black believes that other cities could replicate Rochester's achievement. "If folks in other communities would recognize that excess supply is causing some of the increase in health care costs in their community, they ought to be able to sit down as a group and make some decisions. These aren't easy decisions, and politically some of them are difficult, but this is a better way to manage some of the issues in health care than some of the alternative solutions."

22 What Works Best in Practice?

Reducing the duplication of facilities and service lines would certainly cut the amount of unnecessary and inappropriate care delivered. But, as discussed in Chapter 7, there are many areas of medicine where it's not clear how much care or what kind of care is appropriate. In their previously cited papers on variations in care (Chapter 8), Elliot Fisher and his colleagues emphasize that "the differences in spending across HRRs [hospital referral regions] were largely due to more frequent use of the hospital as a site of care, more frequent physician visits, greater use of medical subspecialists, and more frequent diagnostic tests and minor procedures."[1] Quality of care was not higher in regions where more of these services were delivered. But, without a lot of additional evidence that shows what works and what doesn't work in practice, it's impossible to know which services, specialty as well as primary care, can be safely eliminated.

Although there are plenty of primary-care guidelines based on solid evidence, Bruce Bagley, medical director of quality improvement for the American Academy of Family Physicians (AAFP), points out that many basic questions need to be answered. For example, he says, there is no evidence to support particular intervals for calling back patients with hypertension for checkups; similarly, physicians don't know which kind of therapy is best for treating bronchitis, and no studies have been done on the long-term effectiveness of widely used antidepressant drugs.

In fact, as noted earlier, most medications have been subjected neither to long-term studies nor to comparative effectiveness trials. The lack of such research not only renders patients vulnerable to unforeseen harms but makes it difficult for physicians and patients to decide which drug to use.

Some health policy experts have recently proposed the establishment of a comparative effectiveness research center that would evaluate existing research and fund new trials where more evidence is needed. As envisioned by Gail Wilensky, a health economist and former administrator of the Centers for Medicare and Medicaid Services, this center—which would receive public and private funding—would do comparative studies of prescription drugs, devices, and procedures.[2]

Such research could produce valuable results. For example, one large study recently found that patients with sciatica fared equally well after two years, whether or not they had back surgery.[3] But, to cover the broad spectrum of issues that doctors face daily, and to have a real impact on practice, comparative effectiveness research would have to engage the vast majority of physicians.

Practical Clinical Trials   One promising method of doing comparative studies in the real world is the "practical clinical trial." PCTs are "trials for which the hypothesis and study design are formulated based on information needed to make a [clinical] decision," according to an article written by officials of CMS and the Agency for Healthcare Quality and Research.[4] "The PCTs address practical questions about the risks, benefits, and costs of an intervention as they would occur in routine clinical practice."

While PCTs can be randomized controlled trials or observational studies, the authors note, they differ from conventional research in several important ways: First, they compare clinically relevant, alternative interventions. Second, they're conducted across heterogeneous practice settings with a diverse population of patients. Nobody is excluded from a study because he or she doesn't fit within preconceived parameters. And third, PCTs collect data on a broad range of health outcomes. Endpoints may include, along with morbidity and mortality, patient satisfaction, functional health status, and cost-effectiveness.

Some very large, randomized PCTs have contributed significantly to medical knowledge. Examples include the ALLHAT study funded by the National Institutes of Health, which showed the superiority of cheap diuretics to other drugs for treating hypertension; a Veterans Administration study that proved there is no benefit to arthroscopic surgery for osteoarthritis of the knee;[5] and an international trial showing that commonly used glucose-insulin-potassium infusions have no effect on mortality or cardiac arrest in patients who've had heart attacks.[6]

PCTs are not necessarily less expensive than conventional clinical trials. For example, the seven-year, forty-two-thousand-patient ALLHAT study cost about $120 million.[7] But techniques to conduct PCTs at relatively low cost were developed a decade ago,[8] and it's expected that the spread of electronic health records will further lower the cost and reduce the data collection burden on participating physicians.

Grassroots Networks   The greatest hope for this type of research lies in the recent expansion of practice-based research networks (PBRNs). Consisting mostly of primary-care physicians, these networks help physicians develop evidence on matters that are relevant to everyday practice. They also aid doctors in implementing clinical guidelines and enable them to test those protocols in real practice settings.

For example, the American Academy of Pediatrics' PBRN conducted a study on febrile infants to find out how pediatric practice in office settings differed from the guideline for that condition. Later published in the *Journal of the American Medical Association*, the study found that pediatricians who observed the sick children closely over a few days had outcomes that were just as good as those who complied with the guideline, which stressed the use of tests, antibiotics, and hospitalization.[9]

J. W. Hendricks, a pediatrician in Tulsa, Oklahoma, who participated in this trial, notes that it may lead to an expansion of the guideline. "If you have the ability to recheck this kind of patient and are confident that you can do it, that's probably OK," he says. "So observation has now become an acceptable test."

PBRNs also try to improve current modes of care for which there's little evidence. For example, Linda Stewart, a family physician in Baton Rouge, Louisiana, participated in a government-funded study on the treatment of otitis media. Conducted by the predecessor of the AAFP National Research Network in collaboration with primary-care networks in seven other countries, the study showed that U.S. physicians were prescribing antibiotics to children with ear infections for far longer than their counterparts abroad with no better outcomes.

Stewart believes that the published study "changed the whole concept of how we deal with otitis media. It certainly changed what I do. This kind of research—practical research coming out of offices like mine, where we really are in the trenches with our patients—has a lot to offer to the future of medicine."

Long History   Practice-based research networks first took root in the United States in the1970s. Starting in the early 1990s, the

Agency for Health Care Policy and Research began to fund some PBRN studies. In 2000, the renamed Agency for Health Care Research and Quality (AHRQ) increased that support, encouraging the formation of new networks.[10] Because of stepped-up federal funding and the spread of electronic health records, observers say, the number of networks and their membership has increased substantially in recent years.

Today, roughly ten thousand American physicians participate in PBRNs. The AHRQ-funded PBRN Resource Center has counted 111 U.S. networks, including 4 for nurses. Of the twelve thousand clinicians in the 81 networks registered with the center, 85–90 percent are primary-care physicians.[11]

PBRNs are regional, statewide, or national. Among the latter are the AAFP National Research Network, which includes about three hundred family physicians in forty-five states; the American Academy of Pediatric's Pediatric Research in Office Settings (PROS) network, with around two thousand physicians; and the Practice Partner Research Network, with over five hundred providers (most of them doctors) in thirty-seven states.[12]

Most of the regional PBRNs were launched by and remain closely linked to universities. But these PBRNs are different from university-affiliated clinical trial networks that test new drugs for pharmaceutical firms. Whereas physicians in the latter networks are paid thousands of dollars for each patient they recruit,[13] PBRN members receive little or nothing for their work. These physicians rarely have clinical-trial training or get patients' consent themselves. Instead, research assistants enroll patients when a trial requires it.

Most PBRN funding comes from government agencies such as AHRQ, the Centers for Disease Control, and the National Institutes of Health. But medical societies, universities, and private foundations also support PBRNs. For example, the Robert Wood Johnson Foundation has given $5 million to a dozen PBRNs to do research on altering patient health behavior.[14]

Translating Research into Practice   Traditionally, PBRNs have focused on describing what primary-care physicians do and how it could be improved. For example, a study initiated by a physician in CareNet, a PBRN affiliated with the University of Colorado Health Sciences Center, showed that, in 13 percent of visits, physicians couldn't find the clinical information they needed in their charts. The study generated a paper that was published in the *Journal of the American Medical Association*.[15] CareNet is also one of a few PBRNs that have done groundbreaking research on ambulatory medical errors.[16]

While academicians conduct most PBRN studies, many of the ideas for them come from practicing clinicians. And the PROS network submits every study proposal to representatives of the American Academy of Pediatricians' state chapters. "As the academics talk to the physicians, a study may get modified significantly so it's answering more focused questions and is designed in a way that practitioners can do the study," Hendricks says.

This "bottom up" approach, however, has yielded to a "top down" orientation as government agencies and some private foundations have placed greater emphasis—and funding—on what AHRQ calls "translating research into practice." In a nutshell, this means finding out how to get physicians to follow "evidence-based" practice guidelines so that more patients will receive recommended care.

With support from AHRQ and the Robert Wood Johnson Foundation, for example, the ten-year-old ACORN network in Virginia is focusing its efforts on quality improvement, especially in preventive care. While most of ACORN's current studies are randomized controlled trials, the network is also trying to help physicians in the intervention groups do a better job on preventive screening tests and counseling patients about issues such as diet, exercise, and smoking cessation.

Not all of the results, however, support the top-down view of things. Steven Woolf, MD, a professor of family medicine at Virginia Commonwealth University who's involved in ACORN, recalls that a smoking-cessation guideline that called for intensive counseling at every visit proved no more effective than the usual brief advice. "We decided to test telephone quit lines in the AHRQ-funded randomized controlled trial and are seeing much more dramatic effects," he says.

Why Guidelines Don't Always Work

Evidence-based guidelines are often based on studies conducted in academic medical centers or other specialized settings. These trials usually limit participation to certain subsets of patients. The results may not be relevant to primary-care physicians, either because their patients are different from those in the trial or because the resources available to the clinicians who participated in the study are not found in typical practices.

PBRNs constitute "living laboratories" to test the premises of these guidelines in the real world. "Doctors want to improve care and participate in discovering things that are practical for them," notes Perry Dickinson, MD, a professor of family medicine at the University of Colorado Health Sciences Center. "A lot of the published research doesn't work for the practicing clinician. When they can help guide the research so it's more practical and more meaningful to them, they see that as a real plus."

Paul Hicks, a family physician who belongs to CareNet, agrees that practicing physicians must be involved in guideline development. "Research that's based in a lab or tertiary-care settings is not the wave of the future," he says. "As evidence-based medicine becomes a prerequisite for anybody practicing medicine, we're looking for answers to questions that are important to us. There's no better way to make a study generalizable to people in your population than when it's done among patients in your own practice."

Some physicians are willing to put in extra time on these studies. For example, Hendricks says he spends an hour or two a week extra on PROS trials. Linda Stewart took ten to fifteen minutes to do the paperwork on each of her patients with otitis media. But most doctors don't want to be slowed down. So some networks have found ways to lessen the burden, including extensive use of research assistants and patient surveys.

Pros and Cons of Using EHRs   One way to facilitate physician involvement is to use electronic health records (EHRs) for data collection. Carolyn Clancy, MD, the director of AHRQ, has written about using information technology to accelerate evidence-based-medicine research. With the help of EHRs, Clancy and a colleague theorize, "enrollment in prospective studies, including randomized controlled trials, could be expedited, as could data collection and management. These types of developments can greatly reduce the time necessary to fill gaps in the evidence base."[17]

In an interview, Clancy said that this approach could be used in practice-based research networks. "We see that as a critical part to building the infrastructure to do this kind of work on comparative effectiveness, as well as accelerating the implementation of what we know works. That rolls right off my tongue. But trying to make sure this can be done in a way that does not add time to a doctor's day is really the big trick here. I think it can be done, but it's going to take some work to make that happen."

Among the challenges, she noted, is the fact that EHRs are not designed for clinical research. "It's not clear that for all questions, electronic medical records have precisely the same elements as an electronic research record."

AHRQ has invested heavily in the Practice Partner Research Network (PPRNet), which consists of physicians using a single brand of EHR.[18] Initially, AHRQ funded studies to find out whether the information system could be used to improve care, including primary and secondary prevention of cardiovascular disease.[19] Currently, AHRQ is paying for PPRNet to measure improvement on eighty-four different quality indicators.[20]

PPRNet makes very small demands on physicians in terms of data collection. Once each quarter, explains Steve Ornstein, MD, the network's director, the practices extract a limited set of de-identified data from their EHRs and ship it off to Ornstein at the Medical University of South Carolina in Charleston, South Carolina, where he's a professor of family medicine. He and his associates analyze the data and then send the doctors detailed, graphical reports on their performance. Some of the practices use a special program to re-identify the data by patient and insert it into spread sheets. Similar to chronic-disease registries, these spread sheets prompt the doctors to take action on individual patients who need services.

Ornstein disagrees with those who say that EHRs can't be used for research. "It depends on what kind of data you want to get. If you want to get vital signs, meds, labs, and diagnoses, you can do that with an EHR. But if you want to get data on 'did the patient appear pale' or 'what did the doctor-patient interaction look like,' an EHR can't do that. It depends on the question you want to ask."

Linda Stewart believes EHRs could be a big boon to practical research. "Even if you didn't want to be the one doing the research but your information could be pulled out of the EHR and used as a resource, that would be valuable," she says.

Motivations of Physicians   Why do physicians participate in PBRNs? Richard Wasserman, a pediatrician and director of PROS, lists several reasons: "First, they're curious about what they do and whether it works. Second, they have a need for affiliation. For some physicians, being in practice is very isolating, and this allows them to share something with other practitioners. The final thing is altruism: it's a way to contribute to the discipline of medicine and the promotion of child health."

James Galliher, research director of the AAFP National Research Network, emphasizes family physicians' interest in practical solutions. "The physicians in the network do this because they believe that the research results may have an effect on the way they practice and, hopefully, will have short-term or long-term benefits for patients."

One drawback of the AAFP network, Galliher says, is that not all of the doctors in any given group may participate. "What we've observed is that to improve care, you have to improve systems, not just individual behaviors. As we move into randomized clinical trials, where we're assessing interventions, it becomes more important to have buy-in by the practice as a whole. And some physicians aren't willing to do that."

Another problem with current PBRNs is that they're mostly limited to primary care. While a few specialty networks exist, not much work is going into answering the questions related to the use of hospitals, specialists and procedures that were posed at the beginning of this chapter.

Carolyn Clancy thinks that practical clinical trials could be done in hospitals, looking at the outcomes of patients who saw different numbers of specialists or who were admitted to the intensive care unit at different points in their stay. Observational studies in practice research networks could also answer questions about the frequency of follow-up visits, she says. A network of several group-model HMOs, she adds, have been doing this kind of research for years. "For some of these questions, you may actually have some retrospective data you could draw upon."

Bottom Up versus Top Down   The Medicare Modernization Act of 2003 gave AHRQ authority to perform comparative effectiveness research, but the agency received only $15 million for this purpose in 2004—just enough to do some systematic literature reviews and to publish the results in consumer guides.[21] The main thrust of AHRQ's current work with PBRNs, as mentioned earlier, is "translating research into practice." The National Institutes of Health has awarded an increasing number of grants to PBRNs for similar studies. But some PBRN leaders fear that, if the National Institutes of Health dangles money in front of

PBRNs to get them directly involved in clinical research, it could hijack their movement by changing its focus.

James Mold, MD, for example, heads the Oklahoma Research Network, which consists of 240 clinicians in mostly small, rural family practices. The twelve-year-old PBRN, which is closely affiliated with the University of Oklahoma, receives funding from government agencies, foundations, and the AAFP. Its current studies focus on how rural physicians can implement clinical guidelines and what problems they encounter.

Mold views the National Institutes of Health's top-down approach to the research it funds as a danger sign. "The trouble is the NIH doesn't quite understand the potential or purpose of PBRNs yet, and it's thinking that what they're good for is to identify patients who qualify for clinical trials," Mold says. "That could be useful, but that's not what PBRNs will be best at." Doctors will feel used, he says, because they may not get paid much for the work, "and even if they do, they'll lose a lot of value that they now get from the bottom-up approach."

The fears about the National Institutes of Health may be groundless. But Kevin Peterson, MD, an associate professor of family medicine at the University of Minnesota, believes that the top-down thinkers and the bottom-up advocates will have to compromise to get the most out of PBRNs. On one hand, "clinical research without any connection to practice can become arcane," Peterson says. "On the other hand, clinical practice without any connection to research becomes obsolete. As we begin to take our technology and merge those two, we're going to have a healthier American health information system."

Using PCTs to Find New Evidence   Recent articles in the trade press have talked about PBRNs "coming of age," but actually they're more like an awkward adolescent who's trying to decide what to do with his life. Their work to date is indeed promising; in fact, the Institute of Medicine has called them "a significant underpinning for studies in primary care."[22] But at present, the government's top priority is to get PBRNs to promote clinical guidelines to physicians. While there's nothing wrong with that, what's being missed is the opportunity to use the practice networks to find out what really lies behind all those variations in care.

Under our reform model, primary-care physicians and specialists alike would be encouraged to participate in PBRNs. While doctors wouldn't be forced to do studies, their group practices could reward those who did with bonuses for "good citizenship."

It would be relatively easy for the primary-care groups to participate in practical clinical trials. They'd all have EHRs, so they could generate data automatically for some studies. The software would have to be customized for other trials; but large groups would have staff technicians who could do that work. And, as Steven Woolf of ACORN suggests, the government could put pressure on software vendors to develop EHRs with greater research capabilities.

Physicians, however, would not want to engage in studies that took a lot of time to enroll patients and read them their rights. As Clancy and her colleagues have suggested, "Consent procedures that are both adequate and efficient will need further exploration, because the number of PCTs that can be performed may be limited by the operational burden they impose."[23]

Even if physicians were willing to engage in these studies for no fee, this expansion of the research enterprise would cost a substantial amount. Since industry isn't going to support it, and Congress isn't going to vote more money for it, the best bet for funding PCTs probably lies with the National Institutes of Health. While this would mean shifting some funds from basic to applied research, I'd argue that it would be money well spent. Not only would we find out how to provide better care but we'd be able to save large sums by eliminating waste.

The counterargument is that more money is needed to support basic research that will lead to new cures and save lives. But that doesn't mean we have to devote all research dollars to the development of new drugs and other new technologies. We have to keep investigating the basis for medical interventions, because the underuse, misuse, and overuse of existing services can kill or hurt people just as surely as the lack of new cures does.

Michael Millenson, in his landmark book *Demanding Medical Excellence*, makes a similar point: "Research medicine and everyday medicine often seem to exist in separate worlds. The public thrills to stories about a pill that may slow the aging process. But in everyday medicine we are just now examining the best way to perform hip-replacement surgery that hundreds of thousands of Americans who are aging undergo annually at a cost of nearly $3 billion. In biomedicine, research into menopause captivates Baby Boomer women. In everyday medicine we are just beginning to collect reliable information on alternatives to the 560,000 hysterectomies performed each year, mostly on women who have not yet reached menopause."[24]

It's time to find out what really works and what doesn't. As we do, the answers will aid us in another essential task: figuring out what we can afford. That's part of the job of technology assessment, the subject of the final two chapters.

23 Must Technology Break the Bank?

In every advanced country, regardless of what kind of health care system it has, the cost of care has been relentlessly advancing for many years. The growth in global affluence accounts for much of this increased spending, but costs are rising faster than wealth everywhere. According to the Princeton health economist Uwe Reinhardt, a 1 percent cost increase in per-capita GDP will push up health costs between 1.2 and 1.4 percent, depending on the nation. "In the U.S., that ratio has been about 1.4. So every time income rises 10 percent, health care spending rises 14 percent," he says. "That's the big cost driver."

Clearly, a great deal of inefficiency and waste can be cut out of the U.S. system if we give providers the correct financial incentives, eliminate unnecessary administrative expenses, and resist the pressures of the medical-industrial complex. Interconnected health information systems would also reduce redundancies and help ensure that the right care was provided to the right patients at the right time. But, even though these changes would cut health spending substantially, it would soon resume its inexorable forward march.

This chapter and the next analyze the technology factor from two perspectives: how to determine what should be in a standard benefit package, and how we can encourage beneficial advances without bankrupting the system.

Technology's Impact Health economists attribute about half of the rise in costs to "technology," which is a catchall term covering all kinds of medical advances.[1] Technology can range from new drugs and medical devices to new tests and procedures. What most of these things have in common is that they lead to an increase in the volume and intensity of care. This higher intensity level accounts for part of technology's impact on raising costs. The rest comes in the form of excess medical price growth in everything from patented drugs and PET scanners to the people who are hired to run and maintain the new equipment.[2]

Three other aspects of technology tend to drive up costs: First, new technologies don't always replace old ones. The introduction of MRI and CT scanners didn't put X-ray machines out of business, and coronary artery bypass grafts didn't go away after angioplasties became commonplace. Although about 1.2 million angioplasties were done in 2002—quadruple the number of operations just a decade earlier—cardiothoracic surgeons also performed 515,000 coronary artery bypass grafts in the United States that year.[3] (That's nearly double the number done in 1991.) So while coronary artery bypass grafts have been declining of late, they've certainly not been replaced.

Second, there is a tendency for doctors to perform new procedures more often when they're less invasive and patients are more willing to undergo them. When minimally invasive gallbladder operations came along in the late 1980s, for example, they were much less expensive and dangerous than open surgery, but the number of procedures rose so much that the total cost increased.[4] The same has been true of angioplasties, especially since the advent of stents that keep arteries open after the procedure.[5]

Third, many new technologies lend themselves to "extensions." In some instances, as with cataract removal, the technology improves and is gradually applied to a wider group of people who can benefit from it. Sometimes, a new drug or treatment is applied to patients who won't benefit. For example, the Food and Drug Administration (FDA) approved Vioxx as an alternative to nonsteroidal anti-inflammatory drugs that caused stomach bleeding in some patients. But, partly as a result of heavy television advertising, many doctors soon began prescribing these expensive drugs to all arthritis patients who wanted them, whether or not they had gastric bleeding.[6] The result was to drive up costs—and, incidentally, to expose patients to the cardiac risk of Vioxx and other COX-2 inhibitors.

Interactions with Other Factors   Population growth and aging also increase consumption of health care, including new technologies. Reinhardt doesn't consider aging a major factor, because the demographic change is occurring slowly. But other experts point out that more and more people are living longer and longer.[7] During all those additional years, they're bound to use more health care, even if they're relatively healthy until near the end.[8]

Another important factor is the growth of "treated disease prevalence," or the number of patients with a particular disease who are treated. In a seminal 2005 paper, economist Kenneth Thorpe of Emory University and his colleagues show that the rise in treated disease prevalence, rather than the increase in the average cost per case, resulted in the majority of spending growth from 1987 to 2002. Underlying this trend, the researchers say, is the expansion of technology and a rise in population risk factors.[9]

The most prominent of those risk factors is obesity, Thorpe says. From 1980 to 2000, the percentage of U.S. adults classified as obese doubled to 30 percent, and obese people now account for about 12 percent of all health spending. Among the conditions obese people are more likely than others to have are diabetes, heart disease, cerebrovascular disease, back problems, and depression.

If the incidence of obesity had merely leveled off in 1980, Thorpe says, national health spending would be 15 percent lower than it is today. Because of this statistic, he suggests that current proposals to contain health care costs may be off base. We should focus much more of our efforts on changing health behavior, he says.[10]

The Wonders of Technology   While Thorpe is undoubtedly right, anyone trying to assemble a standard benefit package must proceed from the assumption that better health behavior will be a long-term goal. And, since resources are limited, it seems logical that developers of such a package would consider the costs of new technologies as well as their benefits. Yet experts disagree widely on this subject. One school of thought holds that we should limit the availability of new technology to keep costs down. Another camp argues that technology is wonderful, we must have more of it, and we can easily afford it.

David Cutler, a health economist at Harvard University, presented the technology-is-wonderful view in an influential paper (co-authored with Mark McClellan, who later headed the Centers for Medicare and Medicaid Services),[11] and a subsequent book, *Your Money or Your Life*. Cutler's argument, in essence, is that some technologies create benefits worth many times their cost, because they either extend life or improve the quality of life.

In the *Health Affairs* study, he and McClellan analyze the impact of technology by looking at how medical advances affected the treatment of five conditions: heart attack, low birth weight, depression, cataracts, and breast cancer. They conclude that if a year of life were valued at $100,000, the economic worth of improved treatments for four out of five of these conditions would be several times greater than their costs. (For depression and cataracts, they translate this value into increased quality of life for specified periods of time.) Because new breast cancer treatments haven't reduced mortality much, they say that the costs and the benefits of those interventions are about equal.

In his book, Cutler argues that improvements in medical treatments of low-birth-weight babies and patients with heart disease together account for about 40 percent of our nine-year increase in longevity since 1950. Using the method outlined above, he calculates that the benefits of those two advances alone are worth as much as all of the growth in health costs in the past half-century. Therefore, he concludes that "medical care as a whole is worth the cost."[12]

A Smarter Approach   Alan Garber, MD, a Stanford health economist, notes that the value of a technology cannot be measured without looking at how it's being used. That's why he thinks Cutler is analyzing the problem from the wrong angle. "There's no question that as time has gone on, we're doing better with some diseases," Garber says. "The real question, though, is 'Could we have gotten almost the same benefits for far less money?' If you compare us to the Western European countries, which are spending much less for health care, in broad terms they're doing as well or better than us. So it's not a matter of whether technology is good or bad. The right question is, 'Could we be smarter in how we adopt new technology and how we use it?' "

Other analysts observe that some technologies provide much more benefit than others, relative to their costs. David Eddy, MD, a former senior adviser to Kaiser Permanente who has taught at Duke and Stanford, says, "The task is not to make a global judgment about whether we have too much technology or not enough; it's to sort out which technologies provide real value."

Socioeconomic Quandary   Another problem with the "technology-is-wonderful" view is that it does not address which social classes can afford the new technologies. Working-class people who are uninsured or underinsured obviously cannot. Cutler argues that this is not an issue, because the uninsured receive charity care, the costs of which are passed on to everyone else.[13] But studies have shown that people without insurance receive inferior care and that many die prematurely as a result.[14] So the society that Cutler claims can afford all of this technology fails to provide it to many of its most vulnerable members.

Mark Pauly, another prominent economist, points out that there's no "natural" limit to the share of GDP that health care can commandeer. "All that matters," he writes, "is whether the value of medical spending at the margin is higher or lower than the other spending that it displaces."[15]

But even if we'd rather spend more on health care than on, say, windsurfing, growth in high-tech medical spending is threatening access to basic health care as more and more people lose their insurance. In the end, if U.S. health care goes off the tracks, it won't matter how much the lives we save are worth in dollars compared with the cost of saving them. If the system collapses under the weight of the new technologies, we'll be saving a lot fewer lives.

Should Technology Be Limited?
Daniel Callahan, a medical ethicist and director of international studies at the Hastings Institute, has made a forceful case for limiting the growth and use of health care technology. In his 1998 book *False Hopes*, he argues in favor of a "sustainable medicine" that helps most people live long lives "at a decent level of physical and mental competence." Providing this level of health care to everyone without putting a great stress on society's resources, he says, will require us to curtail our goals for progress and technological innovation.[16]

Making an analogy to environmentalists' idea of sustainable economic growth that doesn't destroy nature, Callahan says we shouldn't take extraordinary measures to keep people alive longer than their "natural" life span. So he would emphasize long-term care and home care and provide less "high-tech rescue" care to the elderly. Similarly, he believes it's a mistake to push our ability to save low-birth-weight infants beyond what can be done now. Further efforts in this direction, he says, "will probably be very expensive and have poor long-term results."[17]

Callahan also points out that a great number of new medical technologies are related not to health but to the desire to make people more "normal" or to raise their self-esteem. Thus, for example, we have cosmetic surgery for long noses and wrinkled skin, and Prozac for those who have even short bouts of depression.[18]

Feeding these demands are the entrepreneurs who profit from satisfying them. And medicine works hand in hand with the market to drive this process forward, Callahan notes. "Because it can create new human possibilities, an expansive medicine is the ideal partner of the market, which must unceasingly find new products to market. And no product is so attractive as one that responds to the fear of death and the desire for health."[19]

Callahan argues that we should prioritize the health of the population, even if that means decreased possibilities for some individuals. Thus he's opposed to the coverage of fertility treatments, which use resources that might be better applied to, say, prenatal care. He'd put more emphasis on public health and less on screening for "low-risk cancer probabilities, or heart disease or other conditions." Such testing should be done, he says, "only when strong evidence exists of a significant benefit for many, not a few."[20]

Don't Blame Technology   Callahan's views are controversial, to say the least. Arthur Caplan, director of the Center for Bioethics at the University of Pennsylvania, terms his approach "naïve and wrongheaded, because we're never going to stop pursuing technology as a matter of policy. You can argue that we should have a steady-state health system, but that's ludicrous. It's politically dead on arrival."

Caplan doesn't even see any way to slow down technological progress. Both the government and private companies, he notes, have invested heavily in medical research, and entrepreneurial firms will continue to capitalize on it. "Where there are opportunities to make money, they'll be investing in technologies that do that. There's no way to stop that, it's going to happen. Everything in our system is constructed to reward enterprise and innovation."

The real problem, Caplan says, is that "we have lots of technology that doesn't do anything; it just costs money." Among the interventions he puts in this category are much end-of-life care and end-stage cancer care, which cost a lot but don't necessarily extend life or improve quality of life.

"People would love to pay for technologies that really work, that really add benefit and reduce pain," he says. "I never heard anybody complain about the high cost of heart transplants or the high cost of cochlear implants or defibrillators. People will pay for those. On the other hand, I don't know why we need ten types of antidepressants. I don't know why patent policy rewards recombining drugs just to get patent extensions. And in the last days of life, we spend a fortune with no real success. Those people should go to hospice or go home at some point in their dying process."

Much of what U.S. health care providers do with technology, writes Victor Fuchs, a Stanford economist, could be termed "flat-of-the-curve" medicine: that is, as the intensity of care rises, the increase in benefit flattens out, as shown by the earlier-mentioned studies on variations in care.[21] The increased intensity may even harm patients. Elliott Fisher and Gilbert Welch of Dartmouth have noted that as patients with milder forms of heart disease have begun to receive angioplasties, some have suffered heart attacks as a result.[22] Similarly, anti-arrythmic drugs for atrial fibrillation and hormone replacement therapy to ward off osteoporosis have hurt patients more than they helped them.[23]

Where Do We Draw the Line?   When anti-arrhythmic drugs and hormone replacement therapy were introduced, their potential for doing harm, of course, wasn't known. Since ineffective treatments can hurt patients, too, the same may be true of many other technologies in current use. Out of forty-nine frequently cited research papers examined in a recent study, for example, forty-five claim that a particular intervention is effective. Of those, seven are contradicted by later studies; seven report effects that are stronger than those demonstrated in later studies; twenty results have been replicated; and eleven are unchallenged. So fewer than half of the claims of effectiveness have been validated.[24]

Despite this track record, the federal government is trying to speed research into practice.[25] For example, the FDA has approved a stent for carotid arteries that could generate hundreds of millions of dollars in sales. While these stents might eliminate the need for carotid endarterectomies, which are hazardous operations, there's also a chance that they could cause blood clots to form, increasing the risk of stroke. Some doctors fear that the neck stents might become commonplace before all of the research results are in[26]—and in fact, the latest study indicates that endarterectomy is safer than stenting.[27]

Other technologies have already become widespread, although there's no clear scientific evidence of their value. For example, CT scanners are being used to detect early signs of lung cancer and to detect heart disease by identifying calcified plaque in the arteries. Experts don't rec-ommend the use of CT machines for these purposes, because the tests haven't been shown to reduce mortality.[28] Yet they're being offered in imaging centers, hospitals, clinics, and even health clubs.[29]

Other expensive technologies approved on the basis of limited trials are only marginally effective. Erbitux for advanced colon cancer, for example, can cost $30,000 for a seven-week course of treatment. Iressa for lung cancer costs $18,000 a month. Yet these drugs extend life by no more than a few months.[30]

The Future Will Be Expensive   Implantable cardioverter de-fibrillators (ICDs) cost about $40,000, including implantation and im-mediate follow-up care.[31] But congestive heart failure patients who have defibrillators are 23 percent less likely to die from sudden cardiac arrest than those who don't have them.[32] So Medicare has expanded its cover-age of ICDs from the relatively small group of cardiac arrest survivors to about five hundred thousand patients with heart failure.[33]

The Centers for Medicare and Medicaid Services (CMS) hasn't yet weighed in on coverage of artificial hearts, which cost about $250,000 each.[34] But the FDA has approved a "temporary" artificial heart that keeps the majority of recipients alive long enough to get heart trans-plants.[35] More recently, the agency allowed a permanent mechanical heart to be implanted in patients who are ineligible for transplants and would die within a month without it. In clinical trials, the approved de-vice has kept patients going for an average of only five months.[36] It seems to be just a matter of time, however, before there are similar devices that enable people to live for years after their hearts fail. When those emerge, the floodgates will open.

Meanwhile, advances in bio-engineering are expected to allow us to regenerate skin, blood, and other organs.[37] Growth factors may be able to program the body to grow new blood vessels to circumvent coronary blockages.[38] And the new science of pharmacogenomics will someday allow drug companies to tailor medications to individuals based on their genetic makeup.[39]

Who would want to stop such miraculous advances? No one. But at the same time, we have to be mindful of their costs. According to a re-cent RAND report on the implications of new technology for Medicare, "ten of the most promising new technologies are forecast to increase spending greatly."[40] Among the most costly will be pacemakers for patients with atrial fibrillation, predicted to cost $1.4 million per year of life saved (in 1999 dollars); permanently implanted left-ventricular assist devices, $512,000 per year of life saved; and anti-angiogenesis drugs for late-stage cancers, $499,000 per year of life saved.

Technology Assessment

U.S. health plans and CMS assess new technologies for clinical effectiveness—but only rarely, cost-effectiveness—in a variety of ways.

Since 1999, CMS has used a group of experts called the Medicare Coverage Advisory Committee (MCAC) to help it decide which new technologies to cover. MCAC evaluates the effectiveness of these interventions compared with established services and medical items. The committee tends to look at technologies that have a large potential impact and that physicians are interested in using.[41]

The Medicare Modernization Act of 2003 required CMS to cut the average length of time to make a national coverage decision from nearly a year to about six months.[42] To get new technologies into circulation faster, CMS has conditioned its approval of some of them on the development of further evidence through registries, clinical trials, and other methods. Among the technologies in this category are ICDs for prophylactic use, PET scans on Alzheimer's patients, and the off-label use of certain chemotherapeutic agents for treatment of colorectal cancer.[43]

The goal, says Steve Phurrough, MD, director of CMS's coverage and analysis group, is to "take the technology or service that we probably would not cover otherwise, and cover it in the context of evidence development."

The Blues' Technology Evaluation Center   While private insurers usually emulate Medicare's coverage policies, they also do their own technology assessments. In this sphere, the Technology Evaluation Center (TEC) of the Blue Cross and Blue Shield Association is very influential. TEC does only twenty to twenty-five evaluations a year, and, like MCAC, usually reviews technologies that could have a big impact on care.[44] Although it doesn't make formal recommendations to the Blues plans around the country, its information about whether something merits coverage carries a lot of weight with those insurers. TEC also works closely with Kaiser Permanente, which factors the center's findings into its own coverage decisions.

Both Kaiser and other health plans also buy technology assessments from a pair of private companies, Hayes Inc. and ECRI. These companies consider a much wider range of technologies than does TEC or MCAC, although they give many of them only a cursory review.[45] Together, all of these evaluation bodies evaluate about 80 percent of new devices and procedures to some extent, points out Jed Weissberg, MD, associate executive director for quality at the Permanente Federation. "The trouble is that there's not enough data to draw any conclusions about most of it," he says. "People are aware it's there and can summarize a couple of case studies and anecdotal reports, but there's not enough data on which to base health policy."

Cost-Effectiveness Analysis   Technology assessment bodies in the United States generally avoid cost-benefit analyses. TEC occasionally does "special reports" on cost-effectiveness "when there are high-profile or controversial issues," says Naomi Aronson, the executive director of TEC. "But it's not something that's a plug-in to a coverage decision.

"We are a clinical-effectiveness assessment program. So we carry on our work independent of any information about cost or coverage. And when you see a cost-effectiveness analysis done, that typically means that the conclusion in the assessment is that health outcomes are improved."

TEC has provided cost-benefit information on the left ventricular assist device and the prophylactic use of ICDs for patients with heart failure. While the latter was found to be more cost effective than the former, Aronson believes that most Blues plans cover both technologies.

This assumption is not surprising, given the legal and public-relations difficulties involved in diverging from the crowd. According to a 2002 survey of health-plan executives, just 40 percent of the plans used formal cost-effectiveness analyses, and these played a fairly minor role in coverage decisions. While only 8 percent of insurers will cover a technology that provides less effective care than the alternatives for lower cost, 93 percent will pay for an intervention that offers greater effectiveness at greater cost.[46]

Alan Garber, who led this study, says that cost-benefit analysis has never been used in the United States as a basis for coverage decisions, except for a brief time in Oregon (on which more will be said later). "The most important obstacle to the formal application of cost-effectiveness analysis to health insurance coverage is that the public is not yet comfortable with it," Garber says. "Until the public is ready, any entity that attempts to use it, whether it's commercial health plans or a federal program, can find itself in a very vulnerable position. Because it's all too easy to portray it as putting dollars above life."

Jed Weissberg says that Kaiser doesn't do cost-effectiveness analyses, because, as a health plan, it has a conflict of interest. "But once we decide that a procedure, device or technique has demonstrated a net beneficial impact on health, then we use our understanding of internal costs and the way our system works to design the dissemination and implementation of that technology."

In other words, Kaiser does not deny patients any technology that's effective. But if something is unlikely to benefit a particular patient, doctors are encouraged to explain why. "We will support our clinicians in their conversations with members to inform them that the chance of benefit is slight, compared with the risk of harm," Weissberg notes. "So we rarely outlaw things; we provide our clinicians with information and try to monitor our own experience as we implement these things in a conscious, clearheaded manner."

NICE and Its Detractors   Despite the demand of insured Americans for access to all available technologies, health-policy experts like Garber, Fuchs, Thorpe, and Eddy recognize that, sooner or later, we'll have to consider costs along with benefits. Garber believes that that day may come when consumers bear so much of the costs that they have to pay attention to health care alternatives. "Eventually, it becomes a matter of considerable importance to the patient to decide whether the care they receive represents good value." He contrasts this consumer-choice model with the European, top-down approach, "in which the cost-effectiveness determines what kinds of care should be provided to people."

Cost-effectiveness analysis is used explicitly in the United Kingdom and the Netherlands. Many other European countries, as well as Canada, Australia, and New Zealand, do cost-benefit evaluations of prescription drugs.[47] But the United Kingdom appears to be ahead of other countries in its efforts to publicize cost-effectiveness analyses. Britain's National

Institute for Clinical Effectiveness (NICE), which was established in 1999, publishes recommendations on drugs, devices, tests, and procedures that are based on cost as well as benefit,[48] and the National Health Service generally follows them.[49]

The track record of NICE has been mixed. It has approved most of the interventions that it has considered,[50] and it beat an ignominious retreat on Relenza, an influenza drug, after its rejection of the moderately effective medication elicited a furious protest from Glaxo Wellcome, Relenza's manufacturer. Drug companies and patient groups, similarly, assailed NICE's refusal to approve beta interferon and glatiramir for treatment of multiple sclerosis.[51] But it has reviewed a wide variety of other technologies without incident, and the British medical establishment accepts its legitimacy.[52]

From the viewpoint of cost control, NICE has been fairly consistent. The multiple sclerosis drugs, for example, would have cost between $70,000 and $157,500 per quality-adjusted year of life saved (QALY). In contrast, all of the recommended services and products cost less than $52,500 per QALY, with one exception: The Institute approved riluzole for motor neuron disease, even though it costs up to $77,000 per QALY. The reason? "Patient values."[53]

Early on, some observers griped about the apparent lack of "patient values" in NICE's rationing decisions.[54] In 2002, NICE formed the Citizens Council to supply public input into those decisions, as well as its clinical guidelines.[55] How much weight NICE's experts give to the advice of the Citizens Council is unclear.

Oregon's Retreat In this country, several health plans post on their Web sites extensive information about why they approved or rejected particular technologies.[56] But, unlike NICE, they don't include cost-benefit analyses, and they have no mechanism for soliciting public comments.

The closest that the United States has come to creating something like NICE is the Oregon Health Plan, which went into effect in February 1994.[57] Yet, although Oregon stated which services the state would cover for an expanded Medicaid population, its approach to rationing was different from that of the United Kingdom. While it initially attempted to use cost-effectiveness analysis, Oregon ultimately prioritized services on the basis of their effectiveness and value to patients, declining to pay for services below a certain point on the list.[58]

The Oregon Health Plan enjoyed a fair amount of success at first. By extending Medicaid coverage to everyone below the poverty line, it covered 125,000 more people, and the percentage of uninsured Oregonians dropped from 18 percent to 11 percent in 1997. Neither doctors nor patients complained about necessary care not being delivered.[59]

But in recent years, like other Medicaid programs across the nation, the Oregon Health Plan has run into a solid wall of budget cuts and public resistance to tax hikes. As a result, after first dropping some more services, Oregon began forcing people off the Medicaid rolls. From 2003 to 2004, the number of those who received the standard Oregon Health Plan benefits dropped from ninety thousand to fifty-four thousand.[60]

Lesson of the Oregon Plan   From the viewpoint of drawing up a standard benefit package, the most important lesson of the Oregon experiment emerged in 1990, when the Oregon Health Services Commission released a list of approved services that were ranked on the basis of cost-effectiveness. Outside reviewers immediately pointed out that "many of the rankings were clinically counterintuitive, assigning higher priorities to some services that were clearly less important than other, lower-ranked services." For example, dental caps for pulp exposure were assigned a higher priority than surgery for ectopic pregnancy, and a certain kind of splint for bone fractures came out higher than an appendectomy. Facing a firestorm of criticism, the commission revised its methodology to make sure that the rankings were based purely on clinical value.[61]

Aside from these incongruities, David Hadorn of RAND declares that cost-effectiveness analysis was bound to fail because of conceptual flaws. Above all, he says, it didn't take into account what he calls the "Rule of Rescue": that is, when the value of a single expensive, life-saving operation is balanced against, say, that of providing pulp caps or prenatal care to dozens of people, human nature will always favor saving the life. "People cannot stand idly by when an identified person's life is visibly threatened if effective rescue measures are available," Hadorn writes.[62]

Why It Hasn't Happened Here   Why hasn't the United States been able to come to terms with the idea of considering cost in benefit decisions, as many other countries have? One reason, says Naomi Aronson of the Technology Evaluation Center, is that there's no scientific, governmental, or social consensus on a cutoff point for cost-effectiveness, such as $50,000 or $100,000 per QALY.

Jed Weissberg of Kaiser Permanente agrees. "There's certainly no public discussion of what that threshold should be. And when I thought about what we should do internally, I realized that we were proud of the fact that we didn't have a threshold—that when things worked, we'd just do them and rely on the mechanism of insurance to spread the costs.

"The best example of that is in the use of replacement enzyme therapies for kids born with genetic diseases. The costs of those run hundreds of thousands of dollars a year. But nobody's going to say you shouldn't put enzyme replacements into a kid, even though there isn't much good information about the outcomes of those kids over a long period of time."

David Eddy, MD, who taught Kaiser's doctors how to develop clinical guidelines and who was chief scientist at the Blues' TEC for twenty years, holds a different view of what's blocking the application of cost-effectiveness analysis in the United States. The reason the public is unwilling to entertain any thought of limits on services, he says, is that "we have imagined ourselves into the position that somehow it is up to someone else to pay the costs. If it is the responsibility of the insurer, or the corporation, or the government, or charity to pay, then why not insist on having everything, no matter what it costs someone else?

"In most care settings, we just keep piling it on. People might howl a bit when their insurance premiums go up or their employers ask them to pay a greater share, but as a country we keep demanding more and more. So in that sense, the actions of society imply that we are willing to pay any cost. On the other hand, nobody's willing to pay the cost himself, and everybody's trying to get someone else to pay. So that says that people believe costs are too high. If costs are too high, you have no option but to look at the things we're spending money on and try to figure out which ones provide value."

24 Toward a Rational System of Rationing

As many observers have pointed out, the United States rations care by ability to pay. Therefore, Americans believe it's ethical to deny some technologies to certain people, Arthur Caplan of the University of Pennsylvania notes. "If you want to get a liver transplant at Cedars-Sinai or the Mayo Clinic, and you don't have insurance or $250,000, you're not going to get it," he says. "We've got a very expensive health-care system, but we have no trouble denying things to people every day."

Nevertheless, we still have trouble with the idea of allowing identifiable individuals to die for lack of care that offers even a slight chance of saving them. Caplan doesn't think that the American public is going to get past this Rule of Rescue soon. Noting that doing so would require a major cultural shift, he says that political and religious leaders would have to mount a campaign comparable to that of the antismoking movement. They'd have to pound home the message that "the best thing to do with technology is to only use it when it stands a reasonable chance of benefit. And a reasonable chance of benefit is not one in a thousand or one in a million or one in a billion."

Since he doesn't believe such a campaign will ever be mounted, Caplan has accepted the idea that we're going to have a multitiered system in which some people get much better health care than others, and that the differences will continue to widen. About the best we can do, he says, is to ensure that everyone has access to a minimum set of health benefits.

Other health care experts, including Uwe Reinhardt and Alan Garber, agree that we're heading to a multitiered system. But there should still be a way to give everyone access to all care that society deems medically necessary, even if that doesn't include every service that might be beneficial. The wealthy would still be able to buy maximum care, and everyone else would receive adequate care.

Implicit and Explicit Rationing   How do we go about this? There are really only two ways: Either we ration care explicitly, which is part of what the United Kingdom does, or we ration it implicitly, as Kaiser Permanente does. The two methods could also be combined. But before we explore that option, let's take a closer look at how the United States rations care today.

Besides rationing by ability to pay, David Eddy pointed out in a recent interview, we also ration care by guideline. In other words, every guideline or agreement among doctors on how to treat patients involves certain tradeoffs. "If anyone ever makes a formulary decision or designs an operational guideline or sets a target for a treatment, an essential part of doing that is drawing a line someplace," he observed. "As soon as you say, 'we recommend these screening tests' or 'these screening tests at these frequencies' or 'these screening tests for these people,' you've drawn a line, and that line does imply some value judgment about what you're willing to do and pay for in order to get a certain amount of benefit. That's just unavoidable."

In an earlier interview in *Medical Economics*, Eddy explained how these decisions play out in the doctor-patient relationship. "Take the annual mammogram," he said. "No one would deny that a mammogram every six months would be better. But we don't tell that to every woman who gets an annual mammogram. We just define the annual mammogram as the standard of care, knowing full well that there's something out there that's better but that costs too much."[1]

While acknowledging that most doctors were not ready to go beyond this, Eddy stated that, under managed care, their responsibility is not only to the individual patient but also to the population of patients who pay for insurance. "To use too many resources on one patient is unfair to other patients who, as result, might be unable to get access to care that they have a right to," he said.

Who Has the Authority to Deny Care?   Eddy's principles have an obvious application to the financially responsible physician groups in our reform model. But as E. Haavi Morreim[2] and others have observed, doctors feel torn between their moral responsibility to serve the patient's best interests and their knowledge that resources are limited. If the patient has little or no insurance, a physician might say, "Let's try a less expensive drug or a less costly treatment, which is nearly as good as the more expensive kind." But if a patient has good insurance, notes Henry Aaron of the Brookings Institution, the physician will try to do everything he can for that patient. "If resources are available, no provider who is not a monster will withhold care that he or she believes promises medical benefit," he observes.[3]

The only way out of this moral bind, Aaron says, is to impose a budget on the provision of care. Every insurance plan has a budget, and it could be argued that a consumer agrees to live within that budget when he or she buys an insurance policy. But Aaron points out that every effort to enforce such limits on individual patients has failed, because the public doesn't believe that health plans have the authority to deny any beneficial care to patients. In fact, they believe that plans deny payments for some care mainly to increase profits.

Nevertheless, if Kaiser Permanente's doctors can gently steer patients to more cost-effective services, other physicians can do the same. And to the extent that the doctors are taking financial responsibility for care, they themselves are stewards of the health care dollar—not on behalf of an HMO but on behalf of all the patients who must be cared for within the limits of their group's budget.

Technology Assessment Board   To build a standard benefit package and deal with new technologies, we'll have to do some explicit rationing as well. That will require a form of technology assessment that includes cost-effectiveness analysis.

Victor Fuchs, the Stanford University economist, has proposed "a large, private center for technology assessment," including cost-benefit analysis, that would be supported by a small levy on all health care spending. Only a centralized body would be able to take a comprehensive approach to technology evaluation, he says. Individual health plans have too small a percentage of the market to make the investment worthwhile. "Government agencies try to fill the void, but the scale of effort is too small, and a private center would be able to avoid the political interference that often intrudes on government-run agencies."[4]

As noted in Chapter 22, economist Gail Wilensky has proposed formation of a "center for comparative effectiveness information." Although this institution would not gather data on cost-effectiveness, it would perform many of the other functions that a national technology assessment board would have to carry out. Wilensky and other experts favor making this an independent, quasi-public body to remove it from both political and commercial influences.[5]

Let's say that the current technology assessment activities of Medicare, the Blues, other plans, and the private technology evaluation companies were absorbed into a single body that operated under a federal mandate but was separate from the government. Under our model, that National Technology Assessment Board would have the authority to draw up a standard benefit package and to drop or add technologies as the evidence on them accumulated. In relation to the utility insurers, it would function in the same way NICE functions with regard to the United Kingdom's National Health Service. The government, while not supervising the technology assessment board, would make its recommendations binding on the utility insurers. Since the insurers would be delegating financial responsibility to the physician groups, those practices would also have to abide by the national board's decisions.

Consumer Council   As mentioned earlier, NICE appoints a Citizens Council that advises the technology experts. David Eddy proposed a similar concept many years ago. In a series of papers, he sketched out the rationale and the method for consumers to participate in technology evaluations. His idea was to assemble a representative group of people, present them with information on the benefits and harms of an intervention, tell them what it would cost, "and observe their choices."[6]

In a recent conversation, Eddy elaborated on this idea, suggesting that the consultative body should consist of several thousand people who would represent a broad cross-section of the population by age, gender, race, geography, and income. Since they'd have to be able to understand basic concepts of medicine and mathematical probability, he adds, they'd have to be of above-average intelligence—a requirement that could be met by picking only people who've had at least some college education.

Eddy also feels strongly that these consumer "judges" should be required to buy their own insurance, with the premiums adjusted according to income and net worth so that everyone feels the same economic pain. That way, he explains, they'd know that the cost of whatever technologies they approved would be reflected in their own insurance premiums.

While this plan makes sense, I don't believe the council members would have to pay the total cost of their insurance to appreciate the cost-benefit ratio of any given technology. Under our reform model, everyone above a certain income level would pay at least 20 percent and possibly as much as half of the insurance cost, depending on their income. And, as taxpayers, they'd be helping to subsidize health care for the poor, the elderly, and the disabled. If they were informed how much their technology choices would raise their health care contributions and their income taxes, they'd have a very good reason to choose wisely.

The situation would be different, however, for the poor, whose insurance would be subsidized by the government, and for the wealthy, who would probably opt out of the standard plan and buy more expensive insurance. So perhaps the technology assessment board should limit membership in this consumer council to those of moderate means, with household incomes, say, of $40,000 to $80,000 a year. Those people, at least, would feel the bite of higher health care costs.

A consumer council would be much easier to implement today than it would have been when Eddy proposed it fifteen years ago, before the Internet became ubiquitous. With the help of high-speed Web access, it would now be vastly simpler to recruit, educate, and poll consumer judges. (However, several hundred might be more manageable than several thousand.) We would, of course, have to pay them for their time, and their terms should probably be limited to a year or two to minimize burnout and attrition. Above all, we'd have to guard their identities to protect them from political and commercial pressures.

What Would the Board Evaluate?   Before we look at what the consumer council would evaluate, we need to understand what the national board itself would assess.

The board might start with a list of all of the services that most health plans covered prior to the changeover to utility insurers. Using insurance data, it would find out which interventions were most expensive in the aggregate. Then it would get actuarial estimates of how much each of these technologies would add to the cost of a benefit package. It would also gather data on the comparative effectiveness and cost of alternative tests, treatments, and procedures, wherever those were available.

The board would then pare down the standard benefit package by asking the consumer council to decide whether it wanted to include certain interventions. This process would avoid the stickiness of setting a dollar threshold for cost-effectiveness; it would leave the determination of relative value up to people who would potentially be the recipients of care.

The same approach could be used for evaluating new technologies, with one important difference: Before determining the cost of a new technology or asking the consumer council to decide whether they wanted it, the national board would have to assess the benefits and risks of the intervention. This assessment is no different from what technology evaluation bodies do now; as Naomi Aronson notes, there's no point in talking about cost-effectiveness until you've established that a technology is effective.

Dividing the Wheat from the Chaff   The consumer council should be asked to evaluate only particular kinds of technology. Among these would be interventions that are high-cost and low-benefit; those that would generate tricky conflicts among different patient values; and those that would be so expensive that they'd limit access to other important technologies or even basic services.

In the first category would be services such as full body scans and growth hormone for naturally short children, as well as fertility treatments, which benefit some people psychologically but not medically. The council should also look at high-cost technologies that are unproven but are starting to come into common use. A good recent example is the use of high-dose chemotherapy with autologous bone marrow transplants to treat metastatic breast cancer; though now largely discredited, this experimental therapy had a lot of support only a few years ago.[7]

One intervention that involves trade-offs among patient values is bariatric surgery for obese patients. With the risks of death and hospital readmission higher than earlier thought,[8] and the annual costs mounting into the billions of dollars, our consumer jury might well decide that this surgery should be reserved only for the morbidly obese. Hip and knee replacements have become increasingly common, and most people believe they have a right to them to improve their quality of life.[9] But if a much more expensive artificial joint were to be invented, the consumer council should weigh in on it.

When it comes to major medical breakthroughs that could bankrupt the system, the council would have a key role to play. For example, it could follow the lead of the Food and Drug Administration today and cover left ventricular assist devices as a bridge to keep people alive until they receive heart transplants. But it might stop short of endorsing permanent left-ventricular assist devices at a cost of $120,000 each.[10]

If the artificial heart ever became feasible as a long-term replacement, our consumer council would have a devil of a time. Clearly, there are far more people with heart failure than there are organs available for transplants. So if we could provide mechanical hearts for all 5 million of those people,[11] we'd be doing a good deed, right? Maybe. But wait—at $250,000 per heart, that would cost $1.25 trillion! That's about two-thirds of what was spent on health care for all Americans in 2005. So, as every other advanced country in the world has already figured out, we'd have to make choices.

A Test for Patient "Experts"   There is no doubt that the consumer council would need a lot of information to make a decision about even a single technology. And it's equally clear that they'd be able to do so only if a range of experts presifted the evidence for them and presented it in terms that educated laypeople could understand.

For example, let's say that the patient judges were asked to decide whether colonoscopy to detect colorectal cancer should be in the standard benefit package. Since Medicare started covering this test for average-risk patients in 2001, there has been a rapid increase in its use.[12] Meanwhile, screening with flexible sigmoidoscopy has dropped precipitously, and the percentage of primary-care physicians who still do the procedure has fallen to 20–25 percent.[13] Fewer doctors do "flex sigs," as they're known, partly because they get paid only $100–$200 for each test.[14] Physicians receive about four times as much for screening colonoscopy, which can cost anywhere from $600 to $2,500 or more,[15] depending on who's paying the bill and where the procedure is done.

The American College of Gastroenterologists, the American Cancer Society, and the U.S. Preventive Services Task Force do not recommend screening colonoscopies in preference to flex sigs, double-contrast barium enema tests, or fecal occult blood tests for screening average-risk people. While fecal occult blood tests have been shown to reduce the mortality rate from colon cancer, and studies strongly suggest the same outcome for flex sigs, less rigorous trials have been done on colonoscopy.[16] Yet it's widely assumed that colonoscopy is effective, and the

Preventive Services Task Force holds that all four forms of colorectal cancer screening are cost-effective compared with no screening.[17]

Conflicting Perspectives   Many experts assert that colonoscopy is the preferred screening tool. "Flex sig sees only the left side of the colon," notes Gavin Harewood, MD, a professor of medicine at the Mayo Clinic. "It's like doing mammography of one breast."

Colonoscopy, however, has a higher complication rate,[18] and it's not clear that it reduces mortality from colon cancer more than the alternatives do. In an article published in 2005, David Ransohoff of the University of North Carolina, Chapel Hill, says that "a combined program of [annual] FOBT [fecal occult blood test] and sigmoidoscopy [every five years] may be as effective as or more effective than a program of colonoscopy screening every 10 years." A gastroenterologist and an authority on colorectal cancer screening, Ransohoff also points out that colonoscopy may not decrease the absolute risk of mortality from colon cancer much more than it increases the cumulative risk of complications.[19]

How could the consumer judges sort through all of these conflicting facts and assertions? The experts would have to provide them with a set of rigidly focused postulates. First, they'd point out that screening colonoscopy is not necessarily more effective in preventing cancer deaths than are flex sigs along with a fecal occult blood test. Furthermore, while screening colonoscopy may be just as cost-effective in the long run, it's currently generating costs of roughly $10 billion a year.[20] And finally, though colonoscopy might reduce the lifetime risk of colorectal cancer from 2.0 percent to 0.8 percent, it also raises the cumulative risk of complications by nearly as much when people are tested at ten-year intervals. Here's how much it would add to the average person's insurance premium, and here's how much it would add to the average tax bill.

Based on these facts, would the consumer council be able to decide whether to cover screening colonoscopy for all patients twenty and older? We have to hope so, because nobody else is in a position to choose among these conflicting patient values.

Hope Springs Eternal   In the long run, neither technology assessment as it's currently done nor methods that include cost-effectiveness analysis will check the growth of technology costs enough to keep health care affordable. The former can weed out only interventions that are ineffective or harmful, and the latter can only inform value judgments that are best made by physicians and patients.

Yet technology assessment can slow down the introduction of some technologies until more evidence is available on their effectiveness. And when we get to "breakthroughs" that can bankrupt the system, a consumer council's members might give their fellow Americans pause if they recommended against adopting the technology, or would approve it only for narrow indications.

We should not be too optimistic about this. Most people want to live at all costs, and most of the population still has enormous faith in the power of medical advances to improve health and extend life. A 2004 study, for example, found that "the public is enthusiastic about cancer screening. This commitment is not dampened by false-positive test results or the possibility that testing could lead to unnecessary treatment."[21]

The other thing people love to hear about is the possibility of increased longevity. But despite numerous stories about the rising number of centenarians, many people say they wouldn't want to live that long. According to a USA Today/ABC News poll, the average American wants to live eighty-seven years, just nine years longer than the current life span of nearly seventy-eight.[22]

Therein lies a small kernel of hope. If we can just content ourselves with a life span that coincides with a level of frailty that nearly all of us will encounter by that age, perhaps there will come a day when the wisest of us will say, "Enough." Then, and only then, will the great engine of technological progress slow to a pace that humanity can afford.

Notes

Introduction

1. Jack Hadley and Peter J. Cunningham, *Perception, Reality, and Health Insurance: Uninsured as Likely as Insured to Perceive Need for Care but Half as Likely to Get Care*, Center for Studying Health System Change, Issue Brief no. 100, October 2005.
2. U.S. Census Bureau, *Income, Poverty, and Health Insurance Coverage in the United States: 2005*, August 2006, 20.
3. Todd Gilmer and Richard Kronick, "It's the Premiums, Stupid: Projections of the Uninsured through 2013," *Health Affairs Web Exclusive*, April 5, 2005, 143–51.
4. Cathy Schoen, Michelle M. Doty, Sara R. Collins, and Alyssa L. Holmgren, "Insured but Not Protected: How Many Adults Are Underinsured?" *Health Affairs Web Exclusive*, June 14, 2005, 289–302.
5. Ibid.
6. P. J. Cunningham and J. H. May, *Tough Trade-offs: Medical Bills, Family Finances, and Access to Care*, Center for Studying Health System Change, Issue Brief no. 85, June 2004; Michelle M. Doty, Jennifer N. Edwards, and Alyssa L. Holmgren, *Seeing Red: Americans Driven into Debt by Medical Bills*, Commonwealth Fund, Issue Brief, August 2005; David U. Himmelstein, Elizabeth Warren, Deborah Thorne, and Steffie Woolhandler, "Illness and Injury as Contributors to Bankruptcy," *Health Affairs Web Exclusive*, February 2, 2005, 63–73.
7. John Leland, "When Even Health Insurance Is No Safeguard," *New York Times*, October 23, 2005.
8. Jon Gabel, Gary Claxton, Isadora Gil, Jeremy Pickreign, Heidi Whitmore, Benjamin Finder, Samantha Hawkins, and Diane Rowland, "Health Benefits in 2005: Premium Increases Slow Down, Coverage Continues to Erode," *Health Affairs*, September/October 2005, 1273–80; Gary Claxton, Jon Gabel, Isadora Gil, Jeremy Pickreign, Heidi Whitemore, Benjamin Finder, Blanca DiJulio, and Samantha Hawkins, "Health Benefits in 2006: Premium Increases Moderate, Enrollment in Consumer-Directed Health Plans Remains Modest," *Health Affairs Web Exclusive*, September 26, 2006, 476–85.
9. Tony Pugh, "Health Cost to Double in Decade," *Philadelphia Inquirer*, February 22, 2006.
10. Uwe Reinhardt, quoted in Howard Larkin, "Downsizing Health Coverage," *Hospitals & Health Networks*, September 2005.

11. Gabel et al., "Health Benefits in 2005."

12. Danny Hakim, "G.M. and Union in a Deal to Cut Health Benefits," *New York Times*, October 18, 2005.

13. Danny Hakim and Jeremy W. Peters, "Union Offers Details of Health Deal with G.M., *New York Times*, October 21, 2005.

14. Mercer Human Resources Consulting, *2005 U.S. Survey of Employer-Sponsored Health Plans*, March 2006.

15. Reed Abelson, "States Are Battling against Wal-Mart over Health Care," *New York Times*, November 1, 2004.

16. Vanessa Fuhrmans, "More Employers Try Limited Health Plans," *Wall Street Journal*, January 17, 2006.

17. Vanessa Fuhrmans, "Few Uninsured Workers Opt for Employers' New Health Plans," *Wall Street Journal*, February 8, 2006.

18. Richard Marosi, "Healthcare Is Migrating South of the Border," *Los Angeles Times*, November 3, 2005.

19. David M. Cutler and Mark McClellan, "Is Technological Change Worth It?" *Health Affairs*, September/October 2001, 11–29; Mark V. Pauly, "Should We Be Worried about High Real Medical Spending Growth in the United States?" *Health Affairs Web Exclusive*, January 8, 2003, 15–27; Sherry Glied, "Are We in a Health Care Crisis?" PBS.org, www.pbs.org/healthcarecrisis/Exprts_intrvw/s_glied.htm; Gina Kolata, "Making Health Care the Engine That Drives the Economy," *New York Times*, August 22, 2006.

20. National Coalition on Health Care, *Building a Better Health Care System: Specifications for Reform*, July 2004.

21. Cathy Schoen, Sabrina K. H. How, Ilana Weinbaum, John E. Craig Jr., and Karen Davis, "Public Views on Shaping the Future of the U.S. Health System," *Commonwealth Fund Report*, August 2006.

22. Ezekiel J. Emanuel and Victor R. Fuchs, "Getting Covered: Choose a Plan Everyone Can Agree On," *Boston Review*, November/December 2005.

23. Robert Pear, "Planned Medicaid Cuts Cause Rift with States," *New York Times*, August 13, 2006.

24. L. M. Nichols, P. B. Ginsburg, R. A. Berenson, R. Christianson, and R. E. Hurley, "Are Market Forces Strong Enough to Deliver Efficient Health Care Systems? Confidence Is Waning," *Health Affairs*, March/April 2004, 8–21.

25. Alain Enthoven, "Market Forces and Efficient Health Care Systems," *Health Affairs*, March/April 2004, 25–27.

26. Wayne J. Guglielmo, "The New Medicare Law: Doctors Cheer," *Medical Economics*, January 9, 2004.

27. Uwe Reinhardt, interview with the author, April 2004.

Chapter 1. How We Got into This Mess

1. Thomas Bodenheimer, "The Political Divide in Health Care: A Liberal Perspective," *Health Affairs*, November/December 2005, 1426–35.

2. Daniel Yankelovich, "The Debate That Wasn't: The Public and the Clinton Plan," *Health Affairs*, Spring 1995, 7–23.

3. Paul Starr, *The Social Transformation of American Medicine* (New York: Basic Books, 1982), 252.

4. Robert Cunningham III and Robert M. Cunningham Jr., *The Blues: A History*

of the Blue Cross and Blue Shield System (DeKalb: Northern Illinois University Press, 1997), 17–18.

5. Starr, *Social Transformation*, 301–6.
6. Cunningham and Cunningham, *Blues*, 12–33.
7. Ibid., 34–37, 44–45.
8. Starr, *Social Transformation*, 267
9. Cunningham and Cunningham, *Blues*, 94.
10. Ibid., 95–96, 97–101; Starr, *Social Transformation*, 330–31.
11. Starr, *Social Transformation*, 311–12.
12. Cunningham and Cunningham, *Blues*, 59.
13. Starr, *Social Transformation*, 346–47.
14. Ibid., 350.
15. Ibid., 364; J. E. Wennberg and J. L. Freeman, "Hospital Use and Mortality among Medicare Beneficiaries in Boston and New Haven," *New England Journal of Medicine* 321, no. 17 (1989): 1168–73.
16. Starr, *Social Transformation*, 369.
17. Cunningham and Cunningham, *Blues*, 149.
18. Starr, *Social Transformation*, 375, 385.
19. Ibid., 381–94; Cunningham and Cunningham, *Blues*, 186–87.
20. Starr, *Social Transformation*, 397–404.
21. Julius B. Richmond and Rashi Fein, *The Health Care Mess: How We Got Into It and What It Will Take to Get Out* (Cambridge, MA: Harvard University Press, 2005), 69–71.
22. Cunningham and Cunningham, *Blues*, 189.
23. Starr, *Social Transformation*, 406, 412.
24. Ibid., 379–80.
25. American Medical Association (AMA), *Physician Characteristics and Distribution in the U.S.* (Chicago: AMA Press, 1997), 10–11.
26. Starr, *Social Transformation*, 400–403.
27. Cunningham and Cunningham, *Blues*, 206–7.
28. Ibid., 207
29. Stuart Altman, "Health System Reform: Let's Not Miss Our Chance," *Health Affairs*, Spring 1994, 69–80.
30. Carol Stevens, "Is There Any Reason Not to Participate in Medicare?" *Medical Economics*, July 6, 1992.
31. Robert Pear, "Doctors Objecting to Planned Cut in Medicare Fees," *New York Times*, November 20, 2005.
32. Michael L. Millenson, *Demanding Medical Excellence: Doctors and Accountability in the Information Age* (Chicago: University of Chicago Press, 1997), 171.
33. Donald W. Moran, "Whence and Whither Health Insurance? A Revisionist History," *Health Affairs*, November/December 2005, 1415–25.
34. Chris Rauber, "Evolution or Extinction?" *Modern Healthcare*, October 19, 1998.
35. Thomas Bodenheimer, "The Major Players Start Dealing," *Nation*, March 22, 1993.
36. Robert Pear, "Congress Is Given Clinton Proposal for Health Care," *New York Times*, October 28, 1993; Adam Clymer, "White House Drops Talk of Capping U.S. Health Spending," *New York Times*, October 29, 1993.
37. American Medical Association, *Physicians and the Changing System: The Preliminary Clinton Reform Plan*, September 1993.

38. Robert Pear, "Health Advisers Plan Exemption for Big Business," *New York Times*, April 26, 1993.

39. Altman, "Health System Reform."

40. Robert Pear and David E. Rosenbaum, "As Health Plan Comes Together, Big Price Tag Comes Into Focus," *New York Times*, April 19, 1993.

41. Ibid.

42. Stephen K. Murata, "What the Clinton Health Plan Means to You," *Medical Economics*, October 25, 1993.

43. Alain C. Enthoven and Sara J. Singer, "A Single-Payer System in Jackson Hole Clothing," *Health Affairs*, Spring 1994, 81–95.

44. Yankelovich, "Debate That Wasn't."

45. Robert J. Blendon, Mollyann Brodie, and John Benson, "What Happened to Americans' Support for the Clinton Plan?" *Health Affairs*, Summer 1995, 7–23.

46. Robert Pear, "Business Group Assails Scope and Cost of Clinton Health Plan," *New York Times*, October 21, 1993; Jeanne Saddler, "Health Mandate Opposed in Chamber Poll," *Wall Street Journal*, April 27, 1994; Saddler, "Mandated Health Coverage Finds Surprising Opponents," *Wall Street Journal*, May 17, 1993.

47. Ken Terry, "Cheaper by the Dozen," *Inc.*, June 1996, 72–76.

48. Shelly S. Brandel and Larry J. Pfannerstill (Milliman USA), *Arizona Health Care Cost Containment Council Issue Paper on Purchasing Pools*, August 27, 2001.

49. Mercer Human Resources Consulting, "Health Benefit Cost Up 11.2% in 2001—Highest Jump in 10 Years," press release, December 10, 2001.

50. Ronald Bangasser (former president of the California Medical Association), interview with the author, December 2004; Jack Zwanziger and Glenn A. Melnick, "Can Managed Care Plans Control Health Costs?" *Health Affairs*, Summer 1996, 186–99.

51. Ken Terry, "Say No to Health Plans? These Doctors Did," *Medical Economics*, August 9, 1999.

52. K. Davis, K. S. Collins, C. Schoen, and C. Morris, "Choice Matters: Enrollees' View of Their Health Plans," *Health Affairs*, Summer 1995, 99–112.

53. Kaiser Family Foundation/Health Educational Research Trust, *2005 Employer Health Benefit Survey: Summary of Findings*, September 14, 2005.

54. Peter Kongstvedt (Accenture), interview with the author, July 2004.

55. Ken Terry, "What's in the Box? Is United Healthcare Delivering on Its Promises?" *Medical Economics*, September 4, 2000.

56. Alison Evans Cuellar and Paul J. Gertler, "How the Expansion of Hospital Systems Has Affected Consumers," *Health Affairs*, January/February 2005, 213–19; Guy Boulton, "Hospitals Control the Market: Health Cost Study Says Insurers Hold a Weak Position," *Milwaukee Journal Sentinel*, June 28, 2006.

57. Bradley C. Strunk, Paul B. Ginsburg, and Jon R. Gabel, "Tracking Health Costs: Hospital Care Surpasses Drugs as the Key Cost Driver," *Health Affairs Web Exclusive*, September 26, 2001, 39–50.

58. Paul B. Ginsburg, "Competition in Health Care: Its Evolution over the Past Decade," *Health Affairs*, November/December 2005, 1512–22.

59. Lewis Sandy, "Homeostasis without Reserve: The Risk of Health System Collapse," *New England Journal of Medicine* 347 (2002): 1971–75.

60. Donald W. Moran, "Whence and Whither Health Insurance? A Revisionist History," *Health Affairs*, November/December 2005, 1415–25.

61. Thomas Bodenheimer, "The Political Divide in Health Care: A Liberal Perspective," *Health Affairs*, November/December 2005, 1426–35.

Chapter 2. 'Round and 'Round on the Reform Carousel

1. John Holahan and Allison Cook, "Changes in Economic Conditions and Health Insurance Coverage, 2000–2004," *Health Affairs Web Exclusive*, November 1, 2005, 498–508.
2. Sara R. Collins, Karen Davis, Michelle M. Doty, Jennifer L. Kriss, and Alyssa L. Holmgren, "Gaps in Health Coverage: An All-American Problem," *Commonwealth Fund Report*, April 2006.
3. Donald W. Moran, "Whence and Whither Health Insurance? A Revisionist History," *Health Affairs*, November/December 2005, 1415–25.
4. Tony Fong, "Cash or Care? Price Is Big Difference in Bush, Dem Health Plans," *Modern Healthcare*, February 9, 2004; Families USA, *The Bush Administration's Fiscal Year 2005 Budget: Analysis of Key Health Care Provisions*, February 4, 2004; Robert Pear, "Health Care, Vexing to Clinton, Is Now at Top of Bush's Agenda," *New York Times*, January 29, 2006.
5. Robert Pear, "Experts See Peril in Bush Health Proposal," *New York Times*, January 28, 2007.
6. Matthew DoBias and Jennifer Lubell, "Back on the Center Stage," *Modern Healthcare*, November 13, 2006.
7. S. Woolhandler, T. Campbell, and D. U. Himmelstein, "Costs of Health Care Administration in the United States and Canada," *New England Journal of Medicine* 349 (2003): 768–75.
8. John Geyman, "Is It Time for National Health Insurance?" *Boston Review*, November/December 2005; "Proposal of the Physicians' Working Group for Single-Payer National Health Insurance," *Journal of the American Medical Association* 290 (2003): 798–805.
9. Henry J. Aaron, "The Costs of Health Care Administration in the United States and Canada—Questionable Answers to a Questionable Question," *New England Journal of Medicine* 349 (2003): 801–3.
10. Henry J. Aaron, interview with the author, April 2004; John C. Goodman, Gerald L. Musgrave, and Devon M. Herrick, *Lives at Risk: Single-Payer National Health Insurance around the World* (Lanham, MD: Rowman & Littlefield, 2004).
11. Karen Davis and Cathy Schoen, "Creating Consensus on Coverage Choices," *Health Affairs Web Exclusive*, April 23, 2003, 199–211.
12. Jeanne M. Lambrew, John D. Podesta, and Teresa L. Shaw, "Change in Challenging Times: A Plan for Extending and Improving Health Coverage," *Health Affairs Web Exclusive*, March 23, 2005, 119–32.
13. Victor R. Fuchs and Ezekiel J. Emanuel, "Health Care Reform: Why? What? When?" *Health Affairs*, November/December 2005, 1399–1414; Emanuel and Fuchs, "Getting Covered: Choose a Plan Everyone Can Agree On," *Boston Review*, November/December 2005.
14. "Wyden Proposes Historic New Health Plan: The Healthy Americans Act," press release, December 2006, http://wyden.senate.gov. Also, see "Healthy Americans Act Section by Section."
15. John Edwards 08, press release, "Universal Health Care Through Shared

Responsibility," February 5, 2007, johnedwards.com/about/issues/health-care-overview.pdf.

16. John M. Broder, "Edwards Details His Health Care Proposal," *New York Times*, February 6, 2007.

17. John Edwards 08, press release, February 5, 2007.

18. Paul Krugman, "Edwards Gets It Right," *New York Times* (February 9, 2007).

19. John Edwards 08 press release, February 5, 2007, p. 4.

20. D. J. Palmisano, D. W. Emmons, G. D. Wozniak, "Expanding Insurance Coverage through Tax Credits, Consumer Choice, and Market Enhancements: The American Medical Association Proposal for Health Insurance Reform," *Journal of the American Medical Association* 291 (2004): 2237–42.

21. Mark V. Pauly, "Keeping Health Insurance Tax Credits on the Table," *Journal of the American Medical Association* 291 (2004): 2255–56.

22. Martin Sipkoff, "The Lure of Tax Reform," *Managed Care* (October 2005).

23. Council for Affordable Health Insurance, press release, "The Bush Health Care Reform Proposal: Good for the Country, Good for States," January 24, 2007; AMA press release, "AMA Applauds Health Care Focus in State of the Union," January 23, 2007; Grace-Marie Turner, president of the Galen Institute, "Lehrer News Hour," PBS-TV, January 25, 2007.

24. White House Press Office, State of the Union Address, January 23, 2007.

25. Sara Rosenbaum, George Washington University, "Lehrer News Hour," PBS-TV, January 25, 2007; also, United Steelworkers, press release, "USW Rejects Bush Health-Care Proposal," January 23, 2007.

26. Robin Toner and Robert Pear, "Bush Revives Some Past Proposals and Offers a New Initiative on Health Insurance," *New York Times*, January 24, 2007.

27. Robert Pear, "Experts See Peril in Bush Health Proposal," *New York Times*, January 28, 2007.

28. Rosenbaum, "Lehrer News Hour."

29. John D. McKinnon and John Harwood, "Bush Bids to Increase Focus on Health Care with Plan on Tax-Based Aid for Consumers, " *Wall Street Journal*, January 22, 2007.

30. Robert Pear, "Experts See Peril in Bush Health Proposal."

31. Paul Krugman, "Gold-Plated Indifference," *New York Times*, January 22, 2007.

32. John F. Cogan, R. Glenn Hubbard, and Daniel P. Kessler, "Making Markets Work: Five Steps to a Better Health Care System," *Health Affairs*, November/December 2005, 1447–57.

33. *Economic Report of the President*, 108th Cong., 2d sess., H. Doc. 108–145 (Washington, DC: U.S. Government Printing Office, 2004), chap. 10, 189.

34. Institute of Medicine, *Insuring America's Health: Principles and Recommendations* (Washington, DC: National Academies Press, 2004), 42–46.

35. Joel B. Finkelstein, "Medicare Reform Opens Up Health Savings Accounts to All," *American Medical News*, December 22–29, 2003.

36. Elizabeth White, "HSAs Likely to Get Early Attention in Individual, Small Group Markets," *BNA's Health Law Reporter*, January 8, 2004; Families USA, *Bush Administration's Fiscal Year 2005 Budget*.

37. "Consumer-Driven Health Plans," in *The InterStudy Competitive Edge, Part II: HMO Industry Report*, October 2003, 73–77.

38. P. Fronstin and S.R. Collins, "The 2nd Annual EBRI/Commonwealth Fund Consumerism in Health Care Survey, 2006: Early Experience With High-

Deductible and Consumer-Driven Health Plans," The Commonwealth Fund, December 2006.

39. Deloitte, "More Employers Turning to Consumer-Driven Plans to Reduce Health Spending," press release, November 15, 2005.

40. Gary Claxton, Jon Gabel, Isadora Gil, Jeremy Pickreign, Heidi Whitemore, Benjamin Finder, Blanca DiJulio, and Samantha Hawkins, "Health Benefits in 2006: Premium Increases Moderate, Enrollment in Consumer-Directed Health Plans Remains Modest," *Health Affairs Web Exclusive*, September 26, 2006, 476–85.

41. America's Health Insurance Plans (AHIP), "HSA Growth Accelerating Among Employers and Consumers," press release, March 9, 2006.

42. Fronstin and Collins, "The 2nd Annual EBRI/Commonwealth Fund Consumerism in Health Care Survey, 2006: Early Experience With High-Deductible and Consumer-Driven Health Plans."

43. Paul Fronstin and Sara A. Collins, *Early Experience with High-Deductible and Consumer-Driven Health Plans: Findings from the EBRI/Commonwealth Fund Consumerism in Health Care Survey*, Commonwealth Fund, Issue Brief no. 288, December 2005.

44. Ken Terry, "What's the Fallout If Patients Pay?" *Medical Economics*, March 7, 2003.

45. Karen Davis, *Will Consumer-Directed Health Care Improve System Performance?* Commonwealth Fund, Issue Brief, August 2004.

46. Robert Galvin, "'A Deficiency of Will and Ambition': A Conversation with Donald Berwick," *Health Affairs Web Exclusive*, January 12, 2005, 1–9.

47. Reed Abelson, "Medicare Says Bonuses Can Improve Hospital Care," *New York Times*, November 15, 2005); Leapfrog Group, "Pay for Performance Improving Health Care Quality and Changing Provider Behavior, but Challenges Persist," press release, November 15, 2005.

48. Mark R. Chassin, Robert W. Galvin, and the National Roundtable on Health Care Quality, "The Urgent Need to Improve Health Care Quality," *Journal of the American Medical Association* 280 (1998): 1000–1005.

49. "Privacy, Compensation Barriers Obstruct Bush's Goal of Electronic Medical Records," *BNA's Health Law Reporter*, January 29, 2004; Markian Hawryluk, "Push Continues for Electronic Health Records," *American Medical News*, June 14, 2004.

50. Marianne Kolbasuk McGee, "High-Tech Cure," *Information Week*, May 3, 2004.

51. "Gingrich: IT Office Will Get Funds," *Health Data Management*, December 3, 2004.

52. David Glendinning, "Health IT Bills Stall in Congress," *American Medical News*, October 23–30, 2006.

53. Richard Hillestadt, James Bigelow, Anthony Bower, Federico Girosi, Robin Meili, Richard Scoville, and Roger Taylor, "Can Electronic Medical Systems Transform Health Care? Potential Health Benefits, Savings, and Costs," *Health Affairs*, September/October 2005, 1103–17; Jan Walker, Eric Pan, Douglas Johnston, Julia Adler-Milstein, David W. Bates, and Blackford Middleton, "The Value of Health Care Information Exchange and Interoperability," *Health Affairs Web Exclusive*, January 19, 2005, 10–25.

54. Ken Terry, "Doctors and EHRs," *Medical Economics*, January 21, 2005; David Gans, John Kralewski, Terry Hammons, and Bryan Dowd, "Medical Groups'

Adoption of Electronic Health Records and Information Systems," *Health Affairs*, September/October 2005, 1323–33. The percentage of hospitals with CPOE systems comes from interviews by the author with Suzanne Delbanco, executive director of the Leapfrog Group, and Tom Handler, an IT consultant with the Gartner Group.

55. Eric W. Ford, Nir Menachemi, and M. Thad Phillips, "Predicting the Adoption of Electronic Health Records: When Will Health Care Be Paperless?" *Journal of the American Medical Informatics Association* 13 (2006): 106–12.

56. The White House, *Executive Order Promoting Quality and Efficient Health Care in Federal Government Administered or Sponsored Health Care Programs*, August 22, 2006.

57. American Medical Association, "AMA on Health Care Transparency Executive Order," press release, August 22, 2006.

58. American College of Physicians, *The Impending Collapse of Primary Care Medicine and Its Implications for the State of the Nation's Health Care*, January 30, 2006, 1.

59. Center for Medicare and Medicaid Services, "Medicare Program; Revisions to Payment Policies under the Physician Fee Schedule for Calendar Year 2006," *Federal Register*, November 21, 2005.

60. Hoangmai H. Pham, Kelly J. Devers, Jessica H. May, and Robert Berenson, "Financial Pressures Spur Physician Entrepreneurism," *Health Affairs*, March/April 2004, 70–81.

61. John K. Iglehart, "The Emergence of Physician-Owned Specialty Hospitals," *New England Journal of Medicine* 352 (2005): 78–84.

62. Dave Carpenter, "A Good Old-Fashioned Building Boom," *Hospitals & Health Networks*, March 2004.

63. Melanie Evans, "Will It Last? Hospital Profits Hit an All-Time High in 2004," *Modern Healthcare*, November 7, 2005.

64. Melanie Evans, "Hospitals' Profitable Year," *Modern Healthcare*, October 30, 2006.

65. Alison Evans Cuellar and Paul J. Gertler, "How the Expansion of Hospital Systems Has Affected Consumers," *Health Affairs*, January/February 2005, 213–19.

66. Melanie Evans and Vince Galloro, "In Good Health, At Least for Now," *Modern Healthcare*, June 12, 2006.

67. Marcia Angell, *The Truth about the Drug Companies: How They Deceive Us and What to Do About It* (New York: Random House, 2004), 3, 48, 52–93.

68. Weiss Ratings Inc., "Nation's HMO Profits Increase 10.7% in 2004," press release, August 8, 2005.

69. UnitedHealth Group, *10K Report for 2005 to the Securities and Exchange Commission*, February 24, 2006, 42.

70. Sarah Leuck and Vanessa Furhmans, "New Medicare Drug Benefit Sparks an Industry Land Grab," *Wall Street Journal*, January 25, 2006; Cinda Becker, "One Question: Credit or Debit?" *Modern Healthcare*, January 16, 2006.

71. Ian Urbina, "In the Treatment of Diabetes, Success Often Does Not Pay," *New York Times*, January 11, 2006.

72. Donald M. Berwick, David R. Calkins, C. Joseph McCannon, and Andrew D. Hackbarth, "The 100,000 Lives Campaign: Setting a Goal and a Deadline for Improving Health Care Quality," *Journal of the American Medical Association* 295 (2006): 324–27; Andis Robeznieks, "Berwick Says 100,000 Lives Campaign Exceeds Goal," *Modern Healthcare Alert*, June 14, 2006.

73. William B. Schwartz, *Life without Disease: The Pursuit of Medical Utopia* (Los Angeles: University of California Press, 1998), 8.

74. George C. Halvorson and George J. Isham, *Epidemic of Care: A Call for Safer, Better, and More Accountable Health Care* (San Francisco: Jossey-Bass, 2003), 1.

75. "Proposal of the Physicians' Working Group for Single-Payer National Health Insurance," *Journal of the American Medical Association* 290 (2003): 798–805.

Chapter 3. The Two Faces of Disease Management

1. Shin-Yi Wu and Anthony Green, *Projection of Chronic Illness Prevalence and Cost Inflation*, RAND Corp., October 2000.

2. M. L. Daviglus, L. Kiang, L. L. Yan, et al., "Relation of Body Mass Index in Young Adulthood and Middle Age to Medicare Expenditures in Older Age," *Journal of the American Medical Association* 292 (2004): 2743–49.

3. Information Technology Association of America (ITAA), "Chronic Care Improvement: How Medicare Transformation Can Save Lives, Save Money, and Stimulate an Emerging Technology Industry," May 2004, www.itaa.org.

4. E. A. McGlynn, S. M. Asch, J. Adams, J. Keesey, J. Hicks, A. DeCristofaro, and E. Kerr, "The Quality of Health Care Delivered to Adults in the United States," *New England Journal of Medicine* 348 (2003): 2635–45.

5. C. D. Saudek, R. L. Derr, and R. R. Kalyani, "Assessing Glycemia in Diabetes Using Self-Monitoring Blood Glucose and Hemoglobin A1c in Diabetes," *Journal of the American Medical Association* 295 (2006): 1688–97.

6. David Nash (chairman of the health policy department at Jefferson Medical College in Philadelphia), interview with the author, December 2005.

7. Laura B. Benko, "Chronic Questions," *Modern Healthcare*, August 8, 2005.

8. Ken Terry, "Disease Management: Continuous Health-Care Improvement," *Business & Health*, April 1995.

9. Ibid.

10. Ken Terry, "Where Disease Management Is Paying Off," *Medical Economics*, July 14, 1997.

11. Edward Wagner, "Promoting Effective Change in Provider Groups to Support Evidence-Based Clinical and Quality Improvement across a Wide Variety of Health Care Settings" (lecture, Epidemiology, Biostatistics and Clinical Research Methods summer session, 2004), http://improvingchroniccare.org/change/index.html.

12. Ken Terry, "Here's What's Coming—Like It or Not," *Medical Economics*, April 27, 1998.

13. Ibid.

14. William R. Gold and Peter Kongstvedt, "How Broadening DM's Focus Helped Shrink One Plan's Costs," *Managed Care*, November 2003.

15. Terry, "Here's What's Coming."

16. Ken Terry, "The Disease Management Boom: How Doctors Are Dealing with It," *Medical Economics*, April 27, 1998.

17. Matthew Weinstock, "Chronic Care: An Acute Problem," *Hospitals & Health Networks*, September 2004.

18. Department of Veterans Affairs, VA *Achievements in Diabetes Care*, Fact Sheet, January 2005.

19. ITAA, "Chronic Care Improvement," 3.
20. American College of Physicians, *Patient-Centered, Physician-Guided Care for the Chronically Ill: The American College of Physicians Prescription for Change* (Philadelphia: American College of Physicians, 2004), 6.
21. Ken Terry, "Do Disease Registries = $$ Rewards?" *Medical Economics*, November 4, 2005; Joel Hyatt (Kaiser Permanente), interview with the author, December 2005.
22. Ashley C. Short, Glen P. Mays, and Jessica Mittler, *Disease Management: A Leap of Faith to Lower-Cost, Higher-Quality Health Care*, Center for Studying Health System Change, Issue Brief no. 69, October 2003.
23. Frank Diamond, "Care Coordination Strikes Right Chord," *Managed Care*, May 2004.
24. Marc L. Berk and Alan C. Monheit, "The Concentration of Health Care Expenditures, Revisited," *Health Affairs*, March/April 2001, 9–18.
25. Jeff Tieman, "Coming of Age: Disease Management Making a Case for Itself Clinically and Financially," *Modern Healthcare*, July 9, 2001.
26. Maureen Glabman, "'Take My Word for It': The Enduring Dispute over Measuring DM's Economic Value," *Managed Care*, April 2006.
27. U.S. Congressional Budget Office, *An Analysis of the Literature on Disease Management Programs*, October 13, 2004.
28. Short, Mays, and Mittler, *Disease Management*.
29. Autumn Dawn Gilbreath, Richard A. Krasuski, Brad Smith, Karl C. Stajduhar, Michael D. Kwan, Robert Ellis, and Gregory L. Freeman, "Long-Term Healthcare and Cost Outcomes of Disease Management in a Large, Randomized, Community-Based Population with Heart Failure," *Circulation* 110 (2004): 3518–26.
30. Bruce Fireman, Joan Barlett, and Joe Selby, "Can Disease Management Reduce Health Care Costs by Improving Quality?" *Health Affairs*, November/December 2004, 63–75.
31. Finlay A. McAlister, Fiona M .E. Lawson, Koon K. Teo, and Paul W. Armstrong, "A Systematic Review of Randomized Trials of Disease Management Programs in Heart Failure," *American Journal of Medicine* 110 (2001): 378–84.
32. Stephen Heffler, Sheila Smith, Sean Keehan, Christine Borger, M. Kent Clemens, and Christopher Truffer, "U.S. Health Spending Projections for 2004–2014," *Health Affairs Web Exclusive*, February 23, 2005, 74–85.
33. Robert S. Galvin and Suzanne Delbanco, "Why Employers Need to Rethink How They Buy Health Care," *Health Affairs*, November/December 2005, 1549–58.
34. Kevin Knight, Enkhe Badamgarav, James M. Henning, Vic Hasselblad, Anacleto D. Gano Jr., Joshua J. Ofman, and Scott R. Weingarten, "A Systematic Review of Diabetes Disease Management Programs," *American Journal of Managed Care* 11 (2005): 242–50.

Chapter 4. Paying for Performance

1. MedVantage Inc., "Pay for Performance Programs for Providers Continue to Increase, Diversify in 2005," press release, November 17, 2005.
2. Laura B. Benko, "Blues Primed to Pay," *Modern Healthcare*, June 27, 2005.
3. Meredith B. Rosenthal, Bruce E. Landon, Sharon-Lise T. Normand, Richard G.

Frank, and Arnold M. Epstein, "Pay for Performance in Commercial HMOs," *New England Journal of Medicine* 355 (2006): 1895–1902.

4. Ken Terry, "Pay for Performance: How Fast Is It Spreading?" *Medical Economics*, November 4, 2005.

5. Center for Medicare and Medicaid Services, "Medicare Begins Performance-Based Payments for Physician Groups," press release, January 31, 2005.

6. CMS, "Medicare Adds Performance-Based Payments for Physicians," press release, October 13, 2006.

7. CMS, "Medicare Pay-for-Performance Demonstration Shows Significant Quality of Care Improvement at Participating Hospitals," press release, May 3, 2005.

8. Ken Terry, "Pay for Performance: A Double-Edged Sword," *Medical Economics*, January 21, 2005.

9. MedVantage, "Pay for Performance Programs."

10. Karen Davis quoted in Leapfrog Group, "Pay for Performance Improving Health Care Quality and Changing Provider Behavior, but Challenges Persist," press release, November 15, 2005.

11. Thomas Bodenheimer, Jessica H. May, Robert A. Berenson, and Jennifer Coughlan, *Can Money Buy Quality? Physician Response to Pay for Performance*, Center for Studying Health System Change, Issue Brief no. 102, December 2005.

12. Ken Terry, "Tackling Pay for Performance," *Medical Economics*, May 6, 2005.

13. Medicare Payment Advisory Commission, *Report to the Congress: Medicare Payment Policy*, March 2005, 1987.

14. Jane Anderson, "IOM: Phase in P4P Slowly; Evaluate Each Step," *Family Practice News*, October 15, 2006.

15. David Glendinning, "Medicare Pay-for-Performance Bill Omits Reimbursement Formula Fix," *American Medical News*, July 25, 2005; Kevin O'Relly, "Panel Sets Primary Care Standards for Medicare Pay-for-Performance," *American Medical News*, September 5, 2005.

16. Cinda Becker, "Right on the Money: CMS Awarding Pay-for-Performance Bonuses," *Modern Healthcare*, November 14, 2005.

17. William Jessee quoted in Terry, "Tackling Pay for Performance."

18. American College of Physicians, "Sweeping Recommendations to Support Pay-for-Performance System," press release, December 15, 2005.

19. Terry, "Tackling Pay for Performance."

20. Terry, "Score One for CMS," *Medical Economics*, June 16, 2006.

21. Ken Terry, "What's in the Box? Is United Healthcare Delivering on Its Promises?" *Medical Economics*, September 4, 2000.

22. Neil Chesanow, "Your Report Card Is About to Go Public," *Medical Economics*, April 12, 1999.

23. Ken Terry, "Better Quality Care, Bigger Paycheck," *Medical Economics*, September 9, 2002.

24. Integrated Healthcare Association, "P4P Program Announces First-Year Results: 'Estimated $50 Million Bonus Payout,'" press release, October 21, 2004.

25. Terry, "Pay for Performance: A Double-Edged Sword;" IHA, "Integrated Healthcare Association Announces New Efficiency Measure in Pay for Performance to Improve Healthcare Quality and Reduce Costs," press release, February 15, 2007.

26. IHA, "Integrated Healthcare Association Announces New Efficiency Measure in Pay for Performance to Improve Healthcare Quality and Reduce Costs."

27. François DeBrantes, national coordinator for BTE, interview with the author, December 2005.

28. Bridges to Excellence, "Physicians, Business, Government and Industry Embrace Common Industry to Improve Health Care: Pay-for-Performance," press release, March 28, 2005.

29. CareFirst Blue Cross Blue Shield, "CareFirst Blue Cross Blue Shield Selects Physicians for Pilot to Enhance Care Quality," press release, May 10, 2005.

30. Chesanow, "Your Report Card Is About to Go Public."

31. Ken Terry, "Physician Report Cards: Help, Ho-Hum, or Horror?" *Medical Economics*, July 21, 2006.

32. Jennifer Hicks Curtis, health services director, WellPoint (parent of Blue Cross of California), speech, Financial Research Associates' P4P Summit, Atlanta, January 23, 2006.

33. Terry, "Pay for Performance: A Double-Edged Sword."

34. Arnold M. Epstein, Thomas H. Lee, and Mary Beth Hamel, "Paying Physicians for High Quality Care," *New England Journal of Medicine* 350 (2004): 406–10.

35. MedVantage Inc., "Pay for Performance Programs for Providers."

36. Agency for Healthcare Quality and Research, "Recommended Starter Set: Clinical Performance Measures for Ambulatory Care," May 2005, www.ahrq.gov/qual/aqastart.htm.

37. Ken Terry, "A Reminder and a Measuring Stick," *Medical Economics*, November 18, 2005.

38. David Glendinning, "Medicare Launches Voluntary Quality Reporting System," *American Medical News*, November 14, 2005.

39. B. E. Landon, S. T. Normand, B. Blumenthal, and J. Daley, "Physician Clinical Performance Assessment: Prospects and Barriers," *Journal of the American Medical Association* 290 (2003): 1183–89; Epstein, Lee, and Hamel, "Paying Physicians for High-Quality Care."

40. Meredith B. Rosenthal, Rushika Fernandopulle, HyunSook Ryu Song, and Bruce Landon, "Paying for Quality: Providers' Incentives for Quality Improvement," *Health Affairs*, March/April 2004, 127–41.

41. Estimate of qualifying physicians' rewards comes from several sources, including ibid. Bangasser (interview, February 2005) said that the IHA plans had set a target of 5 percent but were paying about half of that, and other physicians have told me they're seeing P4P bonuses in the 5 percent range. Also, former IHA director Beau Carter (interview, February 2005) confirmed that most plans are paying less than 10 percent.

42. Bodenheimer et al., *Can Money Buy Quality?*

43. Andrew Siskind (former president of Bristol Park Medical Group, Irvine, CA), interview with the author, February 2005. At a Washington, DC, press conference on November 15, 2005, Carl Volpe, an executive of Wellpoint, parent company of Blue Cross of California, confirmed that Blue Cross's quality incentives had replaced its HMO utilization bonuses.

44. Thomas Bodenheimer, "Primary Care—Will It Survive?" *New England Journal of Medicine* 355 (2006): 861–64.

45. Howard Beckman, interview with the author, November 2004.

46. Laura Landro, "Booster Shot: To Get Doctors to Do Better, Health Plans Try Cash Bonuses," *Wall Street Journal*, September 17, 2004.

47. Integrated Healthcare Association, "California Pay-for-Performance Results Show Improvement in Healthcare Quality," press release, July 5, 2005.

48. Reed Abelson, "Medicare Says Bonuses Can Improve Hospital Care," *New York Times*, November 15, 2005; Abelson, "Bonus Pay by Medicare Lifts Quality," *New York Times*, January 25, 2007; Premier Inc., "Patient Lives Saved As Performance Continues to Improve in Groundbreaking CMS/Premier Pay-for-performance Project," press release, January 26, 2007.

49. Becker, "Right on the Money."

50. Response to a question from the author at a press conference conducted by Premier Inc. on January 26, 2007. Other hospital executives at the conference expressed similar views.

51. Meredith B. Rosenthal, Richard G. Frank, Zhonge Li, and Arnold M. Epstein, "Early Experience with Pay-for-Performance: From Concept to Practice," *Journal of the American Medical Association* 294 (2005): 1789–93.

52. Alice G. Gosfield, "PROMETHEUS Payment: Better for Patients, Better for Physicians," *Journal of Practice Management*, September/October 2006, 100–104. Other details in this section came from Prometheus' inaugural press conference, September 14, 2006, and its Web site (www.prometheuspayment. org).

53. "Results-Based Payment: Beyond Pay for Performance," *Group Practice Journal*, July–August 2005, 22.

54. Institute of Medicine, *Crossing the Quality Chasm: A New Health System for the 21st Century* (Washington, DC: National Academy Press, 2001), 5–6, 181–82.

55. Robert Galvin, "A Deficiency of Will and Ambition: A Conversation with Donald Berwick," *Health Affairs Web Exclusive*, January 12, 2005, 1–9.

Chapter 5. EHRs: Necessary but Not Sufficient

1. Michael O'Toole, quoted in Ken Terry, "A Reminder and a Measuring Stick," *Medical Economics*, November 18, 2005.

2. David Brailer, speech, Health Information Management and Systems Society conference, Dallas, February 17, 2005.

3. Peter Basch, editorial, "Electronic Health Records and the National Health Information Network: Affordable, Adoptable, and Ready for Prime Time?" *Annals of Internal Medicine* 143 (2005): 227–28.

4. "Status of Electronic Medical Record Implementation, 2007." *HIMSS* Leadership Survey: C10 Results Final Report, April 10, 2007, 20.

5. David Gans, John Kralewski, Terry Hammons, and Bryan Dowd, "Medical Groups' Adoption of Electronic Health Records and Information Systems," *Health Affairs*, September/October 2005, 1323–33.

6. Rainu Kaushal, David Blumenthal, Eric G. Poon, et al. "The Costs of a National Health Information Network," *Annals of Internal Medicine* 143 (2005): 165–73.

7. Gans et al., "Medical Groups' Adoption of Electronic Health Records."

8. Robert H. Miller, Christopher West, Tiffany Martin Brown, Ida Sim, and Chris Ganchoff, "The Value of Electronic Health Records in Solo or Small Group Practices," *Health Affairs*, September/October 2005, 1127–37.

9. David Brailer has cited this as "common industry knowledge," and other consultants agree, although they note that the definition of success varies.

10. Ken Terry, "Doctors and EHRs," *Medical Economics*, January 21, 2005.

11. Ibid.

12. Miller et al., "Value of Electronic Health Records."
13. Gans et al., "Medical Groups' Adoption of Electronic Health Records."
14. Ken Terry, "Pay for Performance: A Double-Edged Sword," *Medical Economics*, January 21, 2005.
15. David Brailer quoted in Terry, "EHRs: Where Are We Now?" *Medical Economics*, May 20, 2005.
16. Centers for Medicare and Medicaid Services, "New Regulations to Facilitate Adoption of Health Information Technology," press release, August 1, 2006.
17. Ken Terry, "EHRs: Will Relaxing Stark Bind You Tighter?" *Medical Economics*, February 3, 2006; Terry, "Can Your Hospital Help You Get an EHR?" *Medical Economics*, May 6, 2005.
18. "Medicare Program: Physician Referrals to Health Care Entities with Which They Have Financial Relationships; Exceptions for Certain Electronic Prescribing and Electronic Health Records Arrangements; Proposed Rule," *Federal Register*, October 11, 2005.
19. Terry, "Doctors and EHRs."
20. Ibid.
21. Ken Terry, "Do Disease Registries = $$ Rewards?" *Medical Economics*, November 4, 2005.
22. Robert H. Miller and Ida Sim, "Physicians' Use of Electronic Medical Records: Barriers and Solutions," *Health Affairs*, March/April 2004, 116–26.
23. Jeff Tieman, "Lurching into the Future: Bush Sets 2014 Goals for EMRs, Calls for Incentives," *Modern Healthcare*, May 3, 2004.
24. David Brailer quoted in Ken Terry, "EHRs: The Feds' Big Push," *Medical Economics*, August 20, 2004.
25. William Hersh, "Health Care Information Technology: Progress and Barriers," *Journal of the American Medical Association* 292 (2004): 2273–74.
26. Department of Health and Human Services, *HIT Report at a Glance*, Fact Sheet, July 21, 2004; also, David Brailer's speech at a Washington, D.C. conference to launch the government's health IT initiative on the same date.
27. Department of Health and Human Services, "HHS Awards Contracts to Develop National Health Information Network," press release, November 10, 2005.
28. Department of Health and Human Services, "American Health Information Community Approves First Set of Recommendations," press release, May 17, 2006.
29. Ken Terry, "Get Ready for the New World of Interoperable IT," *MX Magazine*, March/April 2005.
30. Agency for Healthcare Research and Quality, "AHRQ Awards Over $22.3 million in Health Information Technology Implementation Grants," press release, October 6, 2005.
31. Kaushal, Blumenthal, Poon, et al., "Costs of a National Health Information Network."
32. eHealth Initiative and Foundation, "Emerging Trends and Issues in Health Information Exchange," 2005, http://ccbh.ehealthinitiative.org/communities/register_download.mspx.
33. Ken Terry, "The Rocky Road to RHIOs," *Medical Economics*, February 17, 2006; Caroline Broder, "Funding Models Varied for Regional Health Information Organizations," *Healthcare IT News*, May 2, 2005.

34. Liesa Jenkins (executive director, Care Spark), interview with the author, December 2005.

35. Mickey Tripathi (president of Massachusetts e-Health Collaborative), interview with the author, December 2005.

36. Richard Hillestadt, James Bigelow, Anthony Bower, Federico Girosi, Robin Meili, Richard Scoville, and Roger Taylor, "Can Electronic Medical Systems Transform Health Care? Potential Health Benefits, Savings, and Costs," *Health Affairs*, September/October 2005, 1103–17.

37. Clifford Goodman, "Savings in Electronic Medical Record Systems? Do It for the Quality," *Health Affairs*, September/October 2005, 1124–26.

38. Jan Walker, Eric Pan, Douglas Johnston, Julia Adler-Milstein, David W. Bates, and Blackford Middleton, "The Value of Health Care Information Exchange and Interoperability," *Health Affairs Web Exclusive*, January 19, 2005, 10–18.

39. U.S. Government Accounting Office to Representative Jim Nussle, "Health and Human Services' Estimate of Health Care Cost Savings Resulting from the Use of Information Technology," February 16, 2005.

40. Laurence C. Baker, "Benefits of Interoperability: A Closer Look at the Estimates," *Health Affairs Web Exclusive*, January 19, 2005, 22–25.

41. Jaan Sidorov, "It Ain't Necessarily So: The Electronic Health Record and the Unlikely Prospect of Reducing Health Care Costs," *Health Affairs*, July/August 2006, 1079–85.

42. Kaushal, Blumenthal, Poon, et al., "Costs of a National Health Information Network."

43. James M. Walker, "Electronic Medical Records and Health Care Transformation," *Health Affairs*, September/October 2005, 1118–23.

44. Ken Terry, "Re-engineer Your Practice—Starting Today," *Medical Economics*, January 24, 2000.

45. Joseph E. Scherger, "Primary Care Needs a New Model of Office Practice," *British Medical Journal* 330 (2005): 358–59.

46. Joseph E. Scherger, "The End of the Beginning: The Redesign Imperative in Family Medicine," *Family Medicine* 37, no. 7 (2005): 513–16.

47. Ken Terry, "Monitor Patients Online?" *Medical Economics*, July 23, 2001.

48. Robert Lowes, "Phones Driving You Crazy? Try Clinical Messaging," *Medical Economics*, March 19, 2004. This article quotes an analyst saying that 9 percent of doctors e-mail their patients more than five times a week. Also, in Ken Terry, "Patient e-mail: A Growing Trend," *Medical Economics*, October 24, 2003, another expert reports that 10–12 percent of physicians e-mail with patients. Extrapolating from these estimates and adding a margin for growth, the figure probably lies between 10 and 15 percent today.

49. Lowes, "Phones Driving You Crazy?"

50. Ken Terry, "Access Fees: Worth the Risk? What to Charge?" *Medical Economics*, July 23, 2004.

51. Scherger, "End of the Beginning."

52. Ken Terry, "What's the Fallout If Patients Pay?" *Medical Economics*, March 7, 2003.

53. Robert Lowes, "Personal Health Records: What's the Status Now?" *Medical Economics*, February 17, 2006.

54. Ibid.

55. Matt Handley, speech at the Markle Foundation's PHR conference in Washington, DC, October 11, 2005.

56. Ken Terry, *Medical Economics InfoTech Bulletin*, November 24, 2006 (www.memag.com/memag/issue/issueDetail.jsp?id=10814), *InfoTech Bulletin*, December 22, 2006 (www.memag.com/memag/article/articleDetail.jsp?id=392617), and *InfoTech Bulletin*, February 9, 2007 (www.memag.com/memag/issue/issueDetail.jsp?id=11292).

57. Markle Foundation, *Attitudes of Americans Regarding Personal Health Records and Nationwide Electronic Health Information Exchange*, October 2005

58. Markle Foundation, *Americans Want Benefits of Personal Health Records*, June 5, 2003.

59. Markle Foundation, *Attitudes of Americans*.

60. Markle Foundation, *Americans Want Benefits*.

61. Paul C. Tang and David Lansky, "The Missing Link: Bridging the Patient-Provider Health Information Gap," *Health Affairs*, September/October 2005, 1290–95.

62. Senator Bill Frist, speech, Washington, DC, conference to launch the government's health information technology initiative, July 21, 2004.

Chapter 6. Can Consumers Direct Their Own Care?

1. John B. Coombs, James Hereford, and Paul C. LePore, "Listening to the Consumer: A Historical Review," in *Connecting with the New Healthcare Consumer: Defining Your Strategy*, edited by David B. Nash, Mary Pat Manfredi, Barbara Bozarth, and Susan Howell (New York: McGraw-Hill, 2000), 24.

2. Michael L. Millenson, *Demanding Medical Excellence: Doctors and Accountability in the Information Age* (Chicago: University of Chicago Press, 1997), 42, 150.

3. Coombs, Hereford, and LePore, "Listening to the Consumer," 24.

4. Berkeley Rice, "The New Rules on Informed Consent," *Medical Economics*, June 19, 2000.

5. Berkeley Rice, "How Outcomes Research Can Change Health Care," *Medical Economics*, October 11, 1993.

6. Melinda B. Buntin, Cheryl Damberg, Amelia Haviland, Nicole Lurie, Kanika Kapur, and M. Susan Marquis (RAND), *"Consumer Directed" Health Plans: Implications for Health Care Quality and Cost*, California Healthcare Foundation report, June 2005, 23.

7. Donald W. Kemper and Molly Mettler, *Information Therapy: Prescribed Information as a Reimbursable Medical Service* (Boise, ID: Healthwise, 2002), 19–22.

8. Steven Haimowitz, "The Self-Care Trend and the New Healthcare Marketplace," in Nash et al., *Connecting with the New Healthcare Consumer*, 77.

9. Sarah Loughran (Health Grades), and Ann Mond Johnson (Subimo), interviews with the author, August 2005.

10. Med-Vantage Inc., *Provider Pay-for-Performance Incentive Programs: 2004 National Study Results*, March 2005, 26; Beau Carter, a former Med-Vantage executive, told me the percentage of programs associated with report cards is now higher than 30 percent (interview, February 2005).

11. Ken Terry, "The Frog That Roared," *Medical Economics*, November 8, 2004.

12. U.S. Department of Health and Human Services, Centers for Medicare and Medicaid Services, Hospital Compare, www.hospitalcompare.hhs.gov.

13. J. Marvin Bentley, "Government Connections to the New Healthcare Consumer," in Nash et al., *Connecting with the New Healthcare Consumer*, 340.

14. Ibid., 339.

15. "Wisconsin Launches Hospital Quality-Comparison Web Site," *iHealthBeat*, April 12, 2005.

16. myHealthFinder.com Web site, www.myhealthfinder.com.

17. HealthGrades Web site, www.healthgrades.com.

18. Tony Fong, "Priceless," *Modern Healthcare*, March 28, 2005.

19. Centers for Medicare and Medicaid Services, *Helping Patients Get the Best Care for Their Needs*, Fact Sheet, June 1, 2006; Matthew DoBias, "CMS Gets Online Transparency: Payments to Docs, Hospitals Will Be Shown by County," *Modern Healthcare*, June 5, 2006.

20. David Glendinning, "Medicare Begins Posting Physician Price Information Online," *American Medical News*, December 18, 2006.

21. Lucette Lagnado, "California Hospitals Open Books, Showing Huge Price Differences," *Wall Street Journal*, December 27, 2004.

22. Fong, "Priceless."

23. April Fulton, "Health Pricing Transparency Proposal Sparks Hot Debate," *AHIP Coverage*, May/June 2006.

24. Minnesota Health Information Web site, www.minnesotahealthinfo.org.

25. "Aetna, United to Begin Rating Arizona Physicians," *Modernphysician.com*, August 4, 2005. Also, the two plans, which tier physicians, already have very basic scorecards on their Web sites (www.aetna.com and www.uhc.com/findaphysician. htm).

26. Ken Terry, "Physician Score Cards: Help, Ho-Hum, or Horror?" *Medical Economics*, July 21, 2006.

27. Aetna, "Enhanced Physician-Specific Cost and Quality Data Now," press release, August 21, 2006, www.aetna.com/news/2006/pr_20060821.htm.

28. CIGNA, "CIGNA Healthcare Posts More Cost and Quality Information Online," press release, September 20, 2006.

29. Ken Terry, "Here's What's Coming—Like It or Not," *Medical Economics*, April 27, 1998. Lawrence Casalino also told me a story about getting an HMO report card showing that fifty of his patients had not received required mammography or a Pap test. Of those patients, he discovered, forty-six had received the tests, and two of the patients were men.

30. J. B. Dimick, H. G. Welch, and J. D. Birkmeyer, "Surgical Mortality as an Indicator of Hospital Quality: The Problem with Small Sample Size," *Journal of the American Medical Association* 292 (2004): 847–51.

31. R. M. Werner and D. A. Asch, "The Unintended Consequences of Publicly Reporting Quality Information," *Journal of the American Medical Association* 293 (2005): 1239–44.

32. Ashish K. Jha, Zhonghe Li, John Orav, and Arnold E. Epstein, "Care in U.S. Hospitals—the Hospital Quality Alliance Program," *New England Journal of Medicine* 353 (2005): 265–74.

33. M. N. Marshall, P. G. Shekelle, S. Leatherman, and R. H. Brook, "The Public Release of Performance Data: What Do We Expect to Gain? A Review of the Evidence," *Journal of the American Medical Association* 283 (2000): 1866–74.

34. Neil Chesanow, "Your Report Card Is About to Go Public," *Medical Economics*, April 12, 1999.

35. Dale Shaller, Shoshanna Sofaer, Steven D. Findlay, Judith H. Hibbard, David

Lansky, and Suzanne Delbanco, "Consumers and Quality-Driven Health Care: A Call to Action," *Health Affairs*, March/April 2003, 95–101.

36. Ford Fessenden, "Quick, What Do You Give a Heart Attack Patient?" *New York Times*, August 28, 2005.

37. Judith H. Hibbard, Jean Stockard, and Martin Tusler, "Hospital Performance Reports: Impact on Quality, Market Share, and Reputation," *Health Affairs*, July/August 2005, 1150–60.

38. Ibid.

39. Kaiser Family Foundation, *National Survey on Consumers' Experiences with Patient Safety and Quality Information*, November 2004.

40. Thomas H. Lee and Kinga Zapert, "Do High-Deductible Health Plans Threaten Quality of Care?" *New England Journal of Medicine* 353 (2005): 1202–4.

41. Kevin B. O'Reilly, "More States Eye Reporting Infection Rates," *American Medical News*, April 16, 2007.

42. Mark Hochhauser, "Turning the Tables on Consumer-Driven Health Plans," *Managed Care Quarterly* 11, no. 4 (2003): 16–18.

43. Institute of Medicine, *Health Literacy: A Prescription to End Confusion* (Washington, DC: National Academy Press, 2004).

44. Molly Mettler, "The Healthwise Communities Project: Where Healthcare is Practiced by All," in Nash et al., *Connecting with the New Healthcare Consumer*, 378.

45. Jan Hoffman, "Awash in Information, Patients Face a Lonely, Uncertain Road," *New York Times*, August 14, 2005.

46. Solucient, *National Trends in Healthcare Consumerism: The Quality-Conscious Consumer*, September 2004.

47. Mark Hochhauser, "Reason AND Emotion in Health Care Decisions," *Managed Care Quarterly* 12, no. 2 (2004): 18–19.

48. Marcia Angell, *The Truth about the Drug Companies* (New York: Random House, 2004), 125.

49. "TV Ads for Drugs Help Boost Prescriptions, Researchers Say," *Los Angeles Times*, April 27, 2005.

50. John La Puma, "Examining Alternative Medicine: What Consumers Want from Physicians and What Physicians Should Tell Them," in Nash et al., *Connecting with the New Healthcare Consumer*," 494.

51. Ibid., 500.

52. Nortin M. Hadler, *The Last Well Person: How to Stay Well Despite the Health-Care System* (Montreal: McGill-Queen's University Press, 2004), 191.

53. La Puma, "Examining Alternative Medicine," 502.

54. National Center for Health Statistics, www.cdc.gov/nchs/fastats/smoking.htm.

Chapter 7. The Limits of Evidence

1. Centre for Evidence-Based Medicine, University of Toronto, "Glossary of EBM Terms," www.cebm.utoronto.ca/glossary/index.htm#e, quoted in David L. Sackett, Sharon E. Straus, W. Scott Richardson, and William Rosenberg, *Evidence-Based Medicine: How to Practice and Teach EBM*, 2nd ed. (Edinburgh: Churchill Livingstone, 2000), 1.

2. Earl P. Steinberg and Bryan R. Luce, "Evidence-based? Caveat Emptor," *Health Affairs*, January/February 2005, 80–92.

3. S. Hellman and D. S. Hellman, "Of Mice but Not Men: Problems of the Randomized Clinical Trial," *New England Journal of Medicine* 324 (1991): 1585–89.

4. Steinberg and Luce, "Evidence-based?"

5. Terrence M. Shaneyfelt, Michael F. Mayo-Smith, and Johann Rothwangl, "Are Guidelines Following Guidelines? The Methodological Quality of Clinical Practice Guidelines in the Peer-Reviewed Medical Literature," *Journal of the American Medical Association* 281 (1999): 1900–1905.

6. Institute of Medicine, *Crossing the Quality Chasm* (Washington, DC: National Academy Press, 2001), 145.

7. A. O. Berg, "Dimensions of Evidence," *Journal of the American Board of Family Practice* 11, no. 3 (May/June 1998): 216–23; Jay N. Cohn, Sidney O. Goldstein, Barry H. Greenberg, Beverly H. Lorell, Robert C. Bourge, Brian E. Jaski, Sidney O. Gottlieb, Frank McGrew, David L. DeMets, and Bill G. White, "A Dose-dependent Increase in Mortality with Vesnarinone among Patients with Severe Heart Failure," *New England Journal of Medicine* 339 (1998): 1810–16.

8. Cynthia M. Boyd, Jonathan Darer, Chad Boult, Linda P. Fried, Lisa Boult, and Albert W. Wu, "Clinical Practice Guidelines and Quality of Care for Older Patients with Multiple Comorbid Diseases," *Journal of the American Medical Association* 294 (2005): 716–24.

9. Newt Gingrich with Dana Pavey and Anne Woodbury, *Saving Lives and Saving Money: Transforming Health and Healthcare* (Washington, DC: Alexis de Tocqueville Institution, 2003), 57.

10. Michael L. Millenson, *Demanding Medical Excellence: Doctors and Accountability in the Information Age* (Chicago: University of Chicago Press, 1997), 123–25.

11. Alison Grann and Victor R. Grann, "The Case for Randomized Trials in Cancer Treatment: New Is Not Always Better," *Journal of the American Medical Association* 293 (2005): 1001–3.

12. Ricardo Guggenheim, "Putting EBM to Work (Easier Said Than Done)," *Managed Care*, December 2005.

13. M. H. Ebell and A. Shaughnessy, "Information Mastery: Integrating Continuing Medical Education with the Information Needs of Clinicians," *Journal of Continuing Education in the Health Professions* 23 Supp.11 (Spring 2003), S53.

14. Stefan Timmermans and Aaron Mauck, "The Promises and Pitfalls of Evidence-based Medicine," *Health Affairs*, January/February 2005, 18–28.

15. Brent James, "E-Health: Steps on the Road to Interoperability," *Health Affairs Web Exclusive*, January 19, 2005, 26–30.

16. Kaveh G. Shojania and Jeremy M. Grimshaw, "Evidence-based Quality Improvement: The State of the Science," *Health Affairs*, January/February 2005, 138–50.

17. J. Lomas, G. M. Anderson, K. Domnick-Pierre, E. Fayda, M. W. Enkin, and W. J. Hannah, "Do Practice Guidelines Guide Practice?" *New England Journal of Medicine* 321 (1989): 1307–10.

18. The ALLHAT Collaborative Research Group, "Major Outcomes in High-Risk Hypertensive Patients Randomized to Angiotension-Converting Enzyme Inhibitor or Calcium Channel Blocker vs. Diuretic," *Journal of the American Medical Association* 288 (2002): 2981–97.

19. Ken Terry, "Will Evidence-Based Medicine Change How You Practice?" *Medical Economics*, March 8, 1999.

20. James Goodwin, "Chaos, and the Limits of Modern Medicine," *Journal of the American Medical Association* 278 (1997): 1399–1400.

21. E. A. McGlynn, S. M. Asch, J. Adams, J. Keesey, J. Hicks, A. DeCristofaro, and E. Kerr, "The Quality of Health Care Delivered to Adults in the United States," *New England Journal of Medicine* 348 (2003): 2635–45.

22. National Quality Forum standards issued August 3, 2005, www.qualityforum.org/.

23. Ambulatory Care Quality Alliance, "Recommended Starter Set: Clinical Performance Measures for Ambulatory Care," www.ahrq.gov/qual/aqastart.htm.

24. "Medicare's Low-Quality Program," editorial, *American Medical News*, December 5, 2005.

25. David Glendinning, "Medicare Eases Quality Reporting, Warns of Annual Battles Over Pay," *American Medical News*, January 23, 2006; Terris King, deputy director, Office of Clinical Standards and Quality, "Pay for Performance: A Medicare Priority," speech at Pay for Performance Summit, Atlanta, January 23–24, 2006

26. *Joint House-Senate Working Agreement with the AMA*, signed December 16, 2005.

27. Ken Terry, "Score One for CMS," *Medical Economics*, June 16, 2006.

28. Janet Corrigan, interview with the author, May 2006.

29. Jennifer Lubell, "CMS Tries Cash This Time," *Modern Healthcare*, April 9, 2007.

30. Premier Inc., "Premier Inc. Releases Groundbreaking Evidence That Improving Patient Care Can Reduce Costs, Save Lives," press release, June 20, 2006.

Chapter 8. Supply-Induced Demand

1. Katherine Baicker and Amitabh Chandra, "Medicare Spending, the Physician Workforce, and Beneficiaries' Quality of Care," *Health Affairs Web Exclusive*, April 7, 2004, 184–97.

2. Barbara Starfield, Leiyu Shi, Atul Grover, and James Macinko, "The Effects of Specialist Supply on Populations' Health: Assessing the Evidence," *Health Affairs Web Exclusive*, March 15, 2005, 97–107.

3. Edward Salsberg, "The Need for Real Evidence in Physician Workforce Decision Making," *Health Affairs Web Exclusive*, March 15, 2005, 115–18.

4. E. S. Fisher, D. E. Wennberg, T. A. Stukel, D. J. Gottlieb, F. L. Lucas, and E. L. Pinder, "The Implications of Regional Variations in Medicare Spending: Part 1, The Content, Quality, and Accessibility of Care," *Annals of Internal Medicine* 138 (2003): 273–87.

5. E. S. Fisher, D. E. Wennberg, T. A. Stukel, D. J. Gottlieb, F. L. Lucas, and E. L. Pinder, "The Implications of Regional Variations in Medicare Spending: Part 2, Health Outcomes and Satisfaction with Care," *Annals of Internal Medicine* 138 (2003): 288–98.

6. Fisher et al., "Implications of Regional Variations in Medicare Spending: Part I," 286.

7. John E. Wennberg, Elliott S. Fisher, and Jonathan S. Skinner, "Geography and the Debate over Medicare Reform," *Health Affairs Web Exclusive*, February 13, 2002, 96–114; Victor R. Fuchs, "Floridian Exceptionalism," *Health Affairs Web Exclusive*, August 13, 2003, 357–75.

8. J. E. Wennberg and M. M. Cooper, eds., *The Dartmouth Atlas of Health Care 1998* (Chicago: American Hospital Association Press, 1999), 132.

9. J. E. Wennberg, J. L. Freeman, R. M. Shelton, and T. A. Bubolz, "Hospital Use and Mortality among Medicare Beneficiaries in Boston and New Haven," *New England Journal of Medicine* 321 (1989): 1168–73.

10. Wennberg quoted in Ken Terry, "Why Treatment Varies So Greatly," *Medical Economics*, February 10, 1997, 40–56.

11. R. H. Brook, C. J. Kamberg, A. Mayer-Oakes, M. H. Beers, K. Raube, and A. Steiner, *Appropriateness of Acute Medical Care for the Elderly: An Analysis of the Literature*, RAND Publication Series, September 1989.

12. M. R. Chassin, J. Kosecoff, R. E. Park, C. M. Winslow, K. L. Kahn, N. J. Merrick, J. Keesey, A. Fink, D. H. Solomon, and R. H. Brook, "Does Inappropriate Use Explain Geographic Variations in the Use of Health Care Services?" *Journal of the American Medical Association* 258 (1987): 2533–37.

13. T. A. Stukel, F. L. Lucas, and D. E. Wennberg, "Long-term Outcomes of Regional Variations in Intensity of Invasive vs. Medical Management of Medicare Patients with Acute Myocardial Infarction," *Journal of the American Medical Association* 293 (2005): 1329–37.

14. J. N. Weinstein, K. K. Bronner, T. S. Morgan, and J. E. Wennberg, "Trends and Geographic Variations in Major Surgery for Degenerative Diseases of the Hip, Knee, and Spine," *Health Affairs Web Exclusive*, October 7, 2004, 81–89.

15. B. H. Gray, M. K. Gusmano, and S. R. Collins, "AHCPR and the Changing Politics of Health Services Research," *Health Affairs Web Exclusive*, June 25, 2003, 283–307.

16. J. E. Wennberg, "The More Things Change . . . : The Federal Government's Role in the Evaluative Sciences," *Health Affairs Web Exclusive*, June 25, 2003, 308–10.

17. Richard Peto quoted in Christopher Anderson, "Measuring What Works in Health Care," *Science*, February 25, 1994, 1080–81.

18. Gray, Gusmano, and Collins, "AHCPR and the Changing Politics of Health Services Research."

19. Michael L. Millenson, *Demanding Medical Excellence* (Chicago: University of Chicago Press, 1997), 366.

20. See Agency for Healthcare and Research Quality Web site, http://effective-healthcare.ahrq.gov/aboutUs/index.cfm.

21. Karen Migdail (AHRQ communications office), interview with the author, April 2005.

22. "Outcomes/Effectiveness Research: Being Overweight or Underweight Does Not Preclude Elective Noncardiac Surgery for Most Patients," *Research Activities*, no. 207, August 1997, www.ahrq.gov/research/aug97/ra2.htm#head10.

23. Wennberg quoted in Berkeley Rice, "How Outcomes Research Can Change Health Care," *Medical Economics*, October 11, 1993.

24. Ron Winslow, "Videos, Questionnaires Aim to Expand Role of Patients in Treatment Decisions," *Wall Street Journal*, February 25, 1992.

25. Wennberg quoted in Rice, "Outcomes Research."

26. See Foundation for Informed Medical Decision Making Web site, www.fimdm.org/decision_sdms.php.

27. A. M. O'Connor, H. A. Llewellyn-Thomas, and A. B. Flood, "Modifying Unwarranted Variations in Health Care: Shared Decision Making Using Patient Decision Aids," *Health Affairs Web Exclusive*, October 7, 2004, 63–72.

28. John Billings, "Promoting the Dissemination of Decision Aids: An Odyssey in

a Dysfunctional Health Care Financing System," *Health Affairs Web Exclusive*, October 7, 2004, 128–32.

29. O'Conner, Llewellyn-Thomas, and Flood, "Modifying Unwarranted Variations in Health Care."

30. Billings, "Dissemination of Decision Aids."

31. Cynthia Smith, Cathy Cowan, Stephen Heffler, Aaron Catlin, and the National Health Accounts Team, "National Health Spending in 2004: Recent Slowdown Led by Prescription Drug Spending," *Health Affairs*, January/February 2006, 186–96.

Chapter 9. Physicians Go for the Gold

1. Maureen Glabman, "Health Plans Strain to Contain Rapidly Rising Cost of Imaging," *Managed Care*, January 2005.

2. Medicare Payment Advisory Commission (MedPAC), "Issues in Physician Payment Policy," chap. 3 of *Report to the Congress: Medicare Payment Policy*, March 2005, 154.

3. Glabman, "Health Plans."

4. MedPAC, "Issues," 155.

5. Glabman, "Health Plans"; Barbara M. Rothenberg, "Medical Technology as a Driver of Healthcare Costs: Diagnostic Imaging," Blue Cross and Blue Shield Association (BCBSA), October 14, 2003, 2.

6. That MRIs have been used for persistent headaches comes from my conversations with physicians and imaging benefit managers.

7. Kevin B. O'Reilly, "Tests Often Ordered When Not Needed," *American Medical News*, June 19, 2006.

8. Glabman, "Health Plans."

9. According to Katherine Vogt, in "Image Conscious," *American Medical News*, May 17, 2004, the American College of Radiology estimated in 2003 that its members performed 200 million imaging procedures, which represented 70 percent of imaging tests done by radiologists. Using several sources, Glabman ("Health Plans") estimated that 543 million imaging tests were done in 2003. So it appears that radiologists performed about half of these studies. Not all of the rest, however, were done by other kinds of doctors in their offices or facilities; mobile screening, for example, has been gaining in popularity.

10. Vogt, "Image Conscious."

11. Glabman, "Health Plans."

12. BCBSA, "Medical Technology."

13. Christine Gorman and Alice Park, "How New Heart-Scanning Technology Could Save Your Life," *Time*, September 5, 2005.

14. Liz Kowalczyk, "New CT Scanners Offer Faster Diagnoses," *Boston Globe*, April 30, 2006.

15. Lawrence P. Casalino, Hoangmai Pham, and Gloria Bazzoli, "Growth of Single-Specialty Medical Groups," *Health Affairs*, March/April 2004, 82–90.

16. Vogt, "Image Conscious," and my own research.

17. Ken Terry, "The Best Way to Divide Income," *Medical Economics*, April 9, 2004.

18. Marcy Tolkoff, "Exclusive Earnings Survey: How Are You Doing?" *Medical Economics*, October 20, 2006.

19. Glabman, "Health Plans."

20. MedPAC, "Issues," 167.

21. Ibid., 169.

22. BCBSA, "Medical Technology," 6.

23. MedPAC, "Issues," 155.

24. Susan J. Mertes, "The Battle over Imaging: Overutilized or Medically Appropriate and Cost-Effective?" *Group Practice Journal*, June 2005.

25. Kowalczyk, "New CT Scanners Offer Faster Diagnoses."

26. BCBSA "Medical Technology,"2.

27. MedPAC, "Issues," 155. This research is apparently related to the published study, E. S. Fisher, D. E. Wennberg, T. A. Stukel, D. J. Gottlieb, F. L. Lucas, and E. L. Pinder, "The Implications of Regional Variations in Medicare Spending: Part 2, Health Outcomes and Satisfaction with Care," *Annals of Internal Medicine* 138 (2003): 288–98.

28. Glabman, "Health Plans."

29. MedPAC, "Issues," 157.

30. David Glendinning, "CMS Plans to Cut Billions from Medicare Imaging Payments," *American Medical News*, February 27, 2006.

31. MedPAC, "Ambulatory Surgical Center Services," section 3F in *Report to the Congress: Medicare Payment Policy*, March 2004, 188.

32. Craig Jeffries (president of the American Association of Ambulatory Surgery Centers [AAASC]), interview with the author, May 2005.

33. MedPAC, "Ambulatory Surgical Center Services," 190.

34. Ibid., 189.

35. Ibid., 188.

36. Ibid., 189.

37. AAASC, *ASC Physician Ownership and Referral*, Fact Sheet, n.d.

38. MedPAC, "Ambulatory Surgical Center Services," 194.

39. AAASC, "CMS Releases Payment Rates under the Hospital Outpatient Prospective System," press release.

40. MedPAC, "Ambulatory Surgical Center Services," 186.

41. Center for Medicare and Medicaid Services, "CMS Proposes Changes to Policies and Payment for Outpatient Services," press release, August 8, 2006.

42. Reed Abelson, "Hospitals Battle For-Profit Groups for Patients," *New York Times*, October 30, 2002; Mark Taylor, "Physician-owned Enterprises Face Legal Woes," *Modern Healthcare*, August 9, 20; 04.

43. Richard Haugh, "Are You Looking for a Fresh Start with Your MDs?" *Hospitals & Health Networks*, May 2005.

44. Hoangmai H. Pham, Kelly J. Devers, Jessica H. May, and Robert Berenson. "Financial Pressures Spur Physician Entrepreneurism," *Health Affairs*, March/April 2004, 70–81.

45. Myrle Croasdale, "More Physicians Expect Pay for Emergency Call," *American Medical News*, June 6, 2005.

46. American Hospital Association, *Taking the Pulse: The State of America's Hospitals*, 2005, 4.

47. MedPAC, *Report to the Congress: Physician-Owned Specialty Hospitals*, March 2005, 29–32.

48. John K. Iglehart, "The Emergence of Physician-Owned Specialty Hospitals," *New England Journal of Medicine* 352 (2005): 78–84.

49. Leslie Greenwald, Jerry Cromwell, Walter Adamache, Shulamit Bernard,

Edward Drozd, Elisabeth Root, and Kelly Devers, "Specialty Versus Community Hospitals: Referrals, Quality and Community Benefits," *Health Affairs*, January/February 2006, 106–18.

50. David Glendinning, "Lawmakers Weigh Future of Specialty Hospital Referral Ban," *American Medical News*, March 28, 2005.

51. Joel B. Finkelstein, "New Specialty Hospitals on Hold for Now," *American Medical News*, June 6, 2005; CMS, *Payment Provisions in the Traditional Medicare Program That May Be Delayed by the Deficit Reduction Act*, Fact Sheet, January 3, 2006; "Should Doctors Own Hospitals?" *BusinessWeek Online*, February 20, 2006.

52. CMS, "Medicare Issues Final Report to Congress Implementing Strategic Plan for Specialty Hospitals," press release, August 8, 2006.

53. CMS, *Study of Physician-Owned Specialty Hospitals*, Executive Summary, 2005, ii.

54. MedPAC, *Physician-Owned Specialty Hospitals*, 25; U.S. Government Accountability Office to Sens. Charles Grassley and Max Baucus, "Specialty Hospitals: Information on Potential New Facilities," May 19, 2005, 3.

55. Iglehart, "Emergence of Physician-Owned Specialty Hospitals."

56. Aaron Katz, Robert E. Hurley, Kelly Devers, Leslie Jackson Conwell, Bradley C. Strunk, Andrea Staiti, J. Lee Hargraves, and Robert A. Berenson, *Competition Revs Up the Indianapolis Health Care Market*, Center for Studying Health System Change, Community Report no. 1, Winter 2003.

57. Glenn Mays, Laurie E. Felland, Kelly L. McKenzie, Hoangmai H. Pham, and Lydia E. Regopoulos, *Continued Hospital Expansions Raise Cost Concerns in Indianapolis*, Center for Studying Health System Change, Community Report no. 2, June 2005.

58. *The 2005 World Almanac and Book of Facts* (New York: World Almanac Books, 2005).

59. Mays et al., "Continued Hospital Expansions."

60. American Medical Association, "Competition from Specialty Hospitals Promotes High-quality Patient Care," press release, May 24, 2005.

61. CMS, "Study of Physician-Owned Specialty Hospitals," 40–50.

62. E. L. Hannan, J. F. O'Donnell, H. Kilburn Jr., H. R. Bernard, and A. Yazici, "Investigation of the Relationship between Volume and Mortality for Surgical Procedures Performed in New York State Hospitals," *Journal of the American Medical Association* 262 (1989): 503–10.

63. CMS, "Study of Physician-Owned Specialty Hospitals," 49.

64. Chip Kahn, "Give Specialty Hospitals the Hook," *Modern Healthcare*, February 28, 2005.

65. Gail Garfinkel Weiss, "Need a New Source of Revenue? Try Ancillary Services," *Medical Economics*, November 4, 2005.

66. Medical Group Management Association (MGMA), "Orthopedic Group Practices May Have Hit a Plateau, MGMA Report Indicates," press release, November 30, 2005.

Chapter 10. Hospitals Flex Their Muscles

1. American Hospital Association (AHA), *U.S. Registered Community Hospitals: Overview 1999–2003*, Table 3, AHA Hospital Statistics, 2005, 10.

2. Melanie Evans, "Will It Last? Hospital Profits Hit an All-time High in 2004," *Modern Healthcare*, November 7, 2005.

3. Cynthia Smith, Cathy Cowan, Stephen Heffler, Aaron Catlin, and the National Health Accounts Team, "National Health Spending in 2004: Recent Slowdown Led by Prescription Drug Spending," *Health Affairs*, January/February 2006, 186–96.

4. Stephen Heffler, Sheila Smith, Sean Keehan, Christine Borger, M. Kent Clements, and Christopher Truffer, "U.S. Health Spending Projections for 2004–2014," *Health Affairs Web Exclusive*, February 23, 2005, 74–85.

5. Smith et al., "National Health Spending in 2004"; John L. Ashby Jr. and Craig K. Lisk, "Why Do Hospital Costs Continue to Increase?" *Health Affairs*, Summer 1992, 134–47.

6. Reed Abelson, "After a Pause in Merger Activity, Hospitals Are Again Joining Forces," *New York Times*, September 15, 2004.

7. Bernard Wysocki Jr., "FTC Targets Hospital Merger in Antitrust Case," *Wall Street Journal*, January 17, 2005.

8. Ibid.

9. Mark Taylor, "Changing the Balance," *Modern Healthcare*, October 24, 2005.

10. Mary Chris Jaklevic, "What Hospitals 'See' They Get," *Modern Healthcare*, March 6, 2000.

11. Mark Taylor, "Spitzer Probes Alleged Price-Fixing by N.Y. Network," *Modern Healthcare*, December 20–27, 2004.

12. Wysocki, "FTC Targets Hospital Merger."

13. Alison Evans Cuellar and Paul J. Gertler, "How the Expansion of Hospital Systems Has Affected Consumers," *Health Affairs*, January/February 2005, 213–19.

14. Maureen Sullivan quoted in "California Hospital Costs among Fastest Rising in Nation," *BCBS Health Issues*, November 13, 2002.

15. Dave Carpenter, "A Good Old-Fashioned Building Boom," *Hospitals & Health Networks*, March 2004.

16. Dave Carpenter, "The Boom Goes On," *Hospitals & Health Networks*, March 2006.

17. Carpenter, "Good Old-Fashioned Building Boom."

18. Carpenter, "Boom Goes On."

19. Don Babwin, "Building Boom," *Hospitals & Health Networks*, March 2002.

20. Gloria J. Bazzoli, Linda R. Brewster, Gigi Liu, and Sylvia Kuo, "Does U.S. Hospital Capacity Have to Be Expanded?" *Health Affairs*, November/December 2003.

21. Mark Pauly (health economist at the Wharton School), interview with the author, June 2005.

22. Stuart H. Altman, "More Beds for Boomers," *Modern Healthcare*, March 8, 2004.

23. David Shactman, Stuart H. Altman, Efrat Eilat, Kenneth E. Thorpe, and Michael Doonan, "The Outlook for Hospital Spending: Rapid Growth Is Likely to Persist," *Health Affairs*, November/December 2003, 12–26.

24. Bazzoli et al., "Does U.S. Hospital Capacity Have to Be Expanded?"

25. Melanie Evans, "Reaping Rewards: Increased Recruitment, Better Wages Start to Pay Off," *Modern Healthcare*, November 22, 2004; Lillee Gelinas and Chuck Bohlen, *Tomorrow's Work Force: A Strategic Approach*, VHA Research Series, 2002, 4.

26. Melanie Evans, "Coming Up Short: Shortages of Space, Beds, Staff Cause Capacity Crunch," *Modern Healthcare*, October 18, 2004.
27. Evans, "Reaping Rewards."
28. Transcript of New Jersey State Health Planning Board hearing, Orange, NJ, January 7, 2004.
29. Unless otherwise indicated, the material on the closing of the Hospital Center at Orange is from Ken Terry, "Portrait of a Failure," *Medical Economics*, June 3, 2005.
30. *State Staff Report and Recommendations to the State Health Planning Board: Certificate of Need Project Summary on Hospital Center at Orange*, Orange, NJ, January 2004.
31. Letter from Marilyn Dahl, senior assistant commissioner, New Jersey Department of Health and Senior Services, to Mark Chastang, administrator of the Hospital Center at Orange, May 15, 2002.
32. *Certificate of Need Project Summary*.
33. AHA, *U.S. Registered Community Hospitals*.
34. AHA, "State-by-State Analysis Highlights Hospitals' Impact on Communities," press release, May 3, 2004.
35. Lisa W. Foderaro, "Rapidly Shrinking Buffalo Is Left with Half-Empty Hospitals," *New York Times*, April 25, 2005.
36. Richard Perez-Pena, "Hospital Business in New York, Once Prized, Braces for a Crisis," *New York Times*, April 11, 2005.
37. Perez-Pena, "Plan Shows Broad Array of Cuts to Hospitals Statewide," *New York Times*, November 29, 2005.
38. Perez-Pena, "State to Get $1.5 Billion From U.S. to Aid in Hospital Trims," *New York Times*, October 3, 2006.
39. Perez-Pena, "Pataki and Spitzer Back Downsizing of Hospitals," *New York Times*, November 30, 2006.
40. George C. Halvorson, *Strong Medicine* (New York: Random House, 1993), 61–76.

Chapter 11. Why Do Drugs Cost So Much?

1. Bill Berkrot, "Prescription Sleep Aid Use Soaring in US: Study," *Reuters*, October 17, 2005.
2. Michelle Rogers, "Pipeline Promises," *HealthLeaders*, May 2005.
3. Mark Hagland, "Viagra or Bust: Is Pharmacy Cost Crisis Unraveling HMO Utilization Strategy?" *Medicine & Health*, July 13, 1998.
4. Stuart Elliott and Nat Ives, "Selling Prescription Drugs to the Consumer," *New York Times*, October 12, 2004.
5. IMS Health, "IMS Reports Rx Sales Growth Matches All-Time Record," press release, March 31, 1998; IMS Health, "IMS Health Reports 5.4 Percent Dollar Growth in 2005 U.S. Prescription Sales," press release, February 22, 2006.
6. Gardiner Harris, "Drug Makers Seek to Mend Their Fractured Image," *New York Times*, July 8, 2004.
7. Milt Freudenheim, "Drug Prices Up Sharply This Year," *New York Times*, June 21, 2006.
8. Neil Turner, "Pricing Climate Heats Up in U.S. and Europe," *Pharmaceutical*

Executive, July 2004; Jerry Avorn, *Powerful Medicines: The Benefits, Risks, and Costs of Prescription Drugs* (New York: Vintage Books, 2005), 220.

9. IMS Health, "Pricing & Reimbursement Review 2004: Assessing the Impact of Events Affecting Pharmaceutical Markets," July 15, 2005, 12.

10. Robert Pear, "17% Rise in Drug Costs Hit Elderly Hardest, Study Says," *New York Times*, June 27, 2000.

11. Kenneth E. Thorpe, Curtis S. Florence, David H. Howard, and Peter Joski, "The Rising Prevalence of Treated Disease: Effects on Private Health Insurance Spending," *Health Affairs Web Exclusive*, June 27, 2005, 317–25.

12. Aaron Catlin, Cathy Cowan, Stephen Heffler, Benjamin Washington, and the National Health Expenditures Accounts Team, "National Health Spending in 2005: The Slowdown Continues," *Health Affairs*, January/February 2007, 142–51.

13. Gardiner Harris, "Drug Makers Seek to Mend Their Fractured Image," *New York Times*, July 8, 2004.

14. See Pharmaceutical Research and Manufacturers of America (PhRMA) Web site, www.phrma.org/innovation.

15. Ibid., "Reporter's Handbook," citing J. A. DiMasi, R. W. Hansen, and H. G. Grabowski, "The Price of Innovation: New Estimates of Drug Development Costs," *Journal of Health Economics* 22, no. 2 (2003): 151–85.

16. Marcia Angell, *The Truth about the Drug Companies: How They Deceive Us and What to Do About It* (New York: Random House, 2004), 43.

17. Ibid., 48.

18. Avorn, *Powerful Medicines*, 206–7.

19. *PhRMA Annual Membership Survey*, 2005, table 2, www.phrma.org/.

20. Angell, *Truth about the Drug Companies*, 80–81, 90–91. Also, a program that twelve states launched to study the comparative effectiveness of drugs has found no major differences within fifteen therapeutic classes. See Robert Pear and James Dao, "States Trying New Tactics to Reduce Spending on Drugs," *New York Times*, November 21, 2004.

21. Angell, *Truth about the Drug Companies*, 75.

22. Avorn, *Powerful Medicine*, 204, mentions a study funded by the Blue Cross and Blue Shield Association.

23. Hamilton Moses III, E. Ray Dorsey, David H. M. Matheson, and Samuel O. Thier, "Financial Anatomy of Biomedical Research," *Journal of the American Medical Association* 294 (2005): 1333–42.

24. Angell, *Truth about the Drug Companies*, 65.

25. Angell, *Truth about the Drug Companies*, 7, 67–68.

26. Ibid., 69–70.

27. Avorn, *Powerful Medicine*, 200.

28. Ibid., 203.

29. John Abramson, *Overdosed America: The Broken Promise of American Medicine*. (New York, HarperCollins, 2004), 95; Angell, *Truth about the Drug Companies*, 30.

30. PhRMA, *Pharmaceutical Industry Profile 2005*, 2–3.

31. Abramson, *Overdosed America*, 94–95.

32. F. Davidoff, C. D. DeAngelis, J. M. Drazen, et al., "Sponsorship, Authorship, and Accountability," *Journal of the American Medical Association* 286 (2001): 1232–34.

33. Ron Winslow, Sylvia Pagan Westphal, and Heather Won Tesoriero, "Medical

Journal Says Merck Study Left Out Data," *Wall Street Journal*, December 9, 2005.

34. Gardiner Harris, "FDA Announces Strong Warnings for Painkillers," *New York Times*, April 8, 2005.

35. Avorn, *Powerful Medicines*, 71–84, 85–95; Gardiner Harris and Eric Koli, "Lucrative Drug, Danger Signals and the FDA," *New York Times*, June 10, 2005.

36. Alison Young and Chris Adams, "'Off-Label' Drugs Take Their Toll," *Miami Herald*, November 2, 2003.

37. David C. Radley, Stan N. Finkelstein, and Randall S. Stafford, "Off-label Prescribing among Office-Based Physicians," *Archives of Internal Medicine*, 166 (2006): 1021–26.

38. Daren Fonda and Barbara Kiviat, "Curbing the Drug Marketers," *Time*, July 5, 2004.

39. Gardiner Harris, "F.D.A. Failing in Drug Safety, Official Asserts," *New York Times*, November 19, 2004. Also, Robert Langreth, "Trouble Breathing," Forbes.com, April 6, 2006; and Jamie Stengle, AP, "Study Contradicts FDA on Crestor Risks," Yahoo News, May 24, 2005.

40. Barbara Martinez, Anna Wilde Mathews, Joann S. Lublin, and Ron Winslow, "Merck Pulls Vioxx from Market after Link to Heart Problems," *Wall Street Journal*, October 4, 2004.

41. Stephen Langel, "Waxman Report Places FDA Enforcement under Microscope," *Drug Industry Daily Online*, June 27, 2006.

42. Stephen Langel, "Scientists Depict a Broken FDA, Plan PDUFA as a Vehicle for Change," *Drug Industry Daily Online*, July 21, 2006.

43. Angell, *Truth about the Drug Companies*, 208; Abramson, *Overdosed America*, 85.

44. Peter Lurie, Christine M. Almeida, Nicholas Stine, Alexander R. Stine, and Sidney M. Wolfe, "Financial Conflict of Interest Disclosure and Voting Patterns at Food and Drug Administration Drug Advisory Committee Meetings," *Journal of the American Medical Association* 295 (2006): 1921–28.

45. Gardiner Harris, "F.D.A. Rule Limits Role of Advisors Tied to Industry," *New York Times*, March 22, 2007.

46. Angell, *Truth about the Drug Companies*, 209; Abramson, *Overdosed America*, 85–86.

47. Gardiner Harris, "New Drugs Hit The Market, but Promised Trials Go Undone," *New York Times*, March 4, 2006.

48. Angell, *Truth about the Drug Companies*, 29–30.

49. Stephen Langel, "Changes to FDA Postmarket Policies Unlikely Despite Critical Report," *Drug Industry Daily Online*, July 11, 2006.

50. Rich Tomaselli, "Code Red for Direct-to-Consumer Advertising," *Advertising Age*, January 6, 2005.

51. "Advertising; Drug Makers Scramble to Respond to Ad Curbs," *Media & Marketing*, July 6, 2005.

52. American Medical Association, "AMA Calls for Temporary Moratorium on Direct-to-Consumer Advertising of New Prescription Drugs," press release, June 14, 2006.

53. Anna Wilde Mathews, "FDA to Review Drug Marketing to Consumers," *Wall Street Journal*, August 2, 2005.

54. Julie Schmit, "Drug Ad Guidelines Hold a Few Surprises," *USA Today*, August 3, 2005.

55. Thomas Ginsberg, "Drug Ads Pour in for Review," *Philadelphia Inquirer*, February 23, 2006.

56. Troyen A. Brennan, David J. Rothman, Linda Blank, et al., "Health Industry Practices That Create Conflicts of Interest: A Policy Proposal for Academic Medical Centers," *Journal of the American Medical Association* 295 (2006): 429–33.

57. David Blumenthal, "Doctors and Drug Companies," *New England Journal of Medicine* 351 (2004): 1885–90.

58. Ibid.; Angell, *Truth about the Drug Companies*, 126–30.

59. Abramson, *Overdosed America*, 125.

60. Blumenthal, "Doctors and Drug Companies."

61. Angell, *Truth about the Drug Companies*, 141.

62. Abramson, *Overdosed America*, 118–21.

63. Avorn, *Powerful Medicine*, 298–99.

64. Brennan, Rothman, Blank, et al., "Health Industry Practices."

65. Michael Romano, "Fighting Graft—It's Academic," *Modern Healthcare*, January 30, 2006.

66. Andrew Pollack, "Stanford to Ban Drug Makers' Gifts to Doctors, Even Pens," *New York Times*, September 12, 2006.

67. Angell, *Truth about the Drug Companies*, 76; Stuart Elliott and Nat Ives, "Selling Prescription Drugs to the Consumer," *New York Times*, October 12, 2004.

68. Federal Drug Administration, "FDA Approves Prilosec OTC to Treat Frequent Heartburn," press release, June 20, 2003.

69. Diedra Henderson, "Dose of Relief: Are Generic Drugs Just What the Cost-cutters Ordered?" *Boston Globe*, April 30, 2006.

70. Benedict Carey, "Study Finds Little Advantage in New Schizophrenia Drugs," *New York Times*, September 20, 2005.

71. Alex Berenson, "Big Drug Makers See Sales Erode With Their Image," *New York Times*, November 14, 2005.

72. Emily Cox, Andy Behm, and Doug Mager, *2005 Generic Drug Usage Report*, Express Scripts Research Study Findings, www.express-scripts.com/ourcompany/news/outcomesresearch/onlinepublications/study/genericDrugUsageReport2005.pdf.

73. Dar Haddix, "Wall Street Analysis Shows Unexpected Growth in Statin Market," *Drug Industry Daily*, September 27, 2006.

74. Wal-Mart, "Wal-Mart Cuts Prescription Medicines to $4," press release, September 21, 2006.

75. Amy Barrett, Michael Arndt, and Arlene Weintraub, "Prescription for Upheaval: How the Medicare Drug Program Is Tightening the Screws on Big Pharma," *BusinessWeek*, October 17, 2005.

76. Letter from Congressional Budget Office director Douglas Holtz-Eakin to Representative Joe Barton (R-TX), March 4, 2005.

77. Christine Borger, Sheila Smith, Christopher Truffer, Sean Keehan, Andrea Sisko, John Poisal, and M. Kent Clemens, "Health Spending Projections through 2015: Changes on the Horizon," *Health Affairs Web Exclusive*, February 22, 2006, 61–73.

78. Paul Davies, "Medicare Drug Plan: Which Big Pharma Wins?" *Wall Street Journal*, October 11, 2005.

79. Freudenheim, "Drug Prices Up Sharply This Year."

80. Alex Berenson, "Pfizer and Other Drug Makers Report Higher Profits," *New York Times*, October 20, 2006.
81. Robin Toner, "Rival Visions Led to Rocky Start for Drug Benefit," *New York Times*, February 6, 2006.
82. Howard Gleckman, "Plan A: Hook Them with Part D," *Business Week*, January 30, 2006.
83. Toner, "Rival Visions."
84. Robert Pear, "Rules of Medicare Drug Plans Slow Access to Benefits," *New York Times*, February 14, 2006.
85. Centers for Medicare and Medicaid Services, *Total Medicare Beneficiaries with Drug Coverage*, Fact Sheet, June 11, 2005.
86. Richard Wolf, "Drug Plan's Bottom Lines Emerging," *USA Today*, May 23, 2006; editorial, "The Drug Benefit: A Report Card," *New York Times*, June 5, 2006. Wolf's article shows that a majority of beneficiaries were saving money, but a New York Times/CBS News poll in May 2006 found that only 42 percent were, and that 19 percent were spending more than before.
87. Howard Gleckman, "Medicare Surprise: Why Many Seniors Could Temporarily Lose Drug Coverage," *BusinessWeek*, May 1, 2006; Wolters Kluwer Health, "Medicare Part D 'Doughnut Hole' Spurs Seniors to Drop Meds," press release, September 21, 2006.
88. Families USA, *Coverage Through the "Doughnut Hole" Grows Scarcer in 2007*, November 2006.
89. Borger et al., "Health Spending Projections."
90. U.S. House of Representatives Committee on Government Reform, Minority Staff Special Investigations Division, *Medicare Drug Plan Prices Are Higher Than Medicare Drug Card Prices*, February 2006.
91. Families USA, *Expectations Shrinking for Medicare Part D Enrollment*, February 2006.
92. Stephen Langel, "Activists Use Report to Push Increased FDA Funding, State Buying Pools," *Drug Industry Daily Online*, July 12, 2006.
93. David Glendinning, "Medicare Part D Less of a Bargain Than the VA for Prescription Drugs, Study Finds," *American Medical News*, January 23, 2006.
94. Borger et al., "Health Spending Projections."
95. As this book was going to press, Congress was considering bills that would give the FDA more authority over postapproval studies, would limit drug advertising, and would require more transparency in clinical trials. There was no sign, however, that Congress would fail to renew the Prescription Drug User Fee Act.
96. Bridget M. Kuehn, "IOM: Overhaul Drug Safety Monitoring," *Journal of the American Medical Association* 296 (2006): 2075–76.
97. Avorn, *Powerful Medicine*, 376–78.
98. AMA, "AMA Calls for Temporary Moratorium on Direct-to-Consumer Advertising of New Prescription Drugs," press release, June 14, 2005.
99. Catherine D. D'Angelis, Jeffrey M. Drazen, Frank A. Frizelle, et al., "Clinical Trial Registration: A Statement from the International Committee of Journal Editors," *Journal of the American Medical Association* 292 (2004): 1363–64.

Chapter 13. Putting Doctors Together

1. David Lawrence, *From Chaos to Care: The Promise of Team-Based Medicine* (Cambridge, MA: Perseus, 2002), 1–10, 51–66

2. Institute of Medicine (IOM), *Crossing the Quality Chasm: A New Health System for the 21st Century* (Washington, DC: National Academy Press, 2001), 3.

3. Ibid., 92, 103.

4. L. P. Casalino, K. J. Devers, T. K. Lake, M. Reed, and J. J. Stoddard, "Benefits of and Barriers to Large Medical Group Practice in the United States," *Archives of Internal Medicine* 163 (2003): 1958–64.

5. Ibid.; Lawrence, *Chaos to Care*, 12.

6. Lawrence, *Chaos to Care*, 12.

7. Donald Berwick and Sachin Jain, "Systems and Results: The Basis for Quality Care in Prepaid Group Practice," in *Toward a 21st Century Health System: The Contributions and Promise of Prepaid Group Practice*, edited by Alain C. Enthoven and Laura A. Tollen (San Francisco: Jossey-Bass, 2004), 26.

8. Ken Terry, "Doctors and EHRs," *Medical Economics*, January 21, 2005.

9. Kenneth H. Chuang, Harold S. Luft, and R. Adams Dudley, "The Clinical and Economic Performance of Prepaid Group Practice," in Enthoven and Tollen, *Toward a 21st Century Health System*, 46–60.

10. National Committee for Quality Assurance (NCQA) Health Plan Report Card, http://hprc.ncqa.org/index.asp/.

11. Ateev Mehrotra, Arnold M. Epstein, and Meredith B. Rosenthal, "Do Integrated Medical Groups Provide Higher-Quality Medical Care Than Individual Practice Associations?" *Annals of Internal Medicine*, 145 (2006): 826–33.

12. R. R. Gillies, K. E. Chenok, S. M. Shortell, G. Pawlson, and J. J. Wimbush, "The Impact of Health Plan Delivery System Organization on Clinical Quality and Patient Satisfaction," *Health Services Research* 41 (2006): 1181–99.

13. Chuang, Luft, and Dudley, "Clinical and Economic Performance," 55.

14. James C. Robinson, "The Limits of Prepaid Group Practice," in Enthoven and Tollen, *Toward a 21st Century Health System*, 199–212.

15. Robert Lowes, "PPMs: Going . . . Going . . . ," *Medical Economics*, March 5, 2001; Lowes, "How FPA's Implosion Buried Its Doctors," *Medical Economics*, January 25, 1999.

16. Medical Group Management Association (MGMA), *Physician Compensation and Production Survey 2003*, 2003.

17. Ken Terry, "The Best Way to Divide Income," *Medical Economics*, April 9, 2004.

18. Casalino et al., "Benefits and Barriers."

19. MGMA, *Physician Compensation and Production Survey 2003*, 18–20; also, MGMA, "MGMA Reports Nominal Increases in Physician Compensation in 2003," press release, August 11, 2004.

20. Center for Studying Health System Change, "Physicians Lose Ground in Real Income Between 1995 and 2003," press release, June 22, 2006.

21. MGMA press release, August 11, 2004; also, "AMGA, MGMA Data Show 2003 Was Good Year for MD Incomes in Most Specialties," *Physician Compensation Report*, September 2004.

22. Robert Lowes, "The Earnings Freeze—Now It's Everybody's Problem," *Medical Economics*, September 16, 2005.

23. Myrle Croasdale, "Subspecialties Flourishing as IM Residents Shun Primary Care," *American Medical News*, May 16, 2005.
24. American Medical Association (AMA), *Physician Characteristics and Distribution in the US: 2004 Edition* (Chicago: AMA Press, 2004), vi.
25. Uwe Reinhardt, interview with the author, May 2004; V. G. Rodwin, "The Health Care System under French National Health Insurance: Lessons for Health Reform in the United States, *American Journal of Public Health* 93, no. 1 (January 2003): 31–37.
26. David Glendinning, "Medicare Takes AMA Advice, Proposes E&M Pay Boost," *American Medical News*, July 17, 2006.
27. IOM, *Crossing the Quality Chasm*, 98–100.
28. Sam Ho (corporate medical director of PacifiCare), interview with the author, May 2004.
29. Ken Terry, "Taking Back Health Care: Are PODS the Way to Go?" *Medical Economics*, October 14, 1996.
30. *The 2004 World Almanac and Book of Facts* (New York: World Almanac Books, 2004), 376–77.
31. AMA, *Physician Characteristics and Distribution*, 305–10.

Chapter 14. Why Groups Should Take Financial Risk

1. L. P. Casalino, K. J. Devers, T. K. Lake, M. Reed, and J. J. Stoddard, "Benefits of and Barriers to Large Medical Group Practice in the United States" *Archives of Internal Medicine* 163 (2003): 1958–64.
2. Ken Terry, "The Best Way to Divide Income," *Medical Economics*, April 9, 2004.
3. Medical Group Management Association (MGMA), *Physician Compensation and Production Survey 2003*, 2003, 18–20; "AMGA, MGMA Data Show 2003 Was Good Year for MD Incomes in Most Specialties," *Physician Compensation Report*, September 2004.
4. Ken Terry, "Access Fees: Worth the Risk? What to Charge?" *Medical Economics*, July 23, 2004.
5. Robert Lowes, "The Earnings Freeze—Now It's Everybody's Problem," *Medical Economics*, September 16, 2005.
6. Ken Terry, "Can a Small Practice Survive in California?" *Medical Economics*, January 20, 2006.
7. Ken Terry, "Taking Back Healthcare: Are PODS the Way to Go?" *Medical Economics*, October 14, 1996; Terry, "You Can Thrive under Managed Care," *Medical Economics*, April 7, 1997.
8. Ken Terry, "Has Capitation Reached Its High-Water Mark?" *Medical Economics*, February 19, 2001.
9. Michael Parrish, "Will This Medical Brownout Ever End?" *Medical Economics*, October 8, 2001; Ken Terry, "Better Quality Care, Bigger Paycheck," *Medical Economics*, September 9, 2002.
10. Andrew Siskind, interview with the author, December 2004.
11. George C. Halvorson, *Strong Medicine* (New York: Random House, 1993), 193–208.
12. News and Commentary, "Managed Care Backlash Seems to Run Out of Steam," *Managed Care*, December 2004.

13. Ha T. Tu, *More Americans Willing to Limit Physician-Hospital Choice for Lower Medical Costs*, Center for Studying Health System Change, Issue Brief no. 94, March 2005.

14. Ken Terry, "Whose Patient Is It?" *Medical Economics*, February 16, 2007.

15. Institute of Medicine, *Crossing the Quality Chasm: A New Health System for the 21st Century* (Washington, DC: National Academy Press, 2001): 186–88.

16. J. C. Robinson, "Blended Payment Methods in Physician Organizations under Managed Care," *Journal of the American Medical Association* 282 (1999): 1258–63

17. E. Haavi Morreim, *Balancing Act: The New Medical Ethics of Medicine's New Economics* (Washington, DC: Georgetown University Press, 1995), 80.

18. Henry J. Aaron and William B. Schwartz with Melissa Cox, *Can We Say No? The Challenge of Rationing Health Care* (Washington, DC: Brookings Institution Press, 2005), 119.

19. Terry, "Taking Back Health Care."

Chapter 15. A Real-World Model for Reform

1. Medica, "Medica Acquires Patient Choice in Minnesota, Dakotas," press release, March 26, 2004, www.medica.com/; Ann Robinow (vice president and general manager, Patient Choice division of Medica), interview with the author, September 2004.

2. J. B. Christianson, R. Feldman, J. P. Weiner, and P. Drury, "Early Experience with a New Model of Employer Group Purchasing in Minnesota," *Health Affairs*, November/December 1999, 100–114.

3. Ibid.

4. J. B. Christianson and R. Feldman, "Evolution in the Buyers Health Care Action Group Purchasing Initiative," *Health Affairs*, January/February 2002, 76–88; Robinow, interview.

5. Christianson and Feldman, "Evolution"; Robinow, interview; Allan Baumgarten, interview with the author, September 2004.

6. Interviews with Robinow and Minneapolis group leaders.

7. A. Lyles, J. P. Weiner, A. D. Shore, J. Christianson, L. I. Solberg, and P. Drury, "Cost and Quality Trends in Direct Contracting Arrangements," *Health Affairs*, January/February 2002, 89–102.

8. Christianson et al., "Early Experience."

9. Christianson and Feldman, "Evolution"; Robinow, interview; Baumgarten, interview.

10. Christianson et al., "Early Experience."

11. Ibid.

12. Anita J. Slomski, "Who Needs HMOs?" *Medical Economics*, May 12, 1997.

13. Christianson et al., "Early Experience."

14. Slomski, "Who Needs HMOs?"

15. Robinow, interview.

16. Ibid.

17. Slomski, "Who Needs HMOs?"

18. Ibid.; Robinow, interview.

19. Christianson and Feldman, "Evolution."

20. Baumgarten, interview.

21. Robinow, interview.
22. Ibid.
23. Gail Amundsen, medical director, quality, for Health Partners, explained Medica's use of auditors to collect data at a Pay for Performance Summit in Atlanta in March 2006.
24. Lyles et al., "Cost and Quality Trends."
25. Frank Jossi, "Money Matters: A BHCAG Update from the Twin Cities," *Business & Health*, April 1998.
26. Robinow, interview.
27. Patrick Taillefer, interview with the author, September 2004.
28. George C. Halvorson, *Strong Medicine* (New York: Random House, 1993), 120.
29. James C. Robinson, "Consolidation and the Transformation of Competition in Health Insurance," *Health Affairs*, November/December 2004, 11–24.
30. Stephen Heffler, Sheila Smith, Sean Keehan, Christine Borger, M. Kent Clements, and Christopher Truffer, "U.S. Health Spending Projections for 2004–2014," *Health Affairs Web Exclusive*, February 23, 2005, 74–85.
31. Howard Larkin, "Stay Up to Date on Patients' Health Benefits," *Medical Economics*, April 26, 1999.
32. Medical Group Management Association, *MGMA Connexion*, February 2004.
33. James G. Kahn, Richard Kronick, Mary Kreger and David N. Gans, "The Cost of Health Insurance Administration in California: Estimates for Insurers, Physicians, and Hospitals," *Health Affairs*, November/December 2005, 1629–39.
34. Professional services cost $587.4 billion in 2004. Taking 5–7 percent of that and adding it to the $65.8 billion in insurer savings, one gets total savings of $95 billion–$107 billion. While there would be substantial administrative savings in hospitals, nursing homes, and other facilities, as well, they'd undoubtedly find ways to hide those savings if the government set facility prices (see Chapter 19).
35. Vanessa Fuhrmans, "After Streak of Strong Profits, Health Insurers May See Decline," *Wall Street Journal*, July 31, 2006.
36. Laura B. Benko, "Another Healthy Year: Blues Plans See 15% Rise in Net Income for 2005," *Modern Healthcare*, July 17, 2006.
37. Corporate Research Group, "Outlook for Managed Care 2006: CRG Analysts Predict Another Good Year," press release, March 1, 2006; "Who's Earning the Big Bucks at For-Profits?" *Modern Healthcare*, August 1, 2005.
38. Laura B. Benko, "UnitedHealth Sets Off Waves: Proposed Pay Caps for Execs Come Amid Scrutiny," *Modern Healthcare*, April 24, 2006; Eric Dash and Milt Freudenheim, "Chief Executive at Health Insurer Is Forced Out in Options Inquiry," *New York Times*, October 16, 2006.
39. Jonathan G. Bethely, "Health Plans Make More, Spend Less in 2005," *American Medical News*, March 6, 2006.
40. Robinson, "Consolidation."
41. Laura B. Benko, "Anthem Closes $16.4 Billion Deal for WellPoint," *Modern Healthcare*, December 6, 2004.
42. Milt Freudenheim, "United Health to Buy PacifiCare in Push into Medicare," *New York Times*, July 7, 2005.
43. Bob Cook, "AMA Study: Health Plan Market Domination Virtually Complete," *American Medical News*, May 8, 2006.
44. Robinson, "Consolidation."
45. Peter Kongstvedt (Accenture), interview with the author, July 2004.

46. National Committee for Quality Assurance (NCQA), "The Health Plan Employer Data and Information Set," www.ncqa.org/Programs/HEDIS/index.htm.
47. Brian Schilling (NCQA), interview with the author, July 2004.
48. Joan Kostusiak (Aetna), interview with the author, July 2004.
49. NCQA, *The State of Healthcare Quality 2004*, Appendix 2: "HEDIS Effectiveness of Care Measures: Trends, 2000–2003."

Chapter 16. The End of Insurance as We Know It

1. According to the Centers for Medicare and Medicaid Services (CMS), "Payment Rates for 2002 Announced," press release, March 1, 2001, the "floor" amount that CMS would pay Medicare HMOs in 2002 was between $500 and $553 per member per month, depending on county population. The average cost of single coverage in employer-based plans in 2002 was $255, and commercial HMO costs were slightly below that. Jon Gabel, Larry Levitt, Erin Holve, Jeremy Pickreign, Heidi Whitmore, Kelley Dhont, Samantha Hawkins, and Diane Rowland, "Job-Based Health Benefits in 2002: Some Important Trends," *Health Affairs*, September/October 2002, 143–51.
2. Marian Uhlman, "Specialist Care Waning for People on Medicaid," *Philadelphia Inquirer*, March 26, 2005.
3. Robert Pear, "Clinton Considers Stopping Medicaid under Health Plan," *New York Times*, March 29, 1993.
4. Martin Sipkoff, "Managed Medicaid Business Might Be Worth the Difficulties," *Managed Care*, July 2004.
5. Institute of Medicine, *Insuring America's Health* (Washington, DC: National Academies Press, 2004), 80–81.
6. American Hospital Association, *TrendWatch Chartbook 2005*, May 2005, table 4.4, "Aggregate Hospital Payment-to-Cost Ratios for Private Payers, Medicare and Medicaid, 1980–2003," www.ahapolicyforum.org/ahapolicyforum/trend-watch/chartbook2005.html.
7. John Holohan and Arunabh Ghosh, "Understanding the Recent Growth in Medicaid Spending, 2000–2003," *Health Affairs Web Exclusive*, January 26, 2005, 52–62.
8. Laurene A. Graig, *Health of Nations* (Washington, DC: CQ Press, 1999), 167–68.
9. Rudolf Klein, "Britain's National Health Service Revisited," *New England Journal of Medicine* 350 (2004): 937–42; editorial, "Primary Care Trusts: Premature Reorganization, with Mergers, May Be Harmful," *British Medical Journal* 329 (2004): 871–72.
10. As noted in Chapter 5, an electronic health record system costs an average of $33,000 per physician (not counting annual maintenance costs). According to American Medical Association, *Physician Characteristics and Distribution in the US: 2005 Edition* (Chicago, AMA Press, 2005), there were 245,219 primary-care physicians engaged in patient care in 2003. Multiplying the two figures together yields a total of $8.1 billion.

Chapter 17. Getting Down to Nuts and Bolts

1. American Medical Association (AMA), *Physician Characteristics and Distribution in the US: 2004 Edition* (Chicago: AMA Press, 2004), 90–103, 128, 137, 290.
2. Ken Terry, "What's Your Practice Worth?" *Medical Economics*, April 11, 2003.
3. Geoffrey Anders (principal, the Healthcare Group, Plymouth Meeting, PA), interview with the author, December 2004.
4. Ken Terry, "Practice Mergers: What Makes a Winner," *Medical Economics*, October 7, 2005.
5. Mary Ann Bauman (physician in Oklahoma City) and David Ottenbacker (physician in Grand Haven, MI), interviews with the author, April and November 2004.
6. L. P. Casalino, K. J. Devers, T. K. Lake, M. Reed, and J. J. Stoddard, "Benefits of and Barriers to Large Medical Group Practice in the United States," *Archives of Internal Medicine* 163 (2003): 1958–64.
7. David Gans (Medical Group Management Association), interview with the author, June 2006.
8. Ken Terry, "Hospital Hardball," *Medical Economics*, August 9, 2002; Terry, "Will This Stark Workaround Work?" *Medical Economics*, August 4, 2006.
9. Terry, "What's Your Practice Worth?"
10. Norman Kahn Jr., American Academy of Family Physicians, personal communication.
11. AMA, *Physician Characteristics*, 2004.
12. George C. Halvorson, *Strong Medicine* (New York: Random House, 1993), 146.
13. Ken Terry, "Primary Care Feels the Job Squeeze," *Medical Economics*, July 12, 1999. Also, interview with workforce expert Edward Salsberg (Association of American Medical Colleges), December 2004.
14. Ken Terry, "Reengineer Your Practice—Starting Today," *Medical Economics*, January 24, 2000.
15. Future of Family Medicine Leadership Project Leadership Committee, "The Future of Family Medicine: A Collaborative Project of the Family Medicine Community," *Annals of Family Medicine* 2 (2004): S3-S32; American College of Physicians, *The Advanced Medical Home: A Patient-Centered, Physician-Guided Model of Health Care*, policy monograph, 2006.
16. James Merritt, Joseph Hawkins, and Phillip B. Miller, *Will the Last Physician in American Please Turn Off the Lights? A Look at America's Looming Doctor Shortage* (Irving, TX: The MHA Group, 2004). The estimates on time to get a primary-care appointment came from my interviews with physicians and consultants.
17. Ken Terry, "Don't Be Afraid of Same-Day Scheduling," *Medical Economics*, November 5, 2004.
18. Charles M. Kilo, Dennis Horrigan, Marjorie Godfrey, and John Wasson, "Making Quality and Service Pay: Part 1, The Internal Environment," *Family Practice Management*, October 2000.
19. David Lawrence, *From Chaos to Care: The Promise of Team-Based Medicine* (Cambridge, MA: Perseus, 2002), 133–35.
20. Lawrence P. Casalino, "Disease Management and the Organization of Physician Practice," *Journal of the American Medical Association* 293 (2005): 485–88.
21. Terry, "Reengineer Your Practice—Starting Today."

22. Kilo et al., "Making Quality and Service Pay."

23. Edward B. Noffsinger, "Increasing Quality of Care and Access While Reducing Costs through Drop-in Group Medical Appointments," *Group Practice Journal*, January 1999.

24. Siskind, interview.

25. Ken Terry, "Board Recertification Gets Tougher," *Medical Economics*, November 21, 2003.

26. Ibid.

27. Ken Terry, "A New Way to Measure What Residents Learn," *Medical Economics*, March 5, 2004.

Chapter 18. Universal Health Care

1. Kaiser Commission on Medicaid and the Uninsured, *The Uninsured: A Primer*, October 2006, 3.

2. Emmet B. Keeler, "Effects of Cost Sharing on Use of Medical Services and Health," *Journal of Medical Practice Management* 8 (Summer 1992): 317–21.

3. M. Merlis, D. Gould, and B. Mahato, *Rising Out-of-Pocket Spending for Medical Care: A Growing Strain on Family Budgets*, Commonwealth Fund Report 10 (February 2006).

4. Institute of Medicine, *Insuring America's Health: Principles and Recommendations* (Washington, DC: National Academies Press, 2004), 40–41.

5. Families USA, "Paying a Premium: The Increased Cost of Care for the Uninsured," June 8, 2005 (www.familiesusa.org/assets/pdfs/Paying_a_Premium_rev_July_13731e.pdf).

6. Peter Kongstvedt (Accenture), interview with the author, July 2004; John Erb (Deloitte and Touche), interview with the author, July 2004; and interviews by the author with health-plan executives.

7. Institute of Medicine, *Insuring America's Health*, 116.

8. Ibid., 115.

9. American Medical Association, *Physicians and the Changing System: The Preliminary Clinton Reform Plan*, White Paper, September 24, 1993.

10. Institute of Medicine, *Insuring America's Health*, 126–32.

11. Dean Neubauer, "Hawaii: A Pioneer in Health System Reform," *Health Affairs*, Summer 1993, 31–39.

12. Jordan Rau and Evan Halper, "Piecemeal Reforms Win Out," *Los Angeles Times*, November 4, 2004.

13. Pam Belluck, "Massachusetts Sets Health Plan for Nearly All," *New York Times*, April 5, 2006.

14. J. C. Lewin and P. A. Sybinsky, "Hawaii's Employer Mandate and Its Contribution to Universal Access," *Journal of the American Medical Association* 269 (1993): 2538–43.

15. Robbie Dingeman, "Medically Uninsured on Rise in Hawaii," *Honolulu Advertiser*, October 29, 2003.

16. Neubauer, "Hawaii."

17. Ibid.

18. Hawaii Uninsured Project, *Employer Survey: Behaviors and Opinions about Health Insurance for Employees*, 2004.

19. Ibid.

20. John Lewin, interview with the author, July 2004.
21. Dingeman, "Medically Uninsured on Rise in Hawaii."
22. Ibid.; Russo, interview.
23. California Healthcare Foundation, *The Health Insurance Act of 2003: An Overview of SB2*, Fact Sheet, November 2003.
24. Institute for Policy Solutions, *Challenges and Alternatives for Employer Pay-or-Play Program Design*, Executive Summary, March 2005, 6.
25. AP, "Calif. Health Insurance Law Goes to Voters," cited in *Modern Physician*, June 8, 2004.
26. Kaiser Family Foundation/HRET, *California Employer Health Benefits Survey, 2002*, 2002.
27. California Healthcare Foundation, *Health Insurance Act of 2003*.
28. Arindrajit Dube and Michael Reich, *2003 California Establishment Survey: Preliminary Results on Employer-Based Healthcare Reform*, Institute of Labor and Employment, University of California, Los Angeles, September 18, 2003.
29. Heidi Whitmore, Sara R. Collins, Jon Gabel, and Jeremy Pickreign, "Employers' Views on Incremental Measures to Expand Health Coverage," *Health Affairs*, November/December 2006, 1668–78.
30. Laura B. Benko, "California Runs for Coverage," *Modern Healthcare*, September 4, 2006.
31. Clea Benson, "Health Care Bill Appears Doomed: Governor Vows to Veto Medical Insurance Measure, Saying He's Opposed to State-Run Program," *Sacramento Bee*, September 6, 2006.
32. Jennifer Steinhauer, "California Plan for Health Care Would Cover All," *New York Times*, January 9, 2007.
33. Pennsylvania Office of the Governor, "Governor Rendell Unveils Historic 'Prescription for Pennsylvania' to Provide Access to Affordable, Quality Health Care for All Pennsylvanians," press release, January 17, 2007.
34. John Hechinger and David Armstrong, "Massachusetts Seeks to Mandate Health Coverage," *Wall Street Journal*, April 5, 2006.
35. Jeffrey Krasner, "State OK's Disputed Health Plan Rules," *Boston Globe*, September 9, 2006.
36. Pam Belluck, "Massachusetts Sets Health Plan for Nearly All," *New York Times*, April 5, 2006.
37. Commonwealth Health Insurance Connector, "Welcome to the Health Insurance Connector," January 2007, www.massgov/?pageID=hicutilities &L=1&sid=Qhic&U=Qhic_welcome.
38. John E. McDonough, Brian Rosman, Fawn Phelps, and Melissa Shannon, "The Third Wave of Massachusetts Health Care Access Reform," *Health Affairs Web Exclusive*, September 14, 2006, 420–31.
39. Belluck, "Massachusetts Sets Health Plan."
40. John Holahan and Linda Blumberg, "Massachusetts Health Care Reform: A Look at the Issues," *Health Affairs Web Exclusive*, September 14, 2006, 432–43.
41. Reed Abelson, "Bold Goal Confronts Fine Print," *New York Times*, April 7, 2006; Massachusetts Governor's Office, *Q&A on Governor Romney's Health Coverage Plan*, Fact Sheet, April 2006.
42. Massachusetts Governor's Office, *Q&A*.
43. Holahan and Blumberg, "Massachusetts Health Care Reform."
44. Ibid.
45. Julius B. Richmond and Rashi Fein, *The Health Care Mess: How We Got Into It and What It Will Take to Get Out* (Cambridge, MA: Harvard University Press, 2005), 260.

46. Karen Davis and Cathy Schoen, "Universal Coverage: Building on Medicare and Employer Financing," *Health Affairs*, Spring 1994, 8–20.
47. Jack Hadley and John Holahan, "How Much Medical Care Do the Uninsured Use, and Who Pays for It?" *Health Affairs Web Exclusive*, February 12, 2003, 66–81.
48. Jack Hadley and John Holahan, "Covering the Uninsured: How Much Would It Cost?" *Health Affairs Web Exclusive*, June 4, 2003, 250–65.
49. Uwe E. Reinhardt, "Is There Hope for the Uninsured?" *Health Affairs Web Exclusive*, August 27, 2003, 376–90.
50. These estimates are based on data published in 2003. After accounting for health spending growth over the past four years, the cost of covering the uninsured would rise to about $125 billion. But the administrative cost savings would also be higher than the estimate given in the text.
51. Institute of Medicine, "Insuring America's Health,"120.

Chapter 19. Toward Uniform Hospital Pricing

1. American Hospital Association (AHA), *TrendWatch Chartbook 2005*, May 2005, appendix, table 4.4, www.ahapolicyforum.org/ahapolicyforum/trendwatch/chartbook2005.html.
2. Kenneth Thorpe (Emory University), interview with the author, May 2005.
3. Richard Perez-Pena, "Hospital Business in New York, Once Prized, Braces for a Crisis," *New York Times*, April 11, 2005.
4. Center for Medicare and Medicaid Services (CMS), "Medicare Hospital Outpatient Payment System," press release, November 2, 2000.
5. David Shactman, Stuart H. Altman, Efrat Eliat, Kenneth E. Thorpe, and Michael Doonan, "The Outlook for Hospital Spending," *Health Affairs*, November/December 2003, 12–26.
6. Ibid.; National Center for Health Statistics, *Health, United States, 2004* (Hyattsville, MD, 2004), table 125, 273; AHA, *TrendWatch Chartbook 2005*, appendix, table 1.2.
7. John L. Ashby Jr. and Craig K. Lisk, "Why Do Hospital Costs Continue to Increase?" *Health Affairs*, Summer 1992, 134–47.
8. Ibid.
9. Lucette Lagnado, "Hospitals Profit by 'Upcoding' Illnesses," *Wall Street Journal*, April 17, 1997.
10. Brent James, speech at pay-for-performance conference sponsored by the Robert Wood Johnson Foundation, Washington, DC, November 15, 2005.
11. Medicare Payment Advisory Commission, *Physician-Owned Specialty Hospitals*, Report to Congress, March 2005.
12. Paul M. Ginsburg and Joy M. Grossman, "When the Price Isn't Right: How Inadvertent Payment Incentives Drive Medical Care," *Health Affairs Web Exclusive*, August 9, 2005, 376–84.
13. CMS, "CMS Proposes Payment and Policy Changes for Acute Care Hospital Services to Inpatients," press release, April 12, 2006.
14. Ibid.
15. Robert Pear, "White House Alters Plan to Make Large Cuts in Hospitals' Medicare Payments," *New York Times*, August 3, 2006.
16. Jennifer Lubell, "Hospitals See Severity of Situation," *Modern Healthcare*, April 23, 2007.
17. Deborah Chanen, interview with the author, June 2005.

18. Matthew DoBias, "Reshuffling the DRG Deck," *Modern Healthcare*, October 10, 2005.
19. CMS, "CMS Proposes FY2006 Rate Increases for Inpatient Stays in Acute Care Hospitals," press release, April 25, 2005; Ellen Griffith (CMS public affairs department), interview with the author, June 2005.
20. AHA, *TrendWatch: Chartbook 2005*, appendix, table 4.2.
21. CMS, "Medicare Hospital Outpatient Payment System," press release, November 2, 2000.
22. Medicare Payment Advisory Commission, *Outpatient Hospital Services Payment System*, brief, July 13, 2004.
23. CMS, "CMS Proposes Changes to Policies and Payment for Outpatient Services," press release, August 8, 2006.

Chapter 20. Let "Hospitalists" Take Charge

1. Robert Wachter and Lee Goldman, "The Emerging Role of 'Hospitalists' in the American Health Care System," *New England Journal of Medicine* 335 (1996): 514–17.
2. Ken Terry, "The Changing Face of Hospital Practice," *Medical Economics*, August 23, 2002. Fewer than 2 percent of internists were referring to HMO-mandated hospitalist programs in 2000, according to David H. Freed in "Hospitalists: Evolution, Evidence and Eventualities," *Health Care Manager* 23, no. 3 (2004): 238–56.
3. Terry, "Changing Face of Hospital Practice."
4. H. H. Pham, K. J. Devers, S. Kuo, and R. Berenson, "Health Care Market Trends and the Evolution of Hospitalist Use and Roles," *Journal of General Internal Medicine* 20 (2005): 101–7.
5. Robert M. Wachter and Lee Goldman, "The Hospitalist Movement Five Years Later," *Journal of the American Medical Association* 287 (2002): 487–94.
6. Society of Hospital Medicine (SHM), "Society of Hospital Medicine Releases Most Comprehensive Survey Ever on Hospital Medicine," press release, April 30, 2004; Steven Pantilat (SHM president), interview with the author, May 2005. Also, SHM, "Hospital Medicare Specialty Shows 20 Percent Growth," press release, February 22, 2007.
7. SHM, "Society of Hospital Medicine Releases Most Comprehensive Survey Ever."
8. P. K. Lindenauer, S. Z. Pantilat, P. P. Katz, and R. M. Wachter, "Hospitalists and the Practice of Inpatient Medicine: Results of a Survey of the National Association of Inpatient Physicians, *Annals of Internal Medicine* 130 (1999): 343–49.
9. T. H. Hoff, W. F. Whitcomb, K. Williams, J. R. Nelson, and R. Cheesman, "Characteristics and Work Experiences of Hospitalists in the United States," *Archives of Internal Medicine* 161 (2001): 851–58.
10. Terry, "Changing Face of Hospital Practice"; Hoff et al., "Characteristics and Work Experiences of Hospitalists."
11. Robert Wachter, interview with author, May 2005. Also, the SHM 2003 survey found that hospitalists who are compensated on productivity and those employed by local hospitalist groups and multistate companies tended to have a higher number of patient encounters a year.
12. Wachter, interview. But Ronald Greeno of Cogent Healthcare notes that this

range includes many part-time hospitalists. Both the Cogent and Main Line hospitalists follow fifteen to twenty patients at a time, on average.

13. Robert M. Wachter, "An Introduction to the Hospitalist Model," *Annals of Internal Medicine* 130 (1999): 338–42.

14. Terry, "Changing Face of Hospital Practice."

15. Wachter and Goldman, "Hospitalist Movement."

16. Ibid.

17. J. M. Huddleston, K. H. Long, J. M. Naessens, D. Vanness, D. Larson, R. Trousdale, M. Plevak, M. Cabanela, D. Ilstrup, and R. M. Wachter, "Medical and Surgical Comanagement after Elective Hip and Knee Arthroplasty," *Annals of Internal Medicine* 141, no. 1 (2004): 28–38.

18. A. D. Auerbach, R. M. Wachter, P. Katz, J. Showstack, R. B. Baron, and L. Goldman, "Implementation of a Voluntary Hospitalist Service at a Community Teaching Hospital: Improved Clinical Efficiency and Patient Outcomes," *Annals of Internal Medicine* 137 (2002): 859–65; D. Meltzer, W. G. Manning, J. Morrison, M.N. Shah, L. Jin, T. Guth, and W. Levinson, "Effects of Physician Experience on Costs and Outcomes on an Academic General Medicine Service: Results of a Trial of Hospitalists," *Annals of Internal Medicine* 137 (2002): 866–74; editorial, "The Who, What, When, Where, Whom and How of Hospitalist Care," *Annals of Internal Medicine* 137 (2002): 930–31.

19. Lucian L. Leape and Donald M. Berwick, "Five Years after *To Err Is Human*: What Have We Learned?" *Journal of the American Medical Association* 293 (2005): 2384–90; K. T. Kohn, J. M. Corrigan, and M. S. Donaldson, *To Err Is Human: Building a Safer Health System* (Washington, D.C.: National Academy Press; 1999); Drew Altman, Carolyn Clancy, and Robert J. Blendon, "Improving Patient Safety—Five Years after the IOM Report," *New England Journal of Medicine* 351 (2004): 2041–43; R. Koppel, J. P. Metlay, A. Cohen, B. Abaluck, A .R. Localio, S. E. Kimmel, and B. L. Strom, "Role of Computerized Physician Order Entry Systems in Facilitating Medical Errors," *Journal of the American Medical Association* 293 (2005): 1197–203.

20. Robert M. Wachter, "The End of the Beginning: Patient Safety Five Years after 'To Err Is Human,' " *Health Affairs Web Exclusive*, November 30, 2004, 534–45.

21. Ken Terry, "Discharging Primary-Care Doctors from Hospital Rounds," *Medical Economics*, November 25, 1996.

22. Richard B. Freese, "The Park Nicollet Experience in Establishing a Hospitalist System," *Annals of Internal Medicine* 130 (1999): 350–54.

23. Freese, "Park Nicollet Experience."

24. Wachter, interview.

25. D. Hackner, G. Tu, G. D. Braunstein, M. Ault, S. Weingarten, and Z. Mohsenifar, "The Value of a Hospitalist Service: Efficient Care for the Aging Population?" *CHEST* 119 (2001): 580–89.

26. Freese, "Park Nicollet Experience."

27. Richard Afable, speech, pay-for-performance conference, Jefferson Medical College, Philadelphia, July 15, 2005.

28. Wachter and Goldman, "Hospitalist Movement."

29. Christine Borger, Sheila Smith, Christopher Truffer, Sean Keehan, Andrea Sisko, John Poisal, and M. Kent Clemens, "Health Spending Projections Through 2015: Changes On The Horizon," *Health Affairs Web Exclusive*, February 22, 2006, 61–73. John A. Poisal, Christine Truffer, Sheila Smith, Andrea Sisko, Cathy Cowan, Sean Keehan, and Bridget Dickensheets, "Health Spending

Projections Through 2016: Modest Changes Obscure Part D's Impact," *Health Affairs Web Exclusive*, March/April 2007, 242–53.

30. Author's computation.

31. Wachter and Goldman's estimate was based on 10 percent savings. So if 25 percent could be saved, the total figure would be 2.5 times as high.

32. The current number of hospitalists is only two-thirds of the thirty thousand projected by the end of this decade.

Chapter 21. Health Planning and the CON

1. John E. Wennberg, "Practice Variations and Health Care Reform: Connecting the Dots," *Health Affairs Web Exclusive*, October 7, 2004, 140–43; Donald M. Berwick, *Escape Fire: Designs for the Future of Health Care* (San Francisco: Jossey-Bass, 2004), 89; George C. Halvorson, *Strong Medicine* (New York: Random House, 1993), 61–71.

2. Sujit Choudhry, Niteesh K. Choudhry, and Troyen A. Brennan, "Specialty versus Community Hospitals: What Role for the Law?" *Health Affairs Web Exclusive*, August 9, 2005, 361–72.

3. Federal Trade Commission and U.S. Department of Justice, *Improving Health Care: A Dose of Competition*, Executive Summary, July 2004, 22.

4. American Health Planning Association, *The Federal Trade Commission and Certificate of Need Regulation: An AHPA Critique*, January 2005, 7.

5. Choudhry et al., "Specialty versus Community Hospitals."

6. Mike Norbut, "Cutting through the CONfusion," *American Medical News*, February 7, 2005.

7. Paul Starr, *The Social Transformation of American Medicine* (New York: Basic Books, 1982), 402.

8. Norbut, "Cutting through the CONfusion."

9. John Steen (former director of New York City's health planning agency), interview with the author, September 2005.

10. Ibid.; Bonnie DeVinney (director of Finger Lakes Health Services Agency), interview with the author, August 2005.

11. Norbut, "Cutting through the CONfusion."

12. Katherine Vogt, "Michigan Court Refuses to Hear CON Appeal," *American Medical News*, September 26, 2005. Health-care consultants say the same is true for hospital owners all over the country.

13. Steven Stycos, "Shifting Landscape," *Providence Phoenix*, May 6, 2005.

14. John Steen, "Certificate of Need: A Review," American Health Planning Association, www.ahpanet.org/.

15. M. S. Vaughan-Sarrazin, E. L. Hannan, C. J. Gormley, and G. E. Rosenthal, "Mortality in Medicare Beneficiaries Following Coronary Artery Bypass Graft Surgery in States with and without Certificate of Need Regulation," *Journal of the American Medical Association* 288 (2002): 1859–66.

16. Steen, "Certificate of Need."

17. Michael L. Millenson, *Demanding Medical Excellence* (Chicago: University of Chicago Press, 1997), 195.

18. Cited in Paul Starr, *The Social Transformation of American Medicine* (New York: Basic Books, 1982), 414.

19. Christopher J. Conover and Frank A. Sloan, "Does Removing Certificate-of-

Need Regulations Lead to a Surge in Health Care Spending?" *Journal of Health Politics, Policy and Law*, June 1998, 455–81.

20. Cinda Becker, "Volumes Down, Pa. Closes Angio Pilot to New Hospitals," *Modern Physician*, June 1, 2005, http://modernphysician.com/.

21. Pennsylvania Health Care Cost Containment Council, "Utilization, Growth, Profits Surge at Outpatient Surgery Centers; Rehab Hospitals Stage Financial Comeback," press release, August 27, 2004.

22. Carol Stevens, "Are Clouds Closing in on the Rochester Miracle?" *Medical Economics*, April 26, 1993.

23. William J. Hall and Paul F. Griner, "Cost-Effective Health Care: The Rochester Experience," *Health Affairs*, Spring 1993, 58–69.

24. Stevens, "Are Clouds Closing In?"

25. Jim Redmond (spokesman for Excellus Blue Cross and Blue Shield), interview with the author, August 2005. Louis Papa of the county medical society says the uninsured rate is now about 10 percent (interview with the author, August 2005).

26. Boston University Health Policy Institute, "Health Cost Management at the Community Level: Doctors, Hospitals and Industry," *Health Affairs*, Fall 1983, 115–26; Raymond Mayewski (Strong Health), interview with the author, August 2005; William J. Hall and Paul F. Griner, "Cost-Effective Health Care: The Rochester Experience," *Health Affairs*, Spring 1993, 58–69.

27. Mayewski, interview.

28. Stevens, "Are Clouds Closing In?"

29. Howard Berman, letter to the editor, "Rochester Health Care: An Epilogue," *Health Affairs*, Summer 1993, 213.

30. Edgar Black, interview with the author, August 2005; Bonnie DeVinney, e-mail message to the author.

31. With the closing of these two hospitals, Rochester was spared the excess capacity afflicting other upstate New York cities (Redmond, interview). Based on a body of evidence showing that overcapacity raises costs, that suggests that the hospital consolidation contributed to holding local health costs down. See, for example, R. A. Connor, R. D. Feldman, B. E. Dowd, and T. A. Radcliff, "Which Types of Hospital Mergers Save Consumers Money?" *Health Affairs*, November/December 1997, 62–74.

32. Redmond, interview; Howard Beckman (medical director of the Rochester IPA), interview with the author, November 2005.

33. Black interview; Bonnie DeVinney, interview with the author, August 2005.

34. Papa, interview.

35. Leonard E. Redon, "Making Sure Medical System Is Proper Fit for Local Community," *Rochester Democrat and Chronicle*, August 8, 2003, 7A.

36. Community Technology Assessment Advisory Board (CTAAB), "2003 Report to the Community, " www. ctaab.org/; CTAAB, "Summary of CTAAB Recommendations," www.ctaab.org/.

37. Lawrence P. Casalino, Kelly J. Devers, and Linda R. Brewster, "Focused Factories? Physician-Owned Specialty Facilities," *Health Affairs*, November/December 2003, 56–67.

38. Sandra A. Parker, "Let's Talk Ways to Curb Costs," *Rochester Democrat and Chronicle*, December 12, 2004, 33A.

39. CTAAB, "Summary of CTAAB Recommendations."

40. CTAAB, "Applications under Review," Spring 2005.

Chapter 22. What Works Best in Practice?

1. E. S. Fisher, D. E. Wennberg, T. A. Stukel, D. J. Gottlieb, F. L. Lucas, and E. L. Pinder. "The Implications of Regional Variations in Medicare Spending. Part 1: The Content, Quality, and Accessibility of Care," *Annals of Internal Medicine* 138 (2003): 273–87.

2. Gail R. Wilensky, "Developing a Center for Comparative Effectiveness Information," *Health Affairs Web Exclusive*, November/December 2006, 572–85.

3. J. M. Weinstein, D. Tosteson, J. D. Lurie, A.N.A. Tosteson, B. Hanscom, J. S. Skinner, W. A. Abdu, A. S. Hilibrand, S. D. Boden, and R.A. Deyo, "Surgical vs. Nonoperative Treatment for Lumbar Disk Herniation," *Journal of the American Medical Association* 296 (2006): 2441–50.

4. Sean R. Tunis, Daniel B. Stryer, and Carolyn M. Clancy, "Practical Clinical Trials: Increasing the Value of Clinical Research for Decision Making in Clinical and Health Policy," *Journal of the American Medical Association* 290 (2003): 1624–32.

5. Ibid.

6. The CREATE-ECLA Trial Group Investigators, "Effect of Glucose-Insulin-Potassium Infusion on Mortality in Patients with Acute ST-Segmen Elevation Myocardial Infarction," *Journal of the American Medical Association* 293 (2005): 437–46.

7. Tunis, Stryer, and Clancy, "Practical Clinical Trials."

8. C. Baigent, R. Collins, P. Appleby, S. Parish, P. Slieght, and R. Peto, for the ISIS-2 (Second International Study of Infarct Survival) Collaborative Group, "ISIS-2: 10-Year Survival among Patients with Suspected Acute Myocardial Infarction in Randomized Comparison of Intravenous Streptokinase, Oral Aspirin, Both, or Neither," *British Medical Journal* 316 (1998): 1337–43.

9. R. H. Pantell, T. B. Newman, J. Bernzweig, D. A. Bergman, J. I. Takayama, M. Segal, S. A. Finch, and R. C. Wasserman, "Management and Outcomes of Care of Fever in Early Infancy," *Journal of the American Medical Association* 291 (2004): 1203–12.

10. David Lanier, "Primary-Care Practice-Based Research Comes of Age in the United States," *Annals of Family Medicine* 3, Supplement 1 (2005): S2-S4.

11. Ibid.; Brenda Hudson (PBRN Resource Center), interview with the author, March 2006.

12. James Galliher, interview with the author, April 2005; Richard Wasserman, interview with the author, March 2006; Steven Ornstein, interview with the author, March 2006.

13. Marcia Angell, *The Truth about the Drug Companies* (New York: Random House, 2004), 31.

14. Robert Wood Johnson Foundation, "$3 Million in Grants Awarded to Help Primary Care Providers Promote Healthy Behaviors Among Their Patients," press release, July 5, 2005; RWJ Foundation, "$2.1 Million in Grants Awarded to Help Health Care Providers Promote Healthy Behaviors among Their Patients," press release, August 22, 2003.

15. P. C. Smith, R. Araya-Guerra, C. Bublitz, B. Parnes, L. M. Dickinson, R. Van Vorst, J. M. Westfall, W. D. Pace, "Missing Clinical Information During Primary Care Visits," *Journal of the American Medical Association* 293 (2005): 565–71.

16. Perry Dickinson, interview with the author, March 2006; Paul Hicks, interview with the author, March 2006.

17. Carolyn M. Clancy and Kevin Cronin, "Evidence-Based Decision Making: Global Evidence, Local Decisions," *Health Affairs* 24, no. 1 (2005), 151–61.
18. Steven Ornstein, interview with the author, March 2006; Bruce Kleaveland (former chief operating officer of Practice Partner), interview with the author, March 2006.
19. Ornstein, interview; Kleaveland, interview; Agency for Health Care Research and Quality, *Primary Care Practice-based Research Networks*, Fact Sheet, June 2001.
20. Ornstein, interview.
21. Clancy, interview; Clancy, "The New Effective Health Care Program," *Patient Safety & Quality Healthcare*, January/February 2006.
22. Lanier, "Primary-Care Practice-Based Research Comes of Age."
23. Tunis, Stryer, and Clancy, "Practical Clinical Trials."
24. Michael L. Millenson, *Demanding Medical Excellence* (Chicago: University of Chicago Press, 1997), 350.

Chapter 23. Must Technology Break the Bank?

1. Ken Terry, "Technology: The Biggest Health-care Cost-driver of All; Can We Curb its Rise?" *Medical Economics*, March 21, 1994.
2. David Eddy, "Health System Reform: Will Controlling Costs Require Rationing Services?" *Journal of the American Medical Association* 272 (1994): 324–28.
3. American Heart Association (AHA), *Heart Disease and Stroke Statistics*, 2005 update. Comparison with 1992 data from Terry, "Technology."
4. Terry, "Technology."
5. AHA, *Heart Disease and Stroke Statistics*.
6. Alan Garber, interview with the author, October 2005; Mary Duenwald, "One Lesson from Vioxx: Approach New Drugs with Caution," *New York Times*, October 5, 2004.
7. Dana P. Goldman, Baoping Shang, Jayanta Bhattacharya, Alan M. Garber, Michael Hurd, Geoffrey F. Joyce, Darius N. Lakdawalla, Constantjin Panis, and Paul G. Shekelle, "Consequences of Health Trends and Medical Innovation for the Future Elderly," *Health Affairs Web Exclusive*, September 26, 2005, 5–17.
8. Ibid.
9. Kenneth E. Thorpe, Curtis S. Florence, David H. Howard, and Peter Joski, "The Rising Prevalence of Treated Disease: Effects on Private Health Insurance Spending," *Health Affairs Web Exclusive*, June 27, 2005, 317–25.
10. Kenneth Thorpe, interview with the author, October 2005.
11. David M. Cutler and Mark McClellan, "Is Technological Change Worth It?" *Health Affairs*, September/October 2001, 11–29.
12. David M. Cutler, *Your Money or Your Life* (New York: Oxford University Press, 2004), 62–63.
13. Ibid., 11–12.
14. Institute of Medicine, *Insuring America's Health: Principles and Recommendations* (Washington, DC: National Academies Press, 2004), 37.
15. Mark V. Pauly, "Should We Be Worried about High Real Medical Spending Growth in the United States?" *Health Affairs Web Exclusive*, January 8, 2003, 15–27.

16. Daniel Callahan, *False Hopes: Overcoming the Obstacles to a Sustainable, Affordable Medicine* (New York: Simon & Schuster, 1998), 35.

17. Ibid., 254, 256–57.

18. Ibid, 144–45.

19. Ibid., 146.

20. Ibid., 256.

21. Victor R. Fuchs, "More Variation in Use of Care, More Flat-of-the-Curve Medicine," *Health Affairs Web Exclusive*, October 7, 2004, 104–7.

22. Elliott S. Fisher and H. Gilbert Welch, "Avoiding the Unintended Consequences of Growth in Medical Care: How Might More Be Worse?" *Journal of the American Medical Association* 281 (1999): 446–53.

23. Ibid.; Gina Kolata and Melody Petersen, "Hormone Replacement Study a Shock to the Medical System," *New York Times*, July 10, 2002.

24. John P. A. Ioannidis, "Contradicted and Initially Stronger Effects in Highly Cited Clinical Research," *Journal of the American Medical Association* 294 (2005): 218–28.

25. Anna Wilde Mathews, "Are Long Trials Always Needed for New Drugs?" *Wall Street Journal*, April 26, 2004; Bob Carlson, "FDA: Change Is Good," *Biotechnology Review*, March 2004, 27–30.

26. Thomas M. Burton, "Approval of Neck Stent Spurs Debate over Stroke Prevention," *Wall Street Journal*, September 1, 2004.

27. Jean-Louis Mas, Gilles Chatellier, and the EVA-3S Investigators, "Endarterectomy versus Stenting in Patients with Symptomatic Severe Carotid Stenosis," *New England Journal of Medicine* 355 (2006): 1660–71.

28. B. H. Ashar, M. T. Hughes, S. S. Marinopoulos, G. P. Prokopowicz, G. V. Berkenblit, S. D. Sisson, L. A. Simonson, and R.G. Miller, "Current Evidence for the Use of Emerging Radiologic Technologies for Disease Screening," *American Journal of Managed Care* 11 (2005): 385–92; James L. Mulshine and Daniel C. Sullivan, "Lung Cancer Screening," *New England Journal of Medicine* 352 (2005): 2714–20.

29. Vanessa Fuhrmans, "Overuse of Medical Scans Is under Fire," *Wall Street Journal*, January 12, 2005; Alice Park, "Do You Know Your Calcium Score?" *Time*, September 5, 2005.

30. Amy Dockser Marcus, "Price Becomes Factor in Cancer Treatment," *Wall Street Journal*, September 7, 2004; Mathews, "Are Long Trials Always Needed for New Drugs?"

31. Robert A. Berenson, "Getting Serious About Excessive Medicare Spending: A Purchasing Model," *Health Affairs Web Exclusive*, December 10, 2003, 586–602.

32. Gust H. Bardy, Kerry L. Lee, Daniel B. Mark, et al., "Amiodarone or an Implantable Cardioverter-Defibrillator for Congestive Heart Failure," *New England Journal of Medicine* 352 (2005): 225–33.

33. Cinda Becker, "Pending Policy Change to Create Vast New ICD Market," *Modern Physician*, January 21, 2005, http://modernphysician.com/.

34. Zachary A. Goldfarb, "FDA Panel Weighs Artificial-Heart Implants," *Wall Street Journal*, June 17, 2005.

35. Food and Drug Administration, "FDA Approves Temporary Artificial Heart," press release, October 18, 2004.

36. Lawrence K. Altman, "Implantable Heart Device Receives F.D.A. Approval," *New York Times*, September 6, 2006.

37. William B. Schwartz, *Life without Disease: The Pursuit of Medical Utopia* (Los Angeles: University of California Press, 1998), 73–76.
38. Rakesh K. Jain and Peter F. Carmeliet, "Vessels of Death or Life," *Scientific American*, December 2001; Lawrence K. Altman, "Injectable Drug Grows Heart Vessels," *New York Times*, February 24, 1998.
39. William Neaves, "Personalized Medicine in the Postgenome Era," *Cerner Quarterly*, Q4 2005.
40. Goldman et al., "Consequences of Health Trends."
41. Alan M. Garber, "Evidence-Based Coverage Policy," *Health Affairs*, September/October 2001, 62–82.
42. Paul Barr, "Declassifying Coverage," *Modern Healthcare*, March 21, 2005.
43. Steven D. Pearson, Franklin G. Miller, and Ezekiel J. Emanuel, "Medicare's Requirement for Research Participation as a Condition of Coverage," *Journal of the American Medical Association* 296 (2006): 988–91.
44. Steve Phurrough, interview with the author, October 2005; Jed Weissberg, interview with the author, October 2005.
45. Naomi Aronson, interview, October 2005.
46. Alan M. Garber, "Cost-Effectiveness and Evidence Evaluation as Criteria for Coverage Policy," *Health Affairs Web Exclusive*, May 19, 2004, 284–96.
47. Mark Sculpher, Michael Drummond, and Bernie O'Brien, "Effectiveness, Efficiency, and NICE," *British Medical Journal* 322 (2001): 943–44; Garber, interview.
48. Garber, interview.
49. Thomas H. S. Dent and Mike Sadler, "From Guidance to Practice: Why NICE Is Not Enough," *British Medical Journal* 324 (2002): 842–45.
50. James Raferty, "NICE: Faster Access to Modern Treatments? Analysis of Guidance on Health Technologies," *British Medical Journal* 323 (2001): 1300–1303.
51. Richard Smith, editorial, "The Failings of Nice," *British Medical Journal* 321 (2000): 1363–64
52. Dent and Sadler, "From Guidance to Practice."
53. Raferty, "NICE."
54. Smith, " Failings of Nice."
55. NICE, "UK's First Citizens Council Being Established by NICE," press release, August 19, 2002.
56. Aronson, interview.
57. U.S. Dept. of Health and Human Services, *The Oregon Health Plan: An Historical Overview*, February 2004.
58. David Eddy, "Oregon's Methods: Did Cost-effectiveness Analysis Fail?" *Journal of the American Medical Association* 266 (1991): 2135–41; Garber, interview.
59. Kristie Perry Dolan, "How's Oregon's Bold Rationing Program Doing?" *Medical Economics*, July 28, 1997.
60. Wayne J. Guglielmo, "The Oregon Health Plan Hits a Snag," *Medical Economics*, September 17, 2004.
61. David C. Hadorn, "Setting Health Care Priorities in Oregon: Cost-effectiveness Meets the Rule of Rescue," *Journal of the American Medical Association* 265 (1991): 2218–25.
62. Ibid.

Chapter 24. Toward a Rational System of Rationing

1. Ken Terry, "What Is Quality in Health Care?" *Medical Economics*, April 28, 1997.
2. E. Haavi Morreim, *Balancing Act: The New Medical Ethics of Medicine's New Economics* (Washington, DC: Georgetown University Press, 1995), 43–68.
3. Henry J. Aaron, "Should Public Policy Seek to Control the Growth of Health Spending?" *Health Affairs Web Exclusive*, January 8, 2003, 28–36.
4. Victor R. Fuchs, "Health System Reform: A Different Approach," *Journal of the American Medical Association* 272 (1994): 560–63.
5. Gail Wilensky, "Developing a Center for Comparative Effectiveness Information," *Health Affairs Web Exclusive*, November 7, 2006, 572–85; Kathy Buto and Peter Juhn, "Can a Center for Comparative Effectiveness Information Succeed? Perspectives from a Health Care Company," *Health Affairs Web Exclusive*, November 7, 2006, 586–88.
6. David Eddy, "What Care Is 'Essential'? What Services Are 'Basic'?" *Journal of the American Medical Association* 265 (1991): 782–88.
7. Naomi Aronson, interview, October 2005; C. Farquhar, J. Marjoribanks, R. Basser, S. Hetric, and A. Lethaby, "High Dose Chemotherapy and Autologous Bone Marrow or Stem Cell Transplantation Versus Conventional Chemotherapy for Women with Metastatic Breast Cancer," *Cochrane Database of Systematic Reviews* 3 (July 20, 2005): CD003142.
8. Rhonda L. Rundle and Jane Spencer, "Concerns Grow over Weight-Loss Surgery," *Wall Street Journal*, October 19, 2005.
9. David Nash, "Hips and Knees," *Jefferson Medical College Health Policy Newsletter*, September 2005.
10. Dana P. Goldman, Baoping Shang, Jayanta Bhattacharya, Alan M. Garber, Michael Hurd, Geoffrey F. Joyce, Darius N. Lakdawalla, Constantjin Panis, and Paul G. Shekelle, "Consequences of Health Trends and Medical Innovation for the Future Elderly," *Health Affairs Web Exclusive*, September 26, 2005, 5–17.
11. American Heart Association, *Heart Disease and Stroke Statistics*, 2005 update.
12. G. C. Harewood and D.A. Lieberman, "Colonoscopy Practice Patterns Since Introduction of Medicare Coverage for Average-risk Screening," *Clinical Gastroenterology Hepatology* 2, no. 1 (January 2004): 72–77.
13. Figures on screening with flexible sigmoidoscopy are from an unpublished study by Robert Wigton, a professor at the University of Nebraska Medical Center College of Medicine, Omaha, and Patrick Alguire (American College of Physicians), interview with the author, December 2005; American Academy of Family Physicians survey data were supplied by John Pope, professor of clinical family medicine at Louisiana State University in Shreveport, in an interview with the author, December 2005.
14. Pope, interview; Alguire, interview; interviews with other physicians.
15. Centers for Medicare and Medicaid Services, *Medicare RBRVS: The Physician's Guide 2005*, 2005. Private-sector costs are from Robert Wigton, interview with the author, December 2005, and interviews with other physicians.
16. Michael Pignone, Melissa Rich, Steven M. Teutsch, Alfred O. Berg, and Kathleen N. Lohr, "Screening for Colorectal Cancer in Adults at Average Risk: A Summary of the Evidence for the U.S. Preventive Services Task Force," *Annals of Internal Medicine* 137 (2002): 132–41.
17. Michael Pignone, Somnath Saha, Tom Hoerger, and Jeanne Mandelblatt, "Cost-

Effectiveness Analyses of Colorectal Cancer Screening: A Systematic Review for the U.S. Preventive Services Task Force," *Annals of Internal Medicine* 137 (2002): 96–104.

18. Pignone et al., "Screening for Colorectal Cancer."
19. David F. Ransohoff, "Colon Cancer Screening in 2005: Status and Challenges," *Gastroenterology* 128 (2005): 1685–95.
20. Fifty-four percent of the 14.2 million colonoscopies performed in 2002, or 7.67 million, were for screening purposes, according to L. C. Seeff, T. B. Richards, J. A. Shapiro, M. R. Nadel, D. L. Manninen, L. S. Given, F. B. Dong, L. D. Winges, and M. T. McKenna, "How Many Endoscopies Are Performed for Colorectal Cancer Screening? Results from CDC's Survey of Endoscopic Capacity," *Gastroenterology* 127 (2004): 1670–77. If the average cost of Medicare and private-sector colonoscopies was $1,200, including facility fees, the total cost was $9.2 billion, and would probably be more than $10 billion today.
21. Lisa M. Schwartz, Steven Woloshin, Floyd J. Fowler, and H. Gilbert Welch, "Enthusiasm for Cancer Screening in the United States," *Journal of the American Medical Association* 291 (2004): 71–78.
22. Kathleen Fackelmann, "Centenarians Increase in Age and Numbers," *USA Today*, October 24, 2005.

Index